NUTRACEUTICALS IN ARTHRITIS AND PSORIASIS

Management and Prevention of Diseases

AAP Advances in Nutraceuticals

NUTRACEUTICALS IN ARTHRITIS AND PSORIASIS

Management and Prevention of Diseases

Meenakshi Jaiswal, PhD, MPharm
Raj K. Keservani, PhD, MPharm
Rajesh K. Kesharwani, PhD
Swati G. Talele, PhD
Editors

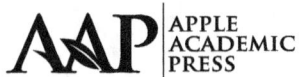

First edition published 2025

Apple Academic Press Inc.
1265 Goldenrod Circle, NE,
Palm Bay, FL 32905 USA
760 Laurentian Drive, Unit 19,
Burlington, ON L7N 0A4, CANADA

CRC Press
2385 NW Executive Center Drive,
Suite 320, Boca Raton FL 33431
4 Park Square, Milton Park,
Abingdon, Oxon, OX14 4RN UK

© 2025 by Apple Academic Press, Inc.

Apple Academic Press exclusively co-publishes with CRC Press, an imprint of Taylor & Francis Group, LLC

Reasonable efforts have been made to publish reliable data and information, but the authors, editors, and publisher cannot assume responsibility for the validity of all materials or the consequences of their use. The authors, editors, and publishers have attempted to trace the copyright holders of all material reproduced in this publication and apologize to copyright holders if permission to publish in this form has not been obtained. If any copyright material has not been acknowledged, please write and let us know so we may rectify in any future reprint.

Except as permitted under U.S. Copyright Law, no part of this book may be reprinted, reproduced, transmitted, or utilized in any form by any electronic, mechanical, or other means, now known or hereafter invented, including photocopying, microfilming, and recording, or in any information storage or retrieval system, without written permission from the publishers.

For permission to photocopy or use material electronically from this work, access www.copyright.com or contact the Copyright Clearance Center, Inc. (CCC), 222 Rosewood Drive, Danvers, MA 01923, 978-750-8400. For works that are not available on CCC please contact mpkbookspermissions@tandf.co.uk

Trademark notice: Product or corporate names may be trademarks or registered trademarks and are used only for identification and explanation without intent to infringe.

Library and Archives Canada Cataloguing in Publication

CIP data on file with Canada Library and Archives

Library of Congress Cataloging-in-Publication Data

CIP data on file with US Library of Congress

ISBN: 978-1-77491-746-6 (hbk)
ISBN: 978-1-77491-747-3 (pbk)
ISBN: 978-1-00354-538-5 (ebk)

ABOUT THE BOOK SERIES: AAP ADVANCES IN NUTRACEUTICALS

Series Editor:
Raj K. Keservani, PhD, MPharm
Faculty of B. Pharmacy, CSM Group of Institutions, Allahabad, India

Rajesh K. Kesharwani, PhD
Nehru Gram Bharati (Deemed to be University), Prayagraj, India

Anil K. Sharma, PhD, MPharm
Department of Pharmacy, School of Medical and Allied Sciences, GD Goenka University, Gurugram, India

In the modern era, mankind has witnessed a paradigm shift with respect to fundamental eating behavior. The lack of physical workouts and busy schedules at offices and in households have promoted the consumption of junk foods, which eventually results in numerous diseases and disorders since the nutritional content from fast food is inadequate. Plumpness and obesity have become a global health threat. The leading causes of death from most developing nations are noncommunicable diseases such as cardiovascular diseases, cancer, arthritis, osteoporosis, and liver toxicity. Patients suffering from such lifestyle ailments are a bit apprehensive towards prolonged use of costly modern therapeutics, which encourages instead the use of alternative approaches for management of such diseases and disorders.

The emerging sector of the nutraceutical industry encompasses products derived from nature, dietary supplements, and functional foods. Nutraceuticals are used for treatment and prevention of a broad range of diseases, such as the common cold, arthritis, sleep-related disorders, cancers, cardiovascular complications, metabolic disorders, and others.

The research on nutraceuticals is increasing day by day, considering the beneficial effects of food or food supplements in the management of diverse diseases. The issue of paramount concern is standardization and establishment of clinical efficacy of nutraceuticals, which is in fact a challenge for researchers around the globe.

This book series aims at realizing the significance of the variety of nutraceuticals for human well-being. The books in the series also emphasize the role of dieticians and nutritionists for the prescription of judicious eating habits. The key food components such as carbohydrates, proteins, and lipids as well as micronutrients (vitamins, minerals) are demonstrated to maintain good health, obviating the need for medicines. Thus, nutraceuticals that are indeed derived from food ingredients are believed to be potential alternative therapeutics.

Asymptomatic diseases/disorders necessitate proper diagnosis. Stressed circumstances have been reported to cause weight loss. Workplace stress is a key variable in the genesis and propagation of metabolic disorders. The nuances of the underlying mechanisms are still to be deciphered. Poor lifestyle trends have been attributed along with the consumption of junk foods in several such instances. Sugar-rich carbonated beverages, the use of contraband drugs, and the consumption of liquor in excess are assigned as risk factors. This book series covers advances and applications in addition to providing the basics of nutraceuticals.

The books in this series are valuable resources for industry professionals to design and develop quality products for end users. In addition, the book series is fortified by ideas of innovation, concept building, manufacturing aspects, quality control, and regulatory status of nutraceuticals.

Ostensibly, business has seen a rise in the nutraceutical consumption in recent years. Pure, safe, efficacious products are the need of the hour globally. There are a number of books on nutraceuticals in the market, yet these are only a few books presenting certain aspects of nutraceuticals therein. This book series offers a holistic view of this promising strategy, which is picking up pace with time. This book series is a unique endeavor to bring manufacturing, research and development, and marketing strategies under a single umbrella.

CURRENT BOOKS IN THE SERIES

- **Micronutrients and Macronutrients as Nutraceuticals**
  Editors: Prakash Chandra Gupta, PhD, Sayan Bhattacharyya, MBBS, MD, Nisha Sharma, PhD, MPharm, Rajesh K. Kesharwani, PhD, and Raj K. Keservani, PhD, MPharm

- **Formulations, Regulations, and Challenges of Nutraceuticals**
  Editors: Tingirikari Jagan Mohan Rao, PhD, Rajesh K. Kesharwani, PhD, Raj. K. Keservani, PhD, and Anil K. Sharma, PhD

- **Food Supplements and Dietary Fibers in Health and Disease**
  Editors: Bhushan R. Rane, PhD, MPharm, Raj K. Keservani, PhD, MPharm, Durgesh Singh, DPhil, Nayan A. Gujarathi, PhD, and Ashish S. Jain, PhD
- **Nutraceuticals in Cancer Prevention, Management, and Treatment**
  Editors: Raj K. Keservani, PhD, MPharm Bui Thanh Tung, PhD, Sippy Singh, DPhil, and Rajesh K. Kesharwani, PhD
- **Advances in Flavonoids for Human Health and Prevention of Diseases**
  Editors: Nisha Sharma, PhD, Deepika Saini, PhD, Rajesh K. Kesharwani, PhD, Prakash Chandra Gupta, and Raj. K. Keservani, PhD
- **The Flavonoids: Extraction and Applications**
  Editors: Deepika Saini, PhD, Rajesh K. Kesharwani, PhD, and Raj K. Keservani, PhD, MPharm
- **Immune-Boosting Nutraceuticals for Better Human Health: Novel Applications**
  Editors: Urmila Jarouliya, PhD, Raj K. Keservani, PhD, MPharm Rajesh K. Kesharwani, PhD, Virendra K. Patel, PhD, and Adi D. Bharti
- **Applications of Functional Foods in Disease Prevention**
  Editors: Raj K. Keservani, PhD, MPharm, and Eknath D. Ahire, MSPharm
- **Plant Metabolites and Vegetables as Nutraceuticals**
  Editors: Raj K. Keservani, PhD, MPharm, Bui Thanh Tung, PhD, Rajesh K. Kesharwani, PhD, MPharm, and Eknath D. Ahire
- **Preventive and Therapeutic Role of Vitamins as Nutraceuticals**
  Editors: Khemchand R. Surana, Eknath D. Ahire, Raj K. Keservani, PhD, MPharm, and Rajesh K. Kesharwani, PhD
- **Nutraceuticals and Bone Health**
  Editors: Deepak Sharma, PhD, Madan Mohan Gupta, PhD, Anil K. Sharma, PhD, MPharm, Raj K. Keservani, PhD, MPharm, and Rajesh K. Kesharwani, PhD
- **Flavonoids as Nutraceuticals**
  Editors: Rajesh K. Kesharwani, PhD, MTech, Deepika Saini, PhD, Raj K. Keservani, PhD, MPharm, and Anil Kumar Sharma, PhD
- **Herbals as Nutraceuticals: Their Role in Healthcare**
  Editors: Raj K. Keservani, PhD, MPharm, Rajeshwar Kamal Kant Arya, PhD, and Rajesh K. Kesharwani, PhD

- **Nutraceutical Fruits: Overview and Disease Prevention**
  Editors: Raj K. Keservani, PhD, MPharm
- **Nutrigenomics and Nutraceuticals**
  Editors: Raj K. Keservani, PhD, MPharm, Eknath D. Ahire,
  Shubham J. Khainar, PhD, Sanjay J. Kshirsagar, PhD, and
  Rajesh K. Kesharwani, PhD
- **Nutraceuticals in Cardiac Health Management**
  Editors: Raj K. Keservani, PhD, MPharm, Rajesh K. Kesharwani, PhD,
  Praveen Kumar Jain, PhD, Bhushan R. Rane, PhD, and
  Nayan A. Gujarathi, PhD
- **Nutraceuticals for the Treatment and Prevention of Sexual Disorders**
  Editors: Raj K. Keservani, PhD, MPharm, Sharangouda J. Patil, PhD,
  and Ivan Aranha, PhD
- **Nutraceuticals in Obesity Management and Control**
  Editors: Raj K. Keservani, PhD, MPharm, and Alka Lohani, PhD
- **The Nature of Nutraceuticals: History, Properties, Sources, and Nanotechnology**
  Editors: Rajesh K. Kesharwani, PhD, Prashant Kumar, PhD, and
  Raj K. Keservani, PhD, MPharm
- **Nutraceuticals in Insomnia and Sleep Problems**
  Editors: Raj K. Keservani, PhD, MPharm, Sayan Bhattacharyya, PhD,
  and Rajesh K. Kesharwani, PhD
- **Nutraceuticals in Respiratory and Pulmonary Diseases**
  Editors: Deepika Saini, PhD, Rajesh K. Kesharwani, PhD, and
  Raj K. Keservani, PhD, MPharm
- **Nutraceuticals in Arthritis and Psoriasis**
  Editors: Meenakshi Jaiswal, PhD, Raj K. Keservani, PhD, MPharm
  Rajesh K. Kesharwani, PhD, and Swati G. Talele, PhD
- **Nutraceuticals for the Treatment and Prevention of Sexual Disorders**
  Editors: Raj K. Keservani, PhD, Sharangouda J. Patil, PhD, and
  Ivan Aranha, PhD
- **Antioxidants as Nutraceuticals**
  Editors: Nayan A. Gujaratih, PhD, Raj K. Keservani, PhD,
  Rajesh K. Kesharwani, PhD, Bhushan R. Rane, PhD, and
  Yogeeta Sameer Goyal, PhD

- **Nutraceuticals in Management and Prevention of Diabetes**
  Editors: Raj K. Keservani, PhD, Prashant Kumar, PhD, and Dheeraj Chitara, PhD
- **Nutraceuticals in Mental Disorder and Brain Health**
  Editors: Raj K. Keservani, PhD, Eknath D. Ahire, PhD, and Shubham J. Khairnar, PhD

ABOUT THE EDITORS

Meenakshi Jaiswal, PhD, MPharm,
Assistant Professor, Department of Pharmacy,
Guru Ghasidas Vishwavidyalaya, Bilaspur, Chhattisgarh, India

Meenakshi Jaiswal, PhD, MPharm, is an Assistant Professor in the Department of Pharmacy at Guru Ghasidas Central University, Bilaspur, Chhattisgarh, India. She has more than 18 years of academic experience at various institute of India. She has presented more than 60 papers at various national and international seminars and conference and attended many workshops. Dr. Jaiswal has published seven Indian patents and has been granted two German patents in her scientific research field. She has supervised more than 35 undergraduate and postgraduate students for their research and project work. Dr. Jaiswal has published books as author as well as book chapters and popular articles in international and national journals. She is a life member of several scientific bodies. She was named Best Faculty in the Field of Chemical Sciences at the 2nd Online International Conference on Advance Interdisciplinary Research (ICAIR 2023), organized by Digvijai Nath Post Graduate College, Gorakhpur, and Science-Tech Institute run by the Manraj Kuwar Singh Educational Society, Lucknow, India. Her research interest includes colon drug targeting, drug delivery systems, and prodrug or conjugates of various antinflammatory drugs. Dr. Jaiswal completed her PhD in Pharmaceutical Science from the Guru Ghasidas Central University, Bilaspur, Chhattisgarh, India.

Raj K. Keservani, PhD
Associate Professor, Faculty of BPharmacy, CSM Group of Institutions,
Prayagraj, Uttar Pradesh, India

Raj K. Keservani, PhD, MPharm, is an Associate Professor in the Faculty of B. Pharmacy at CSM Group of Institutions, Prayagraj, India. He has more than 12 years of academic (teaching) experience from various institutes of India in pharmaceutical education. He has supervised more than 25 undergradate students for their research work and has published 31 peer-reviewed papers in the field of pharmaceutical sciences in national and international journals, one patent, 50 book chapters, three co-authored books, and 40 edited books. He is also active as a reviewer for several international scientific journals. Dr. Keservani is a life member of Society of Pharmaceutical Education and Research (SPER). His research interests include nutraceutical and functional foods, novel drug delivery systems (NDDS), transdermal drug delivery/drug delivery, health science, cancer biology, and neurobiology. Dr. Keservani graduated with a pharmacy degree from the Department of Pharmacy, Kumaun University, Nainital (Uttarakhand), India. He received his Master of Pharmacy (specialization in pharmaceutics) from the School of Pharmaceutical Sciences, Rajiv Gandhi Proudyogiki Vishwavidyalaya, Bhopal, India. He received his PhD degree from IKG Punjab Technical University, Jalandhar, Punjab, India.

Rajesh K. Kesharwani, PhD
Associate Professor, Department of Computer Application,
Nehru Gram Bharati (Deemed to be University), Prayagraj,
Uttar Pradesh, India

Rajesh K. Kesharwani, PhD, MTech, is working as an Associate Professor, Department of Computer Application, Nehru Gram Bharati (Deemed to be University), Prayagraj, India. He has more than 11 years of research and nine years of teaching experience at various institutes of India, imparting bioinformatics and biotechnology education. He has received several awards, including the NASI-Swarna Jayanti Puruskar by The National Academy of Sciences of India. He has supervised one PhD and more than 20 undergraduate and graduate students for their research work. Dr. Kesharwani has authored over 49 peer-reviewed articles, 20 book chapters, and 14 edited books with international publishers. He has been a member of many scientific communities as well as a reviewer for many international journals. He has presented many papers at various national and international conferences. He has been a recipient of a Ministry of Human Resource Development (India) Fellowship and a Senior Research Fellowship from the Indian Council of Medical Research, India. His research fields of interest are medical informatics, protein structure and function prediction, computer-aided drug designing, structural biology, drug delivery, cancer biology, nanobiotechnology, and biomedical sciences. Dr. Kesharwani received his PhD from the Indian Institute of Information Technology, Allahabad, and worked at NIT Warangal for two semesters.

Swati Gokul Talele, PhD
Associate Professor, Department of Pharmaceutics, MGV Pharmacy College, Panchvati, Nashik, Savitribai Phule Pune University, Pune, Maharashtra, India

Swati Gokul Talele, PhD, is currently serving as an Associate Professor in the Department of Pharmaceutics at MGV Pharmacy College, Panchvati, Nashik, Savitribai Phule Pune University, Pune, Maharashtra, India. She has 23 years of experience in research along with teaching. She has published more than 40 research papers in various reputed international and national journals as well as more than 30 review papers. She has also presented research work at several conferences and has received several awards. She has authored the book titled *Natural Excipients* and has many chapters and books that are in progress. She has supervised many MPharm students and is currently associated with many research projects. She has also worked as a college examination officer (CEO) for more than three years and is a member of the university examination committee. Dr. Talele has delivered interactive talks at continuous education programs for registered pharmacists and is a life member of the Association of Pharmacy Teachers of India and a member of the Indian Pharmaceutical Congress Association. Her interests are in the field of nanotechnology, natural polymers, herbal formulations, and radio-labeling-based bio-distribution studies.

CONTENTS

Contributors xvii

Preface xxi

PART I: Nutraceuticals in Arthritis Management and Preventions 1

1. **Role of Glucosamine and Chondroitin Sulfate as Nutraceuticals in Osteoarthritis** 3
   Nishi Gupta, Aimen Salman, Shradhanjali Singh, Amit Kumar Singh, and Shanti Bhushan Mishra

2. **Plant-Based Gum as a Nutraceutical in the Therapy of Arthritis** 27
   Mansi P. Bandawane, Shraddha S. Yeola, Utkarsha P. Patil, Swati G. Talele, Raj K. Keservani, and Laxmikant L. Borse

3. **Role of Nutraceuticals in the Prevention and Treatment of Arthritis** 45
   Pankaj Kumar and Rohit

4. **Arthritis Disease and Omega Polyunsaturated Fatty Acids** 67
   Aarti Tiwari, Satya Prakash Singh, Ajay Kumar Shukla, Vimal Kumar Yadav, Vishnu Prasad Yadav, Shailendra Kumar, Manish Kumar, and Vijay Kumar Yadav

5. **Microalgae and Their Use as Nutraceuticals in Arthritis** 89
   Pankaj Kumar

6. **Modern Nutraceuticals for Treatment of Osteoarthritis** 99
   Bui Thanh Tung, Tran Viet Linh, Nguyen Thuy Ngoc, Trinh Phuong Thao, and Nguyen Duc Thuan

7. **Marine Botanicals as Nutraceuticals for Arthritis** 137
   Pankaj Kumar

PART II: Nutraceuticals in Psoriasis Management and Preventions 163

8. **A Comprehensive Review on Diet and Psoriasis** 165
   Pankaj G. Jain, Afsar S. Pathan, Eknath D. Ahire, Khemchand R. Surana, Raj K. Keservani, and Swati G. Talele

9. **Marine Botanicals as Nutraceuticals for Psoriasis** 183
   Kajal M. Gawade, Bharati S. Garale, Swati G. Talele, Ramdas Dolas, and Laxmikant B. Borse

10. **Microalgae and Their Uses as Nutraceuticals in Psoriasis 205**
    Deepti Dwivedi, Satya Prakash Singh, Ajay Kumar Shukla,
    Shailendra Kumar, and Manish Kumar

11. **Nutraceuticals and Psoriasis: Recent Scientific Evidence in
    Clinical Trials 227**
    Abhish Jadhav, Mrudula Bele, Sahebrao Boraste, Rohan Ahire, Eknath D. Ahire,
    Meenakshi Jaiswal, Raj K. Keservani, and Swati G. Talele

12. **Role of Vitamins and Oils in the Treatment of Psoriasis 245**
    Akshada Atul Bakliwal, Vijay Sharad Chudiwal, Swati Gokul Talele, and
    Gokul Shravan Talele

13. **Nutraceuticals as a Non-Pharmacological Approach for Psoriasis 263**
    Rohit and Pankaj Kumar

14. **Role of Probiotic Supplements in Psoriasis 285**
    Rushikesh D. Patil, Shweta S. Gedam, Swati G. Talele,
    Laxmikant B. Borse, and Abhijeet D. Kulkarni

Index 303

CONTRIBUTORS

Eknath D. Ahire
Department of Pharmaceutics, MET's Institute of Pharmacy, Bhujbal Knowledge City, Adgaon, Nashik, Maharashtra, India

Rohan Ahire
Department of Pharmaceutics, MET's Institute of Pharmacy, Bhujbal Knowledge City, Adgaon, Nashik, Maharashtra, India

Akshada Atul Bakliwal
Department of Pharmaceutics, Sandip Institute of Pharmaceutical Sciences, Mahiravani, Nashik, Maharashtra, India

Mansi P. Bandawane
Department of Pharmaceutics, Sandip Institute of Pharmaceutical Sciences, Nashik, Maharashtra, India

Mrudula Bele
Department of Pharmaceutics, N.D.M.V. P's College of Pharmacy, Nashik, Maharashtra, India

Sahebrao Boraste
Department of Pharmaceutics, Sir Dr. M. S. Gosavi College of Pharmaceutical Education and Research, Nashik, Maharashtra, India

Laxmikant B. Borse
Department of Pharmacology, Sandip Institute of Pharmaceutical Sciences, Nashik, Maharashtra, India

Vijay Sharad Chudiwal
Research Scientist, Pune, Maharashtra, India

Ramdas Dolas
Department of Pharmaceutics, Sandip Institute of Pharmaceutical Sciences, Nashik, Maharashtra, India

Deepti Dwivedi
Institute of Pharmacy, Dr. Ram Manohar Lohia Avadh University, Ayodhya, Uttar Pradesh, India

Bharati S. Garale
Department of Pharmaceutics, Sandip Institute of Pharmaceutical Sciences, Nashik, Maharashtra, India

Kajal M. Gawade
Department of Pharmaceutics, Sandip Institute of Pharmaceutical Sciences, Nashik, Maharashtra, India

Shweta S. Gedam
Sandip Institute of Pharmaceutical Sciences, Nashik, Maharashtra, India

Nishi Gupta
Department of Pharmaceutical Chemistry, United Institute of Pharmacy, Prayagraj, Uttar Pradesh, India

Abhish Jadhav
Department of Pharmaceutics, MET's Institute of Pharmacy, Bhujbal Knowledge City, Adgaon, Nashik, Maharashtra, India

Pankaj G. Jain
Department of Pharmacology, R.C. Patel Institute of Pharmaceutical Education and Research, Shirpur, Maharashtra, India

Meenakshi Jaiswal
Assistant Professor, Department of Pharmacy, Guru Ghasidas Vishwavidyalaya (A Central University), Bilaspur, Chhattisgarh, India

Raj K. Keservani
Associate Professor, Faculty of B. Pharmacy, CSM Group of Institutions, Prayagraj, Uttar Pradesh, India

Abhijeet D. Kulkarni
Sandip Institute of Pharmaceutical Sciences, Nashik, Maharashtra, India

Manish Kumar
Department of Pharmacy, Madhav University, Pindwara, Rajasthan, India

Pankaj Kumar
Professor, Department of Pharmacology, Adesh Institute of Pharmacy and Biomedical Science, Adesh University, Bathinda, Punjab, India

Shailendra Kumar
Institute of Microbiology, Dr. Ram Manohar Lohia Avadh University, Ayodhya, Uttar Pradesh, India

Tran Viet Linh
VNU University of Medicine and Pharmacy, Vietnam National University, Ha Noi, Vietnam

Shanti Bhushan Mishra
Department of Pharmacognosy, United Institute of Pharmacy, Prayagraj, Uttar Pradesh, India

Nguyen Thuy Ngoc
VNU University of Medicine and Pharmacy, Vietnam National University, Ha Noi, Vietnam

Afsar S. Pathan
Department of Pharmacology, R.C. Patel Institute of Pharmaceutical Education and Research, Shirpur, Maharashtra, India

Rushikesh D. Patil
Sandip Institute of Pharmaceutical Sciences, Nashik, Maharashtra, India

Utkarsha P. Patil
Department of Pharmaceutics, Sandip Institute of Pharmaceutical Sciences, Nashik, Maharashtra, India

Rohit
Department of Pharmacy Practice, ISF College of Pharmacy, Moga, Punjab, India

Aimen Salman
Department of Pharmacology, United Institute of Pharmacy, Prayagraj, Uttar Pradesh, India

Ajay Kumar Shukla
Institute of Pharmacy, Dr. Ram Manohar Lohia Avadh University, Ayodhya, Uttar Pradesh, India

Amit Kumar Singh
Department of Pharmaceutics, United Institute of Pharmacy, Prayagraj, Uttar Pradesh, India

Satya Prakash Singh
Institute of Pharmacy, Dr. Ram Manohar Lohia Avadh University, Ayodhya, Uttar Pradesh, India

Contributors

Shradhanjali Singh
Department of Pharmaceutical Chemistry, United Institute of Pharmacy, Prayagraj, Uttar Pradesh, India

Khemchand R. Surana
Department of Pharmaceutical Chemistry, Divine College of Pharmacy, Satana, Maharashtra, India

Gokul Shravan Talele
Department of Pharmaceutical Chemistry, Matoshri College of Pharmacy, Eklahare, Nashik, Maharashtra, India

Swati G. Talele
Department of Pharmaceutics, Sandip Institute of Pharmaceutical Sciences, Mahiravani, Nashik, Maharashtra, India

Trinh Phuong Thao
VNU University of Medicine and Pharmacy, Vietnam National University, Ha Noi, Vietnam

Nguyen Duc Thuan
VNU University of Medicine and Pharmacy, Vietnam National University, Ha Noi, Vietnam

Aarti Tiwari
Institute of Pharmacy, Dr. Ram Manohar Lohia Avadh University, Ayodhya, Uttar Pradesh, India

Bui Thanh Tung
VNU University of Medicine and Pharmacy, Vietnam National University, Ha Noi, Vietnam

Vijay Kumar Yadav
Dr. Bhimrao Ambedkar University, Chhalesar Campus, Agra, Uttar Pradesh, India

Vimal Kumar Yadav
Institute of Pharmacy, Dr. Ram Manohar Lohia Avadh University, Ayodhya, Uttar Pradesh, India

Vishnu Prasad Yadav
Institute of Pharmacy, Dr. Ram Manohar Lohia Avadh University, Ayodhya, Uttar Pradesh, India

Shraddha S. Yeola
Department of Pharmaceutics, Sandip Institute of Pharmaceutical Sciences, Nashik, Maharashtra, India

PREFACE

The inflammatory and painful condition known as arthritis affects multiple joints. Arthritis is characterized by pain and stiffness in the joints, which often increases with age. Osteoarthritis and rheumatoid arthritis are the two most typical forms of the disease. Joint health is maintained by a delicate balancing act between anabolic and catabolic signals, and here is where nutraceuticals come in. There has been a rise in interest in the potential benefits of nutraceuticals for the treatment and, more importantly, the prevention of osteoarthritis due to their regulatory effect on the homeostasis of cartilage metabolism (OA).

Psoriasis is a skin disease that results in red, scaly patches that are itchy and flaky, most often on the scalp, knees, and elbows. Psoriasis is widespread and persistent (chronic), although there is currently no treatment or prevention. Pain, disturbed sleep, and difficulty focusing are all possible results. To that end, nutraceuticals may be considered as a complementary method for psoriasis control. Vitamins and nutritional supplements are often helpful for psoriasis patients, both in reducing symptoms and facilitating the skin's recovery.

The chapters in this book explore elements that deserve consideration in many ways and need to be included in our diet on a regular basis. This book thus lays a very solid foundation for examining the effectiveness and validity of various plant-derived nutraceuticals, which can be used as crucial therapeutic tools in the prevention of arthritis and psoriasis.

This book comprises two parts. Part I details information about nutrients, marine microalgae, and omega polyunsaturated fatty acids in arthritis management. In Part II, botanicals, microalgae, probiotics, and vitamins in the management of psoriasis are discussed.

PART I: NUTRACEUTICALS IN ARTHRITIS MANAGEMENT AND PREVENTION

Shanti Bhushan Mishra and a coworker report the rule of glucosamine and chondroitin sulfate in the management and prevention of osteoarthritis in Chapter 1.

Swati G. Talele et al. emphasize how plant-based gums give nutritional benefits to arthritis in Chapter 2: Plant-Based Gum as a Nutraceutical in the Therapy of Arthritis.

Chapter 3: Role of Nutraceuticals in Prevention and Treatment of Arthritis, written by Pankaj Kumar and Rohit discusses the role of anti-inflammatory nutraceuticals in the prevention of arthritis.

Ajay Kumar Shukla and his co-worker suggest that omega-3 fatty acids may be able to alleviate the symptoms of arthritic illness in Chapter 4.

Pankaj Kumar discusses the dietary benefits of microalgae as well as their use from a medicinal standpoint in the management of rheumatoid arthritis in Chapter 5: Microalgae and Their Use as Nutraceuticals in Arthritis Treatment.

Bui Thanh Tung et al. using nutraceuticals in the treatment of osteoarthritis produces positive results and opens up new avenues for research in the future in Chapter 6: Modern Nutraceuticals for Treatment of Osteoarthritis.

Pankaj Kumar wrote Chapter 7: Marine Botanicals as Nutraceuticals for Arthritis and includes certain nutraceuticals obtained from marine origins that will be useful in the treatment of arthritis.

PART II: NUTRACEUTICALS IN PSORIASIS MANAGEMENT AND PREVENTION

Chapter 8: A Comprehensive Review on Diet and Psoriasis, written by Pankaj G. Jain et al., focuses on insights from psoriasis and what is a good diet for psoriasis. Swati G. Talele and her coworker emphasize the nutritional advantages of marine botanicals in the management of psoriasis in Chapter 9: Marine Botanicals as Nutraceuticals for Psoriasis.

Ajay Kumar Shukla and his associates discuss the potential of microalgae and their bioactive chemicals to treat skin issues such as infections, inflammation, and psoriasis in Chapter 10: Microalgae and Their Uses as Nutraceuticals in Psoriasis.

Abhish Jadhav et al. discuss how nutraceutical supplements can enhance a patient's quality of life and have a positive effect on their general health in Chapter 11: Nutraceuticals and Psoriasis: Recent Scientific Evidence in Clinical Trials.

Akshada Atul Bakliwal et al. discuss in-depth how nutrients and oils can benefit those who have psoriasis in Chapter 12: Role of Vitamins and Oils in the Treatment of Psoriasis.

Nutritional supplements, vitamins, herbal extracts, and phytochemicals are covered in the treatment of psoriasis in Chapter 13: Nutraceuticals: A Non-Pharmacological Approach for Psoriasis, written by Rohit and Pankaj Kumar.

Rushikesh D. Patil and his associates discuss how probiotics can lessen the psoriasis vicinity and severity index of psoriasis sufferers, inhibit the irritation stage of psoriasis, and regulate immune cells in Chapter 14: Role of Probiotic Supplements in Psoriasis.

PART I
NUTRACEUTICALS IN ARTHRITIS MANAGEMENT AND PREVENTIONS

CHAPTER 1

ROLE OF GLUCOSAMINE AND CHONDROITIN SULFATE AS NUTRACEUTICALS IN OSTEOARTHRITIS

NISHI GUPTA,[1] AIMEN SALMAN,[2] SHRADHANJALI SINGH,[1] AMIT KUMAR SINGH,[3] and SHANTI BHUSHAN MISHRA[4]

[1]Department of Pharmaceutical Chemistry, United Institute of Pharmacy, Prayagraj, Uttar Pradesh, India

[2]Department of Pharmacology, United Institute of Pharmacy, Prayagraj, Uttar Pradesh, India

[3]Department of Pharmaceutics, United Institute of Pharmacy, Prayagraj, Uttar Pradesh, India

[4]Department of Pharmacognosy, United Institute of Pharmacy, Prayagraj, Uttar Pradesh, India

ABSTRACT

Osteoarthritis (OA) is a degenerative joint disorder that is characterized by progressive loss of cartilage, periarticular bone changes, and synovial membrane inflammation. Chondroprotectives such as chondroitin sulfate, glucosamine sulfate, hyaluronic acid, collagen hydrolysate, and other supplements play a significant role in OA treatment compared to nonsteroidal anti-inflammatory drugs. Several clinical studies have shown that the specific combination of these micronutrients leads to a more effective reduction of OA symptoms with fewer adverse events. Their chondroprotective effects can be explained by a dual mechanism: (1) as essential components of cartilage and synovial fluid, they promote the anabolic processes of cartilage metabolism; (2) their anti-inflammatory effects can inhibit various inflammatory processes that contribute to cartilage breakdown. These dual mechanisms can slow down cartilage degeneration and help restore joint structure, leading to reduced pain and improved mobility of the affected joint.

1.1 INTRODUCTION

Osteoarthritis (OA), the most recurrent type of arthritis, is distinguished by consistent wear and privation of cartilage in the joints resulting in abrasion between the bones, resulting in pain and swelling. It was long thought that only the cartilage is spurious. Synovium and underlying bone also change, as is now known (Loeser et al., 2012; Felson et al., 2000; Blagojevic et al., 2010). Osteophyte formation takes place after the reaction of periarticular bone, which causes subsidiary diminution in joint movement. It can transpire in any joint but preponderates in weight-endurance joints, such as the knee and hip. In Germany, the ubiquity of recognized osteoarthritis in at least one joint is 27% and more than 50% of the population over 60 agonizes from OA in at least one joint (Heidari et al., 2011). Every year, half a million osteoarthritis cases are responsible for the replacement of joints in the United States of America (Neogi et al., 2013), specifying the burden of OA on patients as well as financially on society. Obesity and the aging of the population are the major risk concerns in the case of OA, with a high prevalence rate from 2000 to 2030 (Hruby et al., 2015).

Progressive effects of continuous mechanical wear and tear on cartilage have been the well-established theory of the pathogenesis of primary osteoarthritis. Thus, "aging" is simply the accumulation of loading cycles over a lifetime of joint use (Aigner et al., 2007). Physiological or superphysiological loading has been the major reason for continuous micro traumata to the cartilage. This entails tedious harm to the extracellular matrix of articular ligament resulting in the deficiency of integrity and function and destruction of the tissue. Obviously, if this is the major scenario, any treatment will largely be futile as moving and loading the joints is inevitable as a consequence of their use. However, this review aims to open up the possibility that age-related changes are less a fate, but rather a challenge for therapeutic intervention which can be taken.

The point of this brief review chapter is to give a report on the pathophysiology of OA. We focus on the pathophysiology and pathogenesis of OA, review some of the current concepts in OA research, and discuss the future of personalized medicine for OA. In the absence of disease-modifying OA drugs (DMOADs), personalized treatment should include lifestyle assessment, physical therapy, and rehabilitation. Even if disease-modifying drugs for OA are on the horizon, it will take years before we have epidemiological data on effectiveness. Therefore, as we eagerly await the development of novel DMOADs, it would be prudent to focus on OA prevention rather than treatment. We will start by providing a report on the global burden of OA and the escalating cost of treatment (Grassel et al., 2020) before discussing the pathophysiology of OA and the need for identifying early inflammatory events and targeting these changes (Primorac et al., 2020) to improve the key symptoms, such as inflammation and pain in OA patients (Hunter et al., 2008).

1.2 THE GLOBAL BURDEN OF OA

OA is the main source of persistent disability universally in people aged over 70 years and has been assigned as a 'fundamentally important illness' by the World Health Organization (WHO). OA is one of the 10 most impairing illnesses in industrialized nations. In the Global Burden of Disease 2010 review, hip and knee OA was positioned as the 11th most elevated contributor to worldwide disability (Heidari et al., 2011). The prevalence of OA is set to increase in line with the expansion in the number of people aged 60 years and older and the rise in weight across the world. In the United States alone, OA is the highest cause of work loss and affects over 20 million people, costing the US economy more than US $100 billion annually (Zhang et al., 2010). OA represents one of the top 5 healthcare costs in Europe (Katz et al., 2021). In the United Kingdom, one-third of people aged 45 and over (8.75 million individuals) have sought treatment for OA, and around half of these individuals have knee OA (a significant portion of those seeking treatment for OA have knee OA). The number of people in the UK with knee OA is estimated to increase to 6.5 million by 2020. Even if an updated report on the global economic burden had been published more recently, it would undoubtedly underestimate the true cost burden to the world's health and social care systems.

As referenced above, as a multifactorial entire joint sickness, OA is a significant contributor to the inflammation and loss of functional capacity in older people. Its prevalence and incidence increase with age, for example, a majority of people over 65 years old are affected by OA (Anderson et al., 2010). Importantly, the trend is continuously rising due to an increase in life expectancy and population aging along with obesity in the next few decades. The functional disability of OA mainly involves activities of daily living related to the weight-bearing joints (hip, knee), such as walking and climbing steps (Guccione et al., 1994). Individuals with OA of weight-bearing joints have to cope with joint pain and a limited range of motion for a significant portion of their lifetime (Corti et al., 2003). However, pain and activity limitation may be intermediate steps over the course of OA, and disability in walking is the final stage necessitating total joint replacement. Similarly, an understanding of the OA pathology will facilitate the development of prevention and treatment strategies aimed at reducing the progressive and symptomatic progression.

1.3 MODIFIABLE AND NON-MODIFIABLE OA RISK FACTORS

Certain elements have been demonstrated to be related to a more serious risk of developing OA. The risk of developing most types of joint pain increases with age, and OA is certainly no exception. Gender is another key risk factor for OA. In fact, most types of joint pain are more common in women, and 60% of individuals with joint pain are women, so perhaps it is not surprising that the female sex also represents a significant risk factor for OA. It has been speculated that leptin might be a systemic or local factor that mediates the metabolic connection between obesity and OA. Leptin and other adipocytokines (adipokines) may be the missing links explaining the gender disparity in the disease.

1.4 INFLAMMATORY ASPECTS OF OA

Inflammation is presently very much acknowledged as a component of osteoarthritis (Jarouliya & Keservani, 2019). Yet, we have had some significant awareness of this for a considerable length of time; we just decided to overlook a portion of the published literature. In a paper published in 1975, George Ehrlich described a group of predominantly menopausal females who presented with a disfiguring and inflammatory OA, some of whom went on to develop changes typical of rheumatoid arthritis (RA). The pioneering work that Ehrlich did in this area was well recognized by the WHO due to the work he carried out for the organization in New York, but his work has earned more respect in recent years and after he died in 2014. Many new studies have shown the presence of synovitis in OA patients and demonstrated a direct relationship between joint inflammation and disease progression.

Aging is a natural and inevitable process characterized by nine hallmarks. These include genomic instability, telomere attrition, epigenetic alterations, loss of proteostasis, deregulated nutrient sensing, mitochondrial dysfunction, cellular senescence, stem cell exhaustion, and altered intercellular communication. Aging and inflammation are major contributing factors to the development and progression of joint and muscle-related conditions.

1.5 MECHANISM OF ARTICULAR CARTILAGE LUBRICATION

Articular ligament is a striking self-greasing system, that can effectively maintain super-oil between two opposing sliding ligament surfaces while enduring high pressures over a wide range of shear rates. Such outstanding lubrication has been systematically researched for many years and theories relevant to articular ligament oil have been proposed based on fluid film (Ji et al., 2019; Crane et al., 2014) or boundary oil. Previously, a more detailed description of articular ligament lubrication has been provided in a review by (Jahn et al., 2016). For the purpose of this mini-review, we focus on the recent findings on the hydration oil mechanism in boundary oil of articular ligament and its implication for the therapeutics of OA. The hydration lubrication mechanism provides a framework for designing highly effective boundary oil systems, which target articular ligaments in OA treatment. Hydration oil occurs in watery and natural media, where the hydration layers are steadily held by either particles or zwitterions they encompass and accordingly try not to be pressed out under pressure. Simultaneously, they remain quickly unwinding and act in a liquid-like reaction to shear (Gaisinskaya et al., 2012; Klein et al., 2013; Ma et al., 2015). Subsequently, more examinations have been performed on ligament grease considering the hydration oil system (Sorkin et al., 2013). Among them, supramolecular cooperative energy in limited oil is considered to provide a sensible model for ligament grease (Seror et al., 2015). Three vital components of articular ligament including hyaluronan, lubricin, and phosphatidylcholine lipid synergize to achieve hydration grease at the exposed phosphocholine groups of the phosphatidylcholine lipid. Consequently, significant oil arises with the shear of such hydration layers surrounding the phosphocholine groups.

1.6 MECHANISM OF SUBCHONDRAL BONE REMODELING

Under physiological circumstances, bone rebuilding constantly keeps up with the metabolic homeostasis and primary respectability of subchondral bone through exact coordination of bone resorption and resulting bone development (Klein, 2013). Aggravations of this cycle bring about subchondral bone irregularities, including bone misfortune and sclerosis, and osteophyte arrangement in the commencement and movement of OA (Zaidi, 2007; Burr & Gallant, 2004; Castaneda et al., 2012). Appropriately, an understanding of the mechanism behind subchondral bone rebuilding is essential for the inhibition of OA progression. Previous research findings have shown that cell communication at the level of progenitors through receptor activator of nuclear factor (NF)-κB ligand (RANKL) functions to couple bone resorption and formation in the remodeling of subchondral bone (Suda et al., 1999). Therefore, identifying pieces of evidence of matricellular communication through transforming growth factor-β1 (TGF-β1) or possibly insulin-like growth factor-1 (IGF-1) (Tang et al., 2009; Qui et al., 2010; Crane & Cao, 2014), and osteoclast-osteoblast communication through semaphorin 4D (Sema4D) and Plexin-B1 have also added new levels to cell communication coupling bone resorption and formation (Negishi et al., 2011). Those various degrees of cell correspondence direct bone rebuilding and adjust subchondral unresolved issue changes in neighborhood ecological and foundational factors during the commencement and movement of OA. Especially, they give ramifications for drug intervention with coupling system of activity to fix subchondral bone irregularities. In accordance with this thought, factors capable of affecting bone remodeling can be targeted as therapeutics for the treatment of subchondral bone in people with OA.

1.7 CURRENT STRATEGIES FOR OA TREATMENT

Current procedures for anticipation and treatment of OA endeavor toward diminishing joint torment while at the same time reestablishing joint capacity, subsequently postponing medical procedure treatment as far as might be feasible. Considering this objective, novel methodologies for OA treatment have yielded a large number of choices, for example, synergetic treatment joining both lubrication and medication intervention, the regulatory balance between bone resorption and growth, and exercise therapy (Figure 1.1). In this part, we will zero in on the new achievement of the aforementioned three therapeutic options in OA treatment.

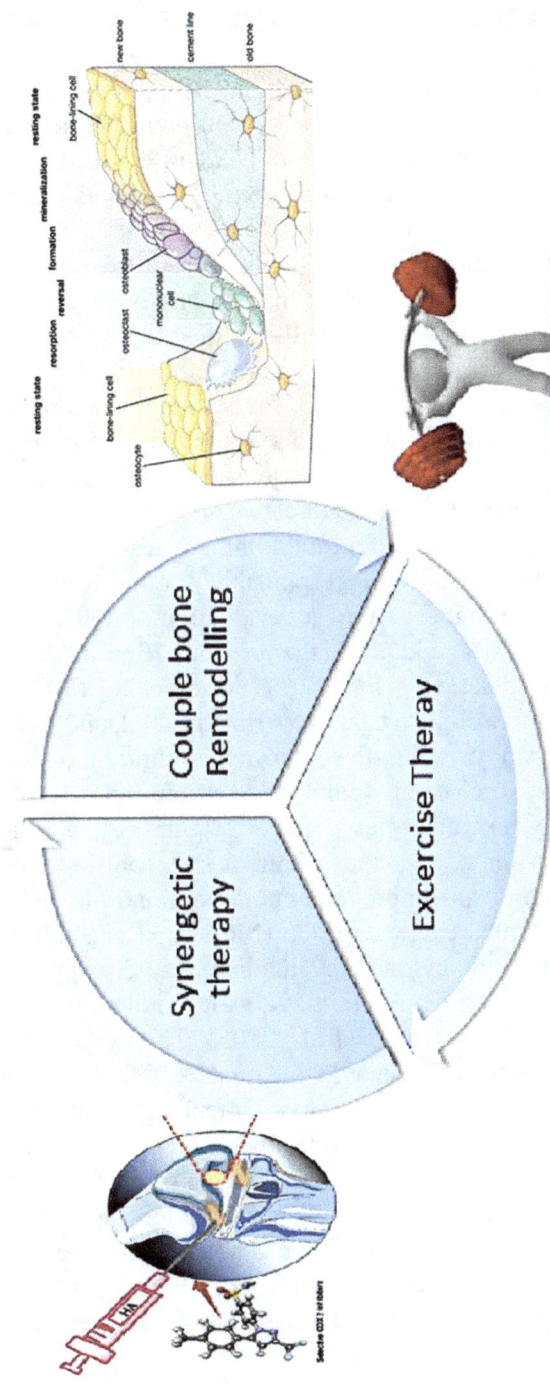

FIGURE 1.1 Strategies involved in the treatment of OA.

1.8 NONPHARMACOLOGICAL AND PREVENTATIVE STRATEGIES

Training, exercise, and weight reduction are pillars in the administration of OA and the advancement of general well-being. Patient education about treatment targets and the significance of changes in lifestyle, exercise, weight reduction, and other measures is supported by two meta-analyses, but the ES for pain relief is small: 0.06 (0.02–0.10).

The recommendation that the initial focus should be on self-improvement and patient-driven treatments rather than on passive treatments delivered by health professionals is based on well-qualified assessment, common sense, and financial considerations (Zhang et al., 2008).

Obesity is a significant risk factor for both the development and progression of tibiofemoral knee OA (both symptomatic and radiographic) (Hart et al., 1992; Felson et al., 1997; Bagge et al., 1991). An association, albeit modest, has also been demonstrated between obesity and OA at various sites like the hip, hand, and patellofemoral joint, suggesting that both mechanical and metabolic factors may be responsible for the link between OA and obesity. In the Framingham study, an evaluation of 800 women showed that a reduction in BMI of ≥ 2 kg/m^2 in the previous 10 years reduced the odds of developing symptomatic OA by > 50% (Felson et al., 1992).

As of late, a huge clinical trial, the Arthritis, Diet, and Activity Promotion Trial (ADAPT) study, randomized 316 overweight or obese older subjects with knee OA to exercise only (combined aerobic and strengthening), dietary weight loss only, exercise plus dietary weight loss, or a healthy lifestyle control group. After a year and a half, despite only modest decreases in body weight, significant improvements in pain and physical function were found in the diet plus exercise group (Messier et al., 2004). A subsequent recent randomized clinical trial, evaluating a rapid weight loss diet among 80 patients with knee OA, found that a weight reduction of 10% improved function by 28% (Christensen et al., 2005). The authors noted that fewer than four patients would need to be treated with a low-energy diet for one patient to achieve a ≥ 50% improvement in the Western Ontario and McMaster Universities Osteoarthritis Index (WOMAC, a measure of joint pain, stiffness, and function) compared to a control diet. To date, there are no longitudinal studies evaluating whether weight loss slows the progression of knee OA, but this effect would appear to be clinically plausible. The pooled effect sizes for improvements in pain (ES = 0.20; CI 0–0.39) and physical disability (ES = 0.23; CI 0.04–0.42) are small with a mean weight loss of 6.1

kg (range 4.7–7.6 kg) (Zhang et al., 2008). There are no published randomized controlled trials (RCTs) for weight loss and hip OA.

Three deliberate audits assessing the impact of activity for hip and knee OA have shown improvement in agony, function, and global appraisal (Roddy & Doherty, 2006). However, data were pooled in these meta-analyzes and included studies of all exercise types, failing to assess the quality of the exercise program. Fewer comparisons between aerobic and strengthening exercises have been made, and both aerobic and strengthening exercises are effective for knee OA (Roddy & Doherty, 2006). Pooled effect sizes for pain relief are in the moderate range for both aerobic (ES = 0.52; CI 0.34–0.70) and muscle strengthening exercises (ES = 0.32; CI 0.23–0.42) for knee OA (Zhang et al., 2008). In a previous Cochrane review assessing exercise in hip and knee OA, there were only two studies totaling 100 participants for hip OA (Fransen et al., 2008). However, in a recent meta-analysis of all individual hip OA trials, exercise was considered more effective, albeit modestly, than usual care (Felson et al., 1992).

Practice treatment for OA of the hip or knee ought to be individualized and patient-focused, considering variables like age, comorbidity, and generally speaking dreariness. Grouping and home activity are equally effective, and patient preference should be taken into consideration. Hydrotherapy is also a helpful adjunct to any exercise program. Adherence is the key indicator of long-term outcomes from exercise in patients with knee or hip OA (Roddy & Doherty, 2006). Improvement in muscle strength and proprioception acquired from exercise programs might reduce the progression of knee and hip OA. The improved proprioception may also reduce the risk of falls.

A recent systematic review showed that acupuncture meeting adequate standards was significantly better than both sham acupuncture and no additional intervention in improving pain and function in patients with chronic knee pain (White et al., 2007). However, there was heterogeneity among the eligible studies, and further research is needed to confirm these findings and provide more information on long-term effects. Another issue is the intensity of provider contact associated with acupuncture and the physiologic effect of needling. Nevertheless, the procedure is reasonably safe and well-tolerated by most, although several sessions are typically required. A summary of the overall evidence showed moderate effect sizes (ES = 0.51; CI 0.23–0.79) for pain, stiffness (ES = 0.41; CI 0.13–0.69), and function (ES = 0.51, CI 0.23–0.79) with a NNT of 4 (CI 3–9) for clinically significant pain relief (Zhang et al., 2008).

In spite of the fact that the evaluation of footwear is suggested in most OA management guidelines, there is a lack of evidence to support this (Roddy & Doherty, 2006). Several observational studies of laterally wedged insoles for medial compartment knee OA have shown symptomatic improvement but not three RCTs. However, in a recent 2-year RCT, the use of laterally wedged insoles was associated with reduced nonsteroidal anti-inflammatory drugs (NSAID) use and better compliance (Pham et al., 2004). Nevertheless, there was no modification of pain, stiffness, or function. There is limited research evaluating medial wedged insoles for lateral compartment knee OA. The only RCT demonstrated improved pain and function with the use of a rearfoot medial wedge compared to a neutral insole in women with valgus lateral compartment knee OA (Hinman & Bennell, 2009). Further research is needed for validation. There have been no controlled studies of footwear in hip OA. The following features have been recommended for footwear for individuals with OA: thick, soft, shock-absorbing sole; minimal heel raise; wide forefoot to allow spreading of the toes during forefoot loading; and deep, soft uppers (Roddy & Doherty, 2006). However, there have been no controlled studies to support this recommendation.

Proof from randomized preliminaries is scanty with respect to the viability of treatments to address malalignment across the knee joint (Felson et al., 2006). In one preliminary, a huge decrease in knee torment was found in those with average compartment OA and varus malalignment, utilizing a neoprene sleeve over the knee. Knee supports that stabilize the knee joint and provide valgus stress have also been shown to improve pain and function in patients with average compartment knee OA. Patellofemoral pain may be caused by shifting or malalignment of the patella (Felson et al., 2006). Patellar realignment with the use of supports or tape may reduce pain. In clinical trials using tape, knee pain was reduced when compared to placebo.

A walking stick can be used to unload painful joints. There are no RCTs to support this, but there was unanimous expert agreement that walking aids can reduce pain in patients with hip and knee OA. This should be held in the contralateral hand at the level of the greater trochanter of the hip (Felson et al., 2006). The use of compression gloves is helpful for stiffness and pain from osteoarthritic involvement of the distal and proximal interphalangeal joints (Barnsley et al., 2005). A variety of splints are also available for the carpometacarpal joint.

1.9 PHARMACOLOGICAL THERAPIES

1.9.1 SIMPLE ANALGESIA

Both paracetamol and non-steroidal anti-inflammatory drugs (NSAIDs) are evidence-based drugs for symptom relief in OA (Bannwarth et al., 2006). Paracetamol is the first-line pharmacologic agent for the treatment of OA recommended by all international guidelines (Zhang et al., 2005; Jordan et al., 2003). A recent meta-analysis suggested that paracetamol is effective for pain relief in OA, albeit with a small effect size (ES = 0.21; 95% CI 0.02–0.41). In the recent Cochrane review, paracetamol demonstrated a statistically significant yet small reduction in pain (ES = 0.13; CI 0.04–0.22) (Towheed et al., 2009). However, there was no improvement in overall WOMAC, suggesting that it should not be expected to have a strong impact on stiffness or function. There was no significant difference in toxicity compared to placebo in short-term trials. Nevertheless, given its relatively favorable side effect profile, it should remain the first-line pharmacologic agent.

NSAIDs are effective agents for the treatment of OA. A meta-analysis suggested that NSAIDs, including COX-2 specific inhibitors, can reduce pain and functional disability in knee OA better than placebo (ES = 0.32; 95% CI 0.24–0.39; ES = 0.29; 95% CI 0.18–0.40, respectively). NSAIDs may be more effective in hip OA, based on a systematic review (ES = 0.69; 95% CI 0.12–1.26). The prolonged use of NSAIDs for OA is not supported. Interestingly, in the meta-analysis including eight trials directly comparing paracetamol and NSAIDs, an aggregated effect size of 0.20 and 0.30 for pain relief and overall WOMAC index, respectively, were observed for oral NSAIDs (Bannwarth et al., 2006). There is high interindividual variability in patient response to both paracetamol and NSAIDs, but there are no recognized clinical predictors of response.

NSAIDs are associated with more adverse events than paracetamol in short-term trials, as confirmed in the new Cochrane systematic review of short-term RCTs [Relative risk (RR) 1.47; 95% CI 1.08–2.00] (Zhang et al., 2008). COX-2-specific inhibitors have been shown to be just as effective as traditional nonselective NSAIDs in patients with OA (Bannwarth et al., 2006). They are associated with significantly fewer upper gastrointestinal (GI) complications, particularly in patients not taking low-dose aspirin, and slightly less dyspepsia compared to conventional NSAIDs. While they are tolerated in most patients with aspirin-induced asthma, they have a pattern of nephrotoxicity and drug interactions similar to those of conventional

NSAIDs (Bannwarth et al., 2006). There is also no evidence that COX-2-specific inhibitors are less harmful to the GI tract than traditional NSAIDs combined with a proton-pump inhibitor (PPI), especially in patients at high risk of developing adverse GI events. Both of these are recommended in patients with increased GI risk (Hooper et al., 2004).

As of late, the cardiovascular dangers of COX-2-specific inhibitors and NSAIDs have been widely featured. A new methodical survey has shown that cardiovascular gambling was expanded with rofecoxib, diclofenac, indomethacin, and most likely meloxicam (McGettigan & Henry, 2006). Significantly, naproxen, with a pooled relative gamble of 0.97 (95% CI 0.87–1.07), neither expanded nor diminished risk (i.e., not cardioprotective as recently suspected). Celecoxib expanded risk at portions higher than 200 mg/day, while at lower dosages, the risk was not expanded. Notwithstanding, the creators suggest alert considering four investigations published since the completion of the meta-analysis (McGettigan & Henry, 2006). They suggest that naproxen appears to be the safest NSAID from a cardiovascular perspective. It should be noted that lumiracoxib was not evaluated in this meta-analysis. In one more systematic review, the overall cardiovascular gamble associated with COX-2-specific inhibitors was not significantly greater than that associated with traditional nonselective NSAIDs (RR = 1.19; 95% CI 0.80–1.75) (Hooper et al., 2004). In a new systematic review and meta-analysis of atherothrombotic complications of COX-2 specific inhibitors and nonselective NSAIDs, the rate of serious vascular events was 1% per annum in COX-2 specific inhibitor-treated patients compared with 0.9% in conventional NSAID-treated patients (RR 1.16; 95% CI 0.97–1.38) (Zhang et al., 2008). However, the heterogeneity in risk among conventional NSAIDs was observed again (i.e., ibuprofen and diclofenac had a modest increase in risk but not naproxen).

It ought to be noted that the European Agency for the Evaluation of Medicinal Products advises that COX-2 specific inhibitors are contraindicated in patients with ischemic coronary illness or stroke and that caution should be exercised in patients with cardiovascular risk factors (Zhang et al., 2008). According to the authors, for a person with a higher risk of developing peptic ulcer disease, a short course of a COX-2-specific inhibitor might be a reasonable choice. Conversely, in one with high cardiovascular risk, if an anti-inflammatory must be used, naproxen along with a PPI might be the safer option. In summary, NSAIDs are effective for symptom relief in OA and should be prescribed at the lowest effective dose for the shortest possible duration.

1.9.2 TOPICAL THERAPY

Momentary utilization of effective NSAIDs is safe and effective in OA of the hand and knee according to a 2004 meta-analysis (Biswal et al., 2006). This was also confirmed in another meta-analysis in 2004 (Lin et al., 2004). However, these were less effective than oral NSAIDs. Additionally, there was possible publication bias as there was significant asymmetry of a funnel plot (Zhang et al., 2008). Their effectiveness in hip OA is uncertain due to the depth of that joint. Four studies have assessed effectiveness at about a month or beyond in knee OA, finding a modest effect (ES = 0.28; 95% CI 0.14–0.42) (Biswal et al., 2006). Effective NSAIDs are generally well tolerated with systemic adverse effects being very rare. However, local adverse events can occur in 10–15% of patients.

Effective capsaicin, the active ingredient of hot chili pepper, exerts its effect by enhancing the release of substance P from unmyelinated C nerve fibers (Rains & Bryson, 1995). It is moderately better than a placebo in reducing the pain of knee OA and may take a few weeks to take effect (Deal et al., 1991). Again, local irritation may occur.

1.9.3 GLUCOSAMINE AND CHONDROITIN

Glucosamine is an aminosaccharide, acting as a preferred substrate for the biosynthesis of glycosaminoglycan chains and, therefore, for the production of aggrecan and other proteoglycans of the ligament (Esko, 1999). Due to the crucial role aggrecans play in providing the ligament its hydrophilicity, compounds enhancing the synthesis of aggrecans may be beneficial in cases of OA, a condition characterized by an increase in matrix underlying protein turnover, with catabolism prevailing over synthesis (Roughley et al., 2014). *In vitro*, glucosamine sulfate (GS) has been shown to reduce prostaglandin E2 (PGE2) production and inhibit nuclear factor kappa B (NFκB) DNA binding in chondrocytes and synovial cells (Kapoor et al., 2012). Glucosamine inhibits gene expression of OA cartilage *in vitro* (Lippiello, 2007). Long-term oral administration of glucosamine sulfate reduces cartilage destruction and upregulation of MMP-3 mRNA in a model of spontaneous osteoarthritis in Hartley guinea pigs (Taniguchi et al., 2013). Glucosamine can prevent cytokine-induced demethylation of a specific CpG site in the IL1b promoter and this is associated with reduced expression of IL1b (Hashimoto et al., 2009). It was suggested that since glucosamine inhibits both anabolic and catabolic genes, the therapeutic effects of glucosamine may be attributed to anticatabolic activities, rather than due to anabolic activities. GS is a stronger inhibitor of gene expression than glucosamine hydrochloride (Uitterlinden et al., 2006).

Glucosamine (an amino sugar) and chondroitin sulfate (a glycosaminoglycan) are generally utilized for the treatment of OA, in spite of the fact that their mechanisms of action are hazy. These are naturally occurring constituents of articular cartilage proteoglycans. A recently updated Cochrane review of glucosamine treatment in knee OA found pain and function improved by 28% and 21% in the Lequesne index, respectively, compared to placebo (Jerosch, 2011). The Lequesne index is a 10-question survey for patients with knee OA, assessing pain, walking distance, and activities of daily living, on a 0–24 scale (Dawson et al., 2005). No improvement in WOMAC pain and function subscales was found. A lack of standardization in glucosamine preparations has contributed to the inconsistency in study outcomes. The new US NIH (National Institutes of Health) supported GAIT (Glucosamine/chondroitin Arthritis Intervention Trial) investigation discovered that the blend of glucosamine hydrochloride and chondroitin sulfate was just more effective than placebo in the subgroup with moderate-to-severe OA (Clegg et al., 2003). In the other groups, the response was similar. However, the study results are difficult to interpret due to the high placebo response, patient selection, and the use of glucosamine hydrochloride. It is unclear if the latter has similar potential clinical benefits as glucosamine sulfate, as most studies demonstrating efficacy for glucosamine in OA have used glucosamine sulfate. The effect size for trials that used glucosamine sulfate was 0.44 (95% CI 0.18–0.70) compared to 0.06 (95% CI 0.08–0.20) for those that used glucosamine hydrochloride (Zhang et al., 2008).

A 2003 meta-analysis assessing chondroitin sulfate for knee OA observed that the treatment was significantly more effective for pain relief compared to a placebo (ES = 0.43; 95% CI 0.32–0.54) (Richy et al., 2003). No dose effect was noted, with 1,200 and 800 mg/day being equally effective. However, in the most recent systematic review, this was less clear. The ES for pain relief was significant (ES = 0.74; 95% CI 0.50–0.99) but there was significant heterogeneity between trials (Reichenbach et al., 2007). While the evidence for glucosamine sulfate and chondroitin sulfate is conflicting, both treatments are safe and well tolerated. Therefore, it is advisable to trial both glucosamine sulfate and chondroitin sulfate to assess response, and patients should be encouraged to continue for at least 90 days as these medications are slow-acting.

1.9.4 INTRA-ARTICULAR THERAPY

The alleviation and potential reduction of knee OA symptoms can be significantly improved by intra-articular corticosteroid injections at 1–3 weeks (ES = 0.72; 95% CI: 0.42–1.02), with a NNT of 4 (Bellamy et al., 2006). Data on long-term effectiveness and impact on function are limited. Strong evidence for intra-articular corticosteroid injections in hip OA is scarce, but the most recent RCT showed improvements in pain and mobility in the steroid-treated group (ES = 0.6) (Anandacoomarasamy et al., 2010). The long-term safety of steroid injections has been supported in a 2-year study (Raynauld et al., 2003). No serious adverse events were reported in the systematic review (Bellamy et al., 2006). Efforts to identify predictors of response, such as biomarkers, have not been consistent. Additionally, there have not been enough head-to-head studies comparing different steroid formulations. While it is impossible to predict individual patient responses, a trial of injections is certainly worthwhile as they are generally well tolerated.

Hyaluronic acid is a high molecular weight glycosaminoglycan present in the synovial fluid of both normal and OA joints. The effectiveness of viscosupplementation with hyaluronic acid injections in knee OA has been suggested to be comparable to NSAIDs and corticosteroid injections. A recent Cochrane review (Bellamy et al., 2006) concluded that hyaluronic acid demonstrated better effectiveness compared to placebo for improvement in pain and function of knee OA. While no head-to-head comparison between specific products has been conducted, viscosupplementation was more consistent from 5 to 13 weeks in terms of pain, range of motion, and WOMAC and Lequesne scores (Bowman et al., 2018; Peck et al., 2021). However, data on effectiveness is conflicting, and overall it likely has modest effects on pain relief. Another meta-analysis in 2005 found no evidence for improved function and no effects on pain compared to saline injections. The conflicting results have been attributed to the inclusion of different controlled trials, differences in outcome measures, and various statistical methods for data synthesis. The evidence for hip OA is much less. Acute local reactions have been reported in 2–8% post-injection.

1.9.5 OPIOID ANALGESIA

A new meta-analysis showed a moderate effect size for pain reduction in OA (ES = 0.78; 95% CI 0.59–0.98) with a mean study duration of 12 weeks. However, there was significant heterogeneity between studies (Zhang et al., 2010). Narcotics are also associated with common adverse events, and the number needed to harm was 5 compared to placebo. The withdrawal rates were higher for stronger opioids (morphine, oxycodone) compared to weaker opioids (tramadol, codeine). There are also no long-term trials of opioids in OA. Nevertheless, they play a significant role, with caution, in the management of patients with chronic, persistent pain for whom surgery is not an option and where other modalities have failed.

1.9.6 OTHER THERAPIES

Diacerein: Rhein, the dynamic metabolite of diacerein, restrains IL1 blend and movement which is ensnared in ligament annihilation (Pelletier et al., 2010). A meta-investigation of controlled clinical examinations for knee and hip OA showed that diacerein was better than fake treatment, like NSAIDs, and showed a persistent impact for as long as 2 months. Further review is expected before comprehensive use.

Reciprocal treatments: Various correlative and alternative medicines are being utilized broadly locally to manage OA pain. These include S-adenosylmethionine (SAMe), methylsulfonylmethane (MSM), dimethyl sulfoxide (DMSO), and green-lipped mussel (GLM). Unfortunately, there has been a lack of good-quality RCTs. A systematic review of DMSO and MSM highlighted significant strategic issues and the need for definitive efficacy trials. In the systematic review of GLM in OA, there were only four RCTs, and three were placebo-controlled. All assessed GLM as adjunctive treatment to regular treatment. The findings of the two studies could not be included due to strategic issues, and further rigorous investigations are required (Brien et al., 2008).

Glucosamine and chondroitin sulfate are currently commonly used for symptom relief in OA. In a landmark clinical trial assessing the disease-modifying potential of glucosamine sulfate, patients were randomly assigned 1,500 mg daily of glucosamine or placebo for three years (Pham et al., 2004). Patients on placebo experienced moderate joint space narrowing, while no significant joint space loss was observed in patients on glucosamine. These findings were corroborated by two other studies. However, the results have since been questioned due to the radiographic technique used to measure joint space width (JSW). The combined results of two RCTs showed an ES of 0.24 for joint space loss reduction (95% CI 0.04–0.43). Radiological outcomes were evaluated in the GAIT study using plain X-rays. There was no statistically significant difference in mean JSW loss observed in any treatment group (glucosamine hydrochloride; chondroitin sulfate; glucosamine hydrochloride + chondroitin sulfate) compared to placebo. A trend was noted in Kellgren — Lawrence grade 2 knees towards improvement compared to placebo. The limitations of the study included a small sample size, variability of JSW measurement, and a slight loss in JSW (Sawitzke et al., 2008).

Chondroitin sulfate gives good outcomes in numerous RCTs as a DMOAD. In a placebo group, a significant decrease in JSW has been observed, with no change in the chondroitin group (800 mg/day) (Pham et al., 2004). Both doxycycline and diacerein have been evaluated in double-blind RCTs. Diacerein was assessed in hip OA in a placebo-controlled RCT and showed significantly lower joint space narrowing in the active arm (Dougados et al., 2001). However, similar effects were not found in the knee OA study (Pham et al., 2004). Doxycycline, evaluated in knee OA, showed less progression in the active arm compared to placebo. It is worth noting that this benefit was only observed in the treated knee and not the opposite knee. Interestingly, in the doxycycline study, there was a discrepancy between suggestive and initial results, possibly indicating different pathways responsible for these outcomes (Dougados et al., 2001). However, this could also be due to the selection of the study population, who were not consistently seeking clinical care for OA. Despite promising results in the search for DMOADs, questions of clinical relevance persist, and further studies are warranted.

1.10 CONCLUSION

GS affects suggestive and underlying results of knee OA. These outcomes ought not to be extrapolated to other glucosamine salts [hydrochloride or arrangements over-the-counter or food supplements] in which no guarantee exists about satisfied, pharmacokinetics, and pharmacodynamics of the tablet.

KEYWORDS

- **chondroitin sulfate**
- **dimethyl sulfoxide**
- **glucosamine sulfate**
- **green-lipped mussel**
- **methylsulfonylmethane**
- **osteoarthritis**

REFERENCES

Aigner, T., Haag, J., Martin, J., & Buckwalter, J. (2007). Osteoarthritis: Aging of matrix and cells – Going for a remedy. *Current Drug Targets, 8*(2), 325–331.

Anandacoomarasamy, A., & March, L. (2010). Current evidence for osteoarthritis treatments. *Therapeutic Advances in Musculoskeletal Disease, 2*(1), 17–28.

Anderson, A. S., & Loeser, R. F. (2010). Why is osteoarthritis an age-related disease? *Best Practice & Research Clinical Rheumatology, 24*(1), 15.

Ateshian, G. A. (2009). The role of interstitial fluid pressurization in articular cartilage lubrication. *Journal of Biomechanics, 42*(9), 1163–1176.

Bagge, E., Bjelle, A., Eden, S., & Svanborg, A. (1991). Factors associated with radiographic osteoarthritis: Results from the population study of 70-year-old people in Goteborg. *Journal of Rheumatology, 18*, 1218–1222.

Bannwarth, B. (2006). Acetaminophen or NSAIDs for the treatment of osteoarthritis. *Best Practice & Research Clinical Rheumatology, 20*, 117–129.

Barnsley, L. (2005). How to treat: Osteoarthritis. *Australian Doctor*, 27–34.

Bellamy, N., Campbell, J., Robinson, V., Gee, T., Bourne, R., & Wells, G. (2006). Intraarticular corticosteroid for treatment of osteoarthritis of the knee. *Cochrane Database of Systematic Reviews, 19*(2), 1–227.

Biswal, S., Medhi, B., & Pandhi, P. (2006). Long-term efficacy of topical nonsteroidal anti-inflammatory drugs in knee osteoarthritis: Meta-analysis of randomized placebo-controlled clinical trials. *Journal of Rheumatology, 33*, 1841–1844.

Blagojevic, M., Jinks, C., Jeffery, A., & Jordan, K. P. (2010). Risk factors for onset of osteoarthritis of the knee in older adults: A systematic review and meta-analysis. *Osteoarthritis and Cartilage, 18*, 24–33.

Bowman, S., Awad, M. E., Hamrick, M. W., Hunter, M., & Fulzele, S. (2018). Recent advances in hyaluronic acid-based therapy for osteoarthritis. *Clinical and Translational Medicine, 7*(6), 1–11.

Brien, S., Prescott, P., Coghlan, B., Bashir, N., & Lewith, G. (2008). A systematic review of the nutritional supplement *Perna canaliculus* (green-lipped mussel) in the treatment of osteoarthritis. *QJM: An International Journal of Medicine, 101*, 167–179.

Burr, D. B., & Gallant, M. A. (2012). Bone remodeling in osteoarthritis. *Nature Reviews Rheumatology, 8*, 665–673.

Castañeda, S., Roman-Blas, J. A., Largo, R., & Herrero-Beaumont, G. (2012). Subchondral bone is a key target for osteoarthritis treatment. *Biochemical Pharmacology, 83*, 315–323.

Christensen, R., Astrup, A., & Bliddal, H. (2005). Weight loss: The treatment of choice for knee osteoarthritis? A randomized trial. *Osteoarthritis and Cartilage, 13*, 20–27.

Clegg, D. O., Reda, D. J., Harris, C. L., Klein, M. A., O'Dell, J. R., Hooper, M. M., et al. (2006). Glucosamine, chondroitin sulfate, and the two in combination for painful knee osteoarthritis. *The New England Journal of Medicine, 354*, 795–808.

Corti, M. C., & Rigon, C. (2003). Epidemiology of osteoarthritis: Prevalence, risk factors, and functional impact. *Aging Clinical and Experimental Research, 15*(5), 359–363.

Crane, J. L., & Cao, X. (2014). Function of matrix IGF-1 in coupling bone resorption and formation. *Journal of Molecular Medicine, 92*, 107–115.

Dawson, J., Linsell, L., Doll, H., Zondervan, K., Rose, P. M. B., Chir, B., & Fitzpatrick, F. R. (2005). Assessment of the Lequesne index of severity for osteoarthritis of the hip in an elderly population. *Osteoarthritis and Cartilage, 13*, 854–860.

Deal, C. L., Schnitzer, T. J., Lipstein, E., Seibold, J. R., Stevens, R. M., Levy, M. D., et al. (1991). Treatment of arthritis with topical capsaicin: A double-blind trial. *Clinical Therapeutics, 13*, 383–395.

Dougados, M., Nguyen, M., Berdah, L., Mazieres, B., Vignon, E., & Lequesne, M. (2001). Evaluation of the structure-modifying effects of diacerein in hip osteoarthritis: ECHODIAH, a three-year, placebo-controlled trial. *Arthritis & Rheumatism, 44*(11), 2539–2547.

Esko, J. D. (1999). Proteoglycans and glycosaminoglycans. In *Essentials of Glycobiology*, pp. 1–17, Cold Spring Harbor Laboratory Press.

Felson, D. T. (2006). Clinical practice. Osteoarthritis of the knee. *The New England Journal of Medicine, 354*, 841–848.

Felson, D. T. (2009). Developments in the clinical understanding of osteoarthritis. *Arthritis Research & Therapy, 11*, 203.

Felson, D. T., Lawrence, R. C., Dieppe, P. A., Hirsch, R., Helmick, C. G., Jordan, J. M., et al. (2000). Osteoarthritis: New insights. Part 1: The disease and its risk factors. *Annals of Internal Medicine, 133*, 635–646.

Felson, D. T., Zhang, Y., Anthony, J. M., Naimark, A., & Anderson, J. J. (1992). Weight loss reduces the risk of symptomatic knee osteoarthritis in women. The Framingham Study. *Annals of Internal Medicine, 116*, 535–539.

Felson, D. T., Zhang, Y., Hannan, M. T., Naimark, A., Weissman, B., Aliabadi, P., et al. (1997). Risk factors for incident radiographic knee osteoarthritis in the elderly: The Framingham Study. *Arthritis & Rheumatism, 40*, 728–733.

Fransen, M., & McConnell, S. (2008). Exercise for osteoarthritis of the knee. *Cochrane Database of Systematic Reviews, 8*(4), CD004376.

Gaisinskaya, A., Ma, L., Silbert, G., Sorkin, R., Tairy, O., Goldberg, R., et al. (2012). Hydration lubrication: Exploring a new paradigm. *Faraday Discussions, 156*, 217–233.

Grässel, S., & Muschter, D. (2020). Recent advances in the treatment of osteoarthritis. *F1000Research, 9*, 1–17.

Gray, M. L., Burstein, D., Kim, Y. J., & Maroudas, A. (2008). Magnetic resonance imaging of cartilage glycosaminoglycan: Basic principles, imaging technique, and clinical applications. *Journal of Orthopaedic Research, 26*, 281–291.

Guccione, A. A., Felson, D. T., Anderson, J. J., Anthony, J. M., Zhang, Y., Wilson, P. W., et al. (1994). The effects of specific medical conditions on the functional limitations of elders in the Framingham Study. *American Journal of Public Health, 84*(3), 351–358.

Guermazi, A., Burstein, D., Conaghan, P., Eckstein, F., Le Graverand-Gastineau, M. P. H., & Keen, H. (2008). Imaging in osteoarthritis. *Rheumatic Disease Clinics of North America, 34*, 645–687.

Hart, D. J., Doyle, D. V., & Spector, T. D. (1999). Incidence and risk factors for radiographic knee osteoarthritis in middle-aged women: the Chingford Study. *Arthritis & Rheumatism, 42*, 17–24.

Hashimoto, K., Oreffo, R. O. C., Gibson, M. B., Goldring, M. B., & Roach, H. (2009). DNA demethylation at specific CpG sites in the IL1B promoter in response to inflammatory cytokines in human articular chondrocytes. *Arthritis & Rheumatism, 60*(11), 3303–3313.

Heidari, B. (2011). Knee osteoarthritis prevalence, risk factors, pathogenesis and features: Part I. *Caspian Journal of Internal Medicine, 2*(2), 205–212.

Hinman, R. S., & Bennell, K. L. (2009). Advances in insoles and shoes for knee osteoarthritis. *Current Opinion in Rheumatology, 21*, 164–170.

Hooper, L., Brown, T. J., Elliott, R., Payne, K., Roberts, C., & Symmons, D. (2004). The effectiveness of five strategies for the prevention of gastrointestinal toxicity induced by non-steroidal anti-inflammatory drugs: Systematic review. *BMJ, 329*, 948.

Hruby, A., & Hu, F. B. (2015). The epidemiology of obesity: A big picture. *Pharmacoeconomics, 33*(7), 673–689.

Hunter, D. J., McDougall, J. J., & Keefe, F. J. (2008). The symptoms of OA and the genesis of pain. *Rheumatic Disease Clinics of North America, 34*(3), 623–643.

Jahn, S., Seror, J., & Klein, J. (2016). Lubrication of articular cartilage. *Annual Review of Biomedical Engineering, 11*(18), 235–258.

Jarouliya, U., & Keservani, R. K. (2019). Pathways leading to child obesity. In D. Bagchi (Ed.), *Global Perspectives on Childhood Obesity: Current Status, Consequences and Prevention* (2nd ed., pp. 137–146). Academic Press. ISBN: 9780128128404.

Jerosch, J. (2011). Effects of glucosamine and chondroitin sulfate on cartilage metabolism in OA: Outlook on other nutrient partners especially omega-3 fatty acids. *International Journal of Rheumatology, 1*, 1–17.

Ji, X., & Zhang, H. (2019). Current strategies for the treatment of early-stage osteoarthritis. *Frontiers in Mechanical Engineering, 5*(57), 1–8.

Jordan, K. M., Arden, N. K., Doherty, M., Bannwarth, B., Bijlsma, J. W., Dieppe, P., et al. (2003). EULAR Recommendations 2003: An evidence-based approach to the management of knee osteoarthritis: Report of a Task Force of the Standing Committee for International Clinical Studies Including Therapeutic Trials (ESCISIT). *Annals of the Rheumatic Diseases, 62*, 1145–1155.

Kapoor, M., Mineau, F., Fahmi, H., Pelletier, J. P., & Pelletier, J. M. (2012). Glucosamine sulfate reduces prostaglandin E2 production in osteoarthritic chondrocytes through inhibition of microsomal PGE synthase-1. *Journal of Rheumatology, 39*(3), 635–644.

Katz, J. N., Arant, K. R., & Loeser, R. F. (2021). Diagnosis and treatment of hip and knee osteoarthritis: A review. *JAMA, 325*(6), 568–578.

Klein, J. (2013). Hydration lubrication. *Friction, 1*, 1–23.

Leeb, B. F., Neumann, K., & Rintelen, B. (2006). A meta-analysis of controlled clinical studies with diacerein in the treatment of osteoarthritis. *Archives of Internal Medicine, 166*(17), 1899–1906.

Lin, J., Zhang, W., Jones, A., & Doherty, M. (2004). Efficacy of topical non-steroidal anti-inflammatory drugs in the treatment of osteoarthritis: Meta-analysis of randomized controlled trials. *BMJ, 329*, 324.

Lippiello, L. (2007). Collagen synthesis in tenocytes, ligament cells, and chondrocytes exposed to a combination of glucosamine HCl and chondroitin sulfate. *Evidence-Based Complementary and Alternative Medicine, 4*(2), 219–224.

Loeser, R. F., Goldring, S. R., Scanzello, C. R., & Goldring, M. B. (2012). Osteoarthritis: A disease of the joint as an organ. *Arthritis & Rheumatism, 64*(6), 1697–1707.

Ma, L., Gaisinskaya-Kipnis, A., Kampf, N., & Klein, J. (2015). Origins of hydration lubrication. *Nature Communications, 6*, 6060.

McGettigan, P., & Henry, D. (2006). Cardiovascular risk and inhibition of cyclooxygenase: A systematic review of the observational studies of selective and nonselective inhibitors of cyclooxygenase 2. *JAMA, 296*, 1633–1644.

Messier, S. P., Loeser, R. F., Miller, G. D., Morgan, T. M., Rejeski, W. J., Sevick, M. A., et al. (2004). Exercise and dietary weight loss in overweight and obese older adults with knee osteoarthritis: The Arthritis, Diet, and Activity Promotion Trial. *Arthritis & Rheumatism, 50*, 1501–1510.

Negishi-Koga, T., Shinohara, M., Komatsu, N., Bito, H., Kodama, T., Friedel, R. H., et al. (2011). Suppression of bone formation by osteoclastic expression of semaphorin 4D. *Nature Medicine, 17*, 1473–1480.

Neogi, T. (2013). The epidemiology and impact of pain in osteoarthritis. *Osteoarthritis and Cartilage, 21*(9), 1145–1153.

Peck, J., Slovek, A., Miro, P., Vij, N., Traube, B., Lee, C., et al. (2021). A comprehensive review of viscosupplementation in osteoarthritis of the knee. *Orthopedic Reviews, 13*(1), 1–11.

Pelletier, J. M., & Pelletier, J. P. (2010). Effects of diacerein at the molecular level in the osteoarthritis disease process. *Therapeutic Advances in Musculoskeletal Disease, 2*(2), 95–104.

Pelletier, J. P., Raynauld, J. P., Beaulieu, A. D., Bessette, L., Morin, F., Delorme, P., et al. (2016). Chondroitin sulfate efficacy versus celecoxib on knee osteoarthritis structural changes using magnetic resonance imaging: A 2-year multicenter exploratory study. *Arthritis Research & Therapy, 18*(256), 1–12.

Pham, J. W., Pellino, J. L., Lee, Y. S., Carthew, R. W., & Sontheimer, E. J. (2004). A Dicer-2-dependent 80s complex cleaves targeted mRNAs during RNAi in Drosophila. *Cell, 117*(1), 83–94.

Pham, T., Maillefert, J. F., Hudry, C., Kieffert, P., Bourgeois, P., Lechevalier, D., et al. (2004). Laterally elevated wedged insoles in the treatment of medial knee osteoarthritis: A two-year prospective randomized controlled study. *Osteoarthritis and Cartilage, 12*, 46–55.

Primorac, D., Molnar, V., Rod, E., Jelec, Z., Cukelj, F., Matisic, V., et al. (2020). Knee osteoarthritis: A review of pathogenesis and state-of-the-art non-operative therapeutic considerations. *Genes, 11*(8), 1–35.

Qiu, T., Wu, X., Zhang, F., Clemens, T. L., Wan, M., & Cao, X. (2010). TGF-β type II receptor phosphorylates the PTH receptor to integrate bone remodeling signaling. *Nature Cell Biology, 12*, 224–234.

Rains, C., & Bryson, H. M. (1995). Topical capsaicin: A review of its pharmacological properties and therapeutic potential in post-herpetic neuralgia, diabetic neuropathy, and osteoarthritis. *Drugs & Aging, 7*, 317–328.

Raynauld, J. P., Wright, C. B., Ward, R., Choquette, D., Haraoui, B., Pelletier, J. M., et al. (2003). Safety and efficacy of long-term intraarticular steroid injections in osteoarthritis of the knee: A randomized, double-blind, placebo-controlled trial. *Arthritis & Rheumatism, 48*(2), 370–377.

Reichenbach, S., Sterchi, R., Scherer, M., Trelle, S., Bürgi, E., Bürgi, U., et al. (2007). Meta-analysis: Chondroitin for osteoarthritis of the knee or hip. *Annals of Internal Medicine, 146*, 580–590.

Richy, F., Bruyere, O., Ethgen, O., Cucherat, M., Henrotin, Y., & Reginster, J. Y. (2003). Structural and symptomatic efficacy of glucosamine and chondroitin in knee osteoarthritis: A comprehensive meta-analysis. *Archives of Internal Medicine, 163*, 1514–1522.

Roddy, E., & Doherty, M. (2006). Changing lifestyles and osteoarthritis: What is the evidence? *Best Practice & Research Clinical Rheumatology, 20*, 81–97.

Roughley, P. J., & Mort, J. S. (2014). The role of aggrecan in normal and osteoarthritic cartilage. *Journal of Experimental Orthopedics, 1*(1), 1–11.

Sawitzke, A. D., Shi, H., Finco, M. F., Dunlop, D. D., Bingham, C. O., Harris, C. L., et al. (2008). The effect of glucosamine and/or chondroitin sulfate on the progression of knee osteoarthritis: A report from the glucosamine/chondroitin arthritis intervention trial. *Arthritis & Rheumatism, 58*(10), 3183–3191.

Scharf, H. P., Mansmann, U., Streitberger, K., Witte, S., Krämer, J., Maier, C., et al. (2006). Acupuncture and knee osteoarthritis: A three-armed randomized trial. *Annals of Internal Medicine, 145*, 12–20.

Seror, J., Zhu, L., Goldberg, R., Day, A. J., & Klein, J. (2015). Supramolecular synergy in the boundary lubrication of synovial joints. *Nature Communications, 6*, 6497.

Shengelia, R., Parker, S. J., Balin, M., George, T., & Reid, M. C. (2014). Complementary therapies for osteoarthritis: Are they effective? *Pain Management Nursing, 14*(4), e274–e288.

Sorkin, R., Kampf, N., Dror, Y., Shimoni, E., & Klein, J. (2013). Origins of extreme boundary lubrication by phosphatidylcholine liposomes. *Biomaterials, 34*, 5465–5475.

Suda, T., Takahashi, N., Udagawa, N., Jimi, E., Gillespie, M. T., & Martin, T. J. (1999). Modulation of osteoclast differentiation and function by the new members of the tumor necrosis factor receptor and ligand families. *Endocrine Reviews, 20*, 345–357.

Tang, Y., Wu, X., Lei, W., Pang, L., Wan, C., Shi, Z., et al. (2009). TGF-β1-induced migration of bone mesenchymal stem cells couples bone resorption with formation. *Nature Medicine, 15*, 757–765.

Taniguchi, S., Ryu, J., Seki, M., Sumino, T., Tokuhashi, Y., & Esumi, M. (2012). Long-term oral administration of glucosamine or chondroitin sulfate reduces the destruction of cartilage and up-regulation of MMP-3 mRNA in a model of spontaneous osteoarthritis in Hartley guinea pigs. *Journal of Orthopedic Research, 30*(5), 673–678.

Towheed, T. E., Maxwell, L., Judd, M. G., Catton, M., Hochberg, M. C., & Wells, G. (2009). Acetaminophen for osteoarthritis. *Cochrane Database of Systematic Reviews, 1*, 1–74.

Tugwell, P. (2010). OARSI recommendations for the management of hip and knee osteoarthritis: Part III: Changes in evidence following systematic cumulative update of research published through January 2009. *Osteoarthritis and Cartilage, 18*(4), 476–499.

Uitterlinden, E. J., Koevoet, J. L. M., Jennikens, Y. M., Zeinstra, S. M. A. B., Degroot, J., Veraar, J. A. N., Weinans, H., & Osch, G. J. V. M. V. (2006). Glucosamine decreases the expression of anabolic and catabolic genes in human osteoarthritic cartilage explants. *Osteoarthritis and Cartilage, 14*(3), 250–257.

White, A., Foster, N. E., Cummings, M., & Barlas, P. (2007). Acupuncture treatment for chronic knee pain: A systematic review. *Rheumatology (Oxford), 46*, 384–390.

Zaidi, M. (2007). Skeletal remodeling in health and disease. *Nature Medicine, 13*, 791–801.

Zhang, W., Doherty, M., Arden, N., Bannwarth, B., Bijlsma, J., Gunther, K. P., et al. (2005). EULAR evidence-based recommendations for the management of hip osteoarthritis: Report of a task force of the EULAR Standing Committee for International Clinical Studies Including Therapeutics (ESCISIT). *Annals of the Rheumatic Diseases, 64*, 669–681.

Zhang, W., Jones, A., & Doherty, M. (2004). Does paracetamol (acetaminophen) reduce the pain of osteoarthritis? A meta-analysis of randomized controlled trials. *Annals of the Rheumatic Diseases, 63*, 901–907.

Zhang, W., Moskowitz, R. W., Nuki, G., Abramson, S., Altman, R. D., Arden, N., et al. (2008). OARSI recommendations for the management of hip and knee osteoarthritis, Part II: OARSI evidence-based, expert consensus guidelines. *Osteoarthritis and Cartilage, 16*, 137–162.

Zhang, W., Nuki, G., Moskowitz, R. W., Abramson, S., Altman, R. D., Arden, N. K., Zeinstra, B. S., Brandt, K. D., Croft, P., Doherty, M., Dougados, M., Hochberg, M., Hunter, D. J., Kwoh, K., Lohman, L. S., & Tugwell, P. (2010). OARSI recommendations for the management of hip and knee osteoarthritis: Part III: Changes in evidence following systematic cumulative update of research published through January 2009. *Osteoarthritis and Cartilage, 18*(4), 476–499.

Zhang, Y., & Jordan, J. M. (2010). Epidemiology of osteoarthritis. *Clinical Geriatrics Medicine, 26*(3), 355–369.

Zhu, J., Liu, Z., Brady, E., Otto-Bliesner, B., Zhang, J., Noone, D., et al. (2017). Reduced ENSO variability at the LGM revealed by an isotope-enabled Earth system model. *Geophysical Research Letters, 44*(13), 6984–6992.

CHAPTER 2

PLANT-BASED GUM AS A NUTRACEUTICAL IN THE THERAPY OF ARTHRITIS

MANSI P. BANDAWANE,[1] SHRADDHA S. YEOLA,[1] UTKARSHA P. PATIL,[1] SWATI G. TALELE,[1] RAJ K. KESERVANI,[2] and LAXMIKANT L. BORSE[3]

[1]Department of Pharmaceutics, Sandip Institute of Pharmaceutical Sciences, Nashik, Maharashtra, India

[2]Associate Professor, Faculty of B. Pharmacy, CSM Group of Institutions, Prayagraj, Uttar Pradesh, India

[3]Department of Pharmacology, Sandip Institute of Pharmaceutical Sciences, Nashik, Maharashtra, India

ABSTRACT

Food or food products that provide clinical or welfare of health, such as inhibition of a disease, are known as nutraceuticals. Herbal nutraceuticals are significant tools in retaining health and as antidotes to nutritionally produced severe and persisting sickness, ensuring optimal health, durability, and standard of living. Arthritis is described as an acute or chronic joint inflammation that often coexists with pain and structural damage. There are moreover 100 distinct types of arthritis with osteoarthritis being the most ordinary source of non-inflammatory arthritis. Arthritis produced due to redness can occur in many settings and can be triggered by neurodegenerative processes (rheumatoid arthritis, psoriatic arthritis, ankylosing spondylitis, etc.), crystal accumulation, incited inflammation (gout, pseudogout, basic calcium phosphate disease), or infections (septic arthritis). This chapter primarily focuses on some natural gums used to treat arthritis. Gum Arabic has anti-inflammatory properties because it is a secondary type of butyrate. The outcomes of Gum Arabic in treating rheumatoid arthritis are beneficial because of its immune-modulating properties. The gum resin distillate of B. serrata includes active components like boswellic acid, which is a potent anti-inflammatory agent and a particular non-corrosive blocker of 5-Lipoxygenase (5-LOX). An exclusive composition that contains both acidic and non-acidic components of Boswellia serrata gum resin possesses efficacy towards anti-osteoarthritis. Cashew gum contains Anacardic acids, which show anti-inflammatory properties, and another plant *C. weitii* (Guggulu) unlocked a recent opening on the practice of this plant in Ayurveda, which is also found to be an anti-inflammatory agent. This chapter emphasizes how plant-based gums will provide nutritional benefits to arthritis.

2.1 INTRODUCTION

The word "Nutraceutical" includes 'Nutrients' and 'Pharmaceuticals.' According to the AAFCO in 1996, 'nutrient' is defined as any feed component that helps and supports life in some way, whereas 'nutraceutical' means any non-poisonous food constituent that is medically approved to provide healthcare benefits including inhibition, treatment, or healthcare (Kathleen et al., 2013). Some food ingredients are isolated or purified and marketed in medicinal forms that are not generally associated with food. Depending on the jurisdiction, products are claimed to improve chronic diseases, enhance health, delay the aging process, or increase life expectancy (Rajasekaran et al., 2008). For the purpose of regulating the nutraceutical industry, the Indian government enacted the Food Safety and Standards Act. Nutraceuticals avoid complications and contain balanced dietary nutrients as foods to ensure they are safe. That's why nutraceuticals are advantageous over other medicines (Baby Chauhan et al., 2013).

Nutraceuticals are gaining popularity for a number of reasons (Praveshkumar et al., 2016; Olaiya et al., 2016):

- The value of health maintenance is a concern that is growing among consumers.
- Nutraceuticals are upgrading health and arresting chronic diseases among those who have become dissatisfied with pharmaceutical agents.
- The healthcare industry is well aware of the fact that our heavily processed food supply, which is made up of crops grown with

chemical fertilizers, pesticides, herbicides, and genetically modified seeds, lacks the nutrients essential for suitable health.
- People who believe prevention is more important than cure.

2.2 ARTHRITIS

Arthritis is elucidated as inflammation of the joint (the word "artho" stands for joint and "itis" represents inflammation). The indications of rheumatoid arthritis (RA) are symmetrical and inflammatory, initially affecting small joints, but eventually affecting other organs, such as the dermis, optics, heart, kidney, and lungs. In Rheumatoid Arthritis joints suffer bone and cartilage destruction, and tendons and ligaments are also weak (Lee, Kim et al., 2017). A patient with arthritis may experience severe pain due to damage to joints and bone erosion. The symptoms of RA include morning rigidity of the damaged joints for > 30 min, drowsiness, an increase in body temperature, weight loss, joints that are tender, swollen, and warm, and rheumatoid nodules under the skin. There are remissions and exacerbations associated with the onset of this disease, normally in the middle age group of 35 to 60 years. It can also affect infants even prior to the age of 16 years, mentioned as Juvenile Rheumatoid Arthritis (JRA), which is close to RA except that the rheumatoid factor is unknown (Fox et al., 2002; McInnes et al., 2011; Chaudhari et al., 2016; Picerno et al., 2015). RA can be distinguished clinically from osteoarthritis (OA) in that the affected joints in Rheumatoid Arthritis are the proximal interphalangeal (PIP) and metacarpophalangeal (MP) joints; Osteoarthritis predominantly influences the distal interphalangeal (DIP) joints. OA is the most general type of arthritis, and it is the result of deterioration alternative to an autoimmune disorder. Osteoarthritis has no results on the pleura, heart, or immune structure. Furthermore, OA generally manifests on one lateral side of the anatomy, in contrast to RA, which is symmetrical. One more difference is that Rheumatoid arthritis patients are afflicted with cautious morning stiffness for ≥1 h. Patients with OA may also experience morning rigidity, but it normally settles or diminishes within 20 to 30 minutes (McGonagle et al., 2015; Piyarulli et al., 2016). Several drugs have been utilized to manage RA, but there are reports regarding the side effects of these drugs. There has been a connection between TNF (inflammatory cytokine) blocking agents and a condition known as leukocytoclastic vasculitis or LCV. Humira and Remicade are apparently hazardous for cancer and serious infections (Gay et al., 2010) (Figure 2.1).

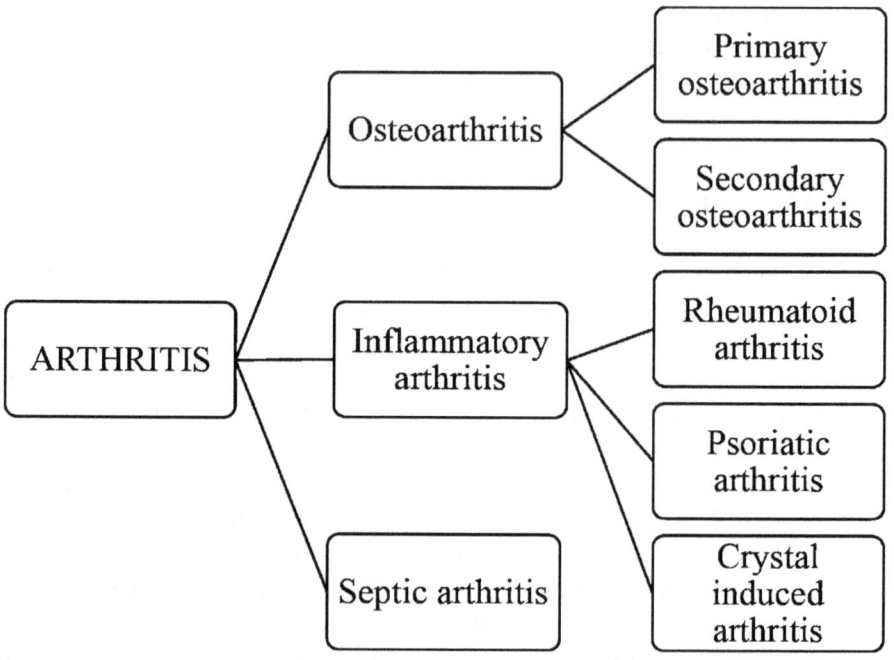

FIGURE 2.1 Structure of arthritis.

2.2.1 RHEUMATOID ARTHRITIS (RA)

Rheumatoid arthritis (RA) occurs in 1% of the adult population. The arachidonic acid pathway produces different arachidonic acid metabolites that are responsible for the depletion of bone and cartilage (Nithyashree et al., 2020). The metabolites of arachidonic acid cause inflammation in the synovium, leading to the inhibition of cell proliferation. Two types of isoforms are produced by cyclooxygenases, namely COX-1 and COX-2. COX-2 is activated in inflammatory situations, and its expression is higher in the synovial tissues of patients with rheumatoid arthritis (Hoxha et al., 2018). The impairment of joints is caused by the multifaceted interaction of immune modulators. Certain cells, such as B cells, T cells, and macrophages (synoviocytes), play a major role in the development of rheumatoid arthritis. B cells produce autoantibodies like anti-citrullinated protein antibodies and rheumatoid factor, which further enhance the inflammatory process (Nithyashree et al., 2020) (Figure 2.2).

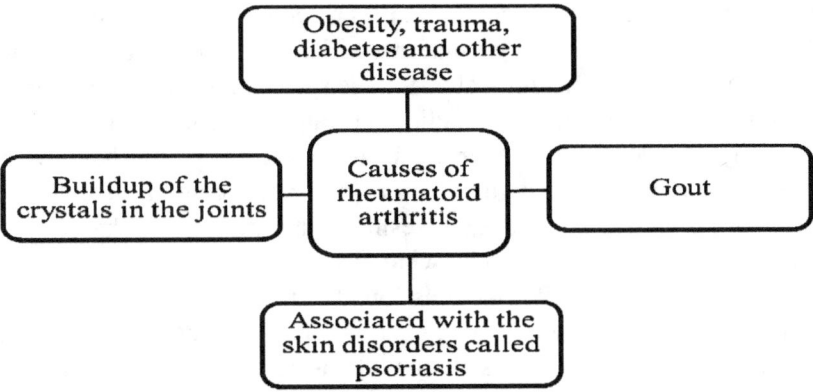

FIGURE 2.2 Causes of rheumatoid arthritis.

2.2.2 OSTEOARTHRITIS

A degenerative disease characterized by structural and functional changes in synovial joints, osteoarthritis is caused by a large range of disorders affecting these joints. Typically, it has been referred to as a disorder of hyaline cartilage. Osteoarthritis involves the whole joint organ, including the semilunar cartilage, subchondral bone, connective tissue, periarticular muscle, and synovium (Pelletier et al., 2001).

2.3 GUMS

Recent trends towards using natural products call for the substitution of artificial additives with naturally occurring additives (Zatz et al., 1989). Today, the whole globe is growing interested in natural drugs and excipients. Natural materials are more advantageous than synthetic ones as they are chemically inactive, harmless, cost-effective, biodegradable, and usually available (Whistler et al., 1996; Kulkarni et al., 2005). In general, natural gum (gums obtained from plants) is a hydrophilic polymer of excessive molecular mass based on monosaccharide units connected by glycosidic bonds. They are usually insoluble in oils or organic solvents including hydrocarbons, ether, or alcohols. Gums are water-soluble and swell up or diffuse in cool water to offer a sticky mixture or gel. Arabinose, galactose, mannose, and glucuronic acid forms are obtained on hydrolysis (Naga Vamsi Krishna et al., 2016).

The gums are classified on the basis of water solubility. They are classified as water-soluble, water-insoluble, and partially soluble gums. Some gums disperse in water and form a translucent colloidal solution (e.g., Gum Arabic).

Some gums, e.g., gum tragacanth, and gum karaya, are insoluble in water; however, they expand into a gel-like mass. The thick translucent solution is obtained by adding sufficient water. Swollen jelly diffuses in water and sets into mixtures by the inclusion of additional water; this phenomenon is formed by partially soluble gums. The term gum-resin refers to resins that have characteristics of both resins and gums. Some gum resins contain a small amount of oil and are known as Oleo-gum resins. Some resin is discharged on the trunk of the tree due to abrasion by wind, fire, lightning, or wounds caused by animals (Davison et al., 1980). Gums found in nature include acacia, Ghatti, karaya, locust bean, Albizia, khaya, guar, tragacanth, and xanthan, which are extracted as exudates or extracts along with the cortex of stems, branches, and roots of numerous plants (Smith et al., 1959). Plant-based polymers have been studied for their appealing forms in various pharmaceutical dosages such as matrix systems for control, film coating agents, buccal films, microparticles, gummy fluid preparations, ophthalmic solutions, suspensions, implants, and their relevance and effectiveness have been demonstrated. Some also have uses as viscosity enhancers, stabilizing agents, disintegrating agents, dissolving agents, surfactants, dispersing agents, gelling agents, hydrogels, and binders (Pandey et al., 2004; Chamarthy et al., 2008).

As carbohydrate biomolecules, gums have the ability to bond with water molecules and form gels. Gums are usually associated with proteins and minerals during their development. Gums are available in various forms, including seed gums, mucilage gums, exudate gums, etc. Plant-based gums have high bioavailability and are therefore among the major essential gums (Mohammad Sadegh Amiri et al., 2021). Due to their high bioavailability property, gums have become very important for human health. Throughout history, people have used plant-derived gums for various purposes. The principal components that make them pertinent for use in distinct applications are adhesive properties, high stability, viscosity, emulsification action, and surface-active properties. In many pharmaceutical preparations, plant-derived gums are considered as a building block of formulations because of their bioavailability, widespread accessibility, safe nature, and reasonable prices. Gums consist of a lot of compounds, like polysaccharides. Gums are derived through different segments of plants. Some gums may be obtained from the seed epidermis, while others come from the leaves and bark of the plants. Gums and mucilage are available in greater quantities in a diversity of animals and plants, marine meadows, fungi, and other microbial sources (Mohammad Sadegh Amiri et al., 2021). Instead, they carry out a number of functions. According to origin, behavior, and chemical structure, Gums can be obtained from (Figure 2.3):

- Plant seed endosperm (guar gum);
- Plant exudates (tragacanth, karaya gum);
- Shrubs and trees (gum Arabic, cashew gum);
- Algae extracts (agar);
- Microbial (xanthan gum);
- Animal source (chitin).

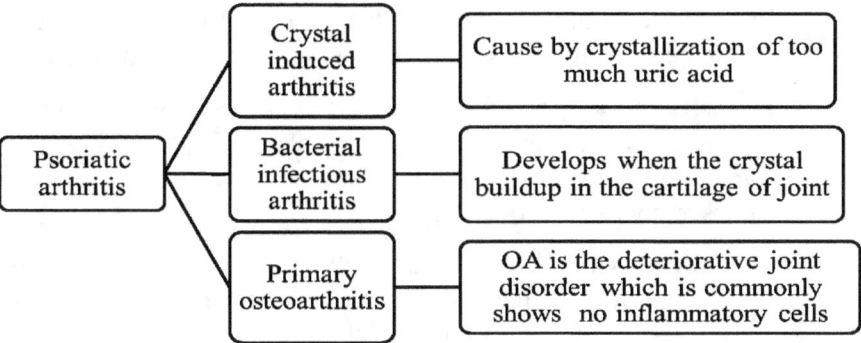

FIGURE 2.3 Natural gums isolated from various origins.

2.3.1 ADVANTAGES OF GUMS

1. **Local Accessibility:** The developing countries are experiencing plant production being promoted by governments, for plants like tragacanth and guar gum due to their wide applications in different industries.

2. **Biocompatible and Non-Poisonous:** All plant materials are carbohydrates consisting of monosaccharide units. Therefore, they are non-toxic.

3. **Economical:** Natural sources are always cheaper to use. The production cost is also much lower compared to artificial substances.

4. **Environmentally Friendly:** These are biodegradable and have no adverse impact on humans.

2.3.2 DISADVANTAGES OF GUMS

1. **Microbial Impurity:** The perspiration capacity available in the gums and mucilage is normally 10% or more, so if they are exposed to

external environmental conditions, there is a possibility of microbial impurities. These can be avoided by the proper use of preservatives and proper handling.

2. **Uncontrolled Rate of Hydration:** The percentage of the chemical constituents in a given plant material may differ due to variations in the collection of natural materials at different times, as well as differences in species, region, and weather patterns. Therefore, it is necessary to develop appropriate monographs on available mucilages.

3. **Viscosity Changes:** Normally, the viscosity of formulations increases when the gums come into contact with water. Due to the complex nature of gums and mucilages, it has been discovered that the viscosity reduces over time.

4. **Amount of Variation:** Gums and mucilages are obtained from natural sources, so their production is dependent on climatic and seasonal conditions (Girish et al., 2009).

2.3.3 GUM ARABIC

Gum Arabic is used as an immunomodulator in a patient with Rheumatoid arthritis.

- **Synonyms:** Acacia gum, chaargund, meska.
- **Biological Source:** It is the gum obtained from the tree *Acacia Senegal*, also known as hard gum. Gum Arabic is a fiber that comes from dried gummy exudates of the stem and branches of the *A. Senegal* plant. Gum Arabic has been found to be a powerful immunomodulator *in vitro*. It has shown therapeutic effects as it increases the level of IL10 in the body, resulting in a decrease in inflammation and pain (Matsumoto et al., 2006).
- **Family:** Fabaceae
- **Subfamily:** Caesalpinioideae

A short-chain fatty acid called butyrate, produced by colonic bacterial aerobic fermentation of gum Arabic, is one of the key products of this fermentation (Kvale et al., 1995). It has potent anti-inflammatory effects, is capable of inhibiting TNF-α expression by stopping NF-KB-DNA binding, and can downregulate immune responses. In addition, butyrate also plays a role in inhibiting histone deacetylase in the cells (Luhrs et al., 2001).

Several studies suggest that HDAC hindrance may reduce inflammatory responses through the acetylation of non-histone proteins. *In vitro* and *in vivo* studies suggest that HDAC inhibitors may cause cell death, resulting in anti-inflammatory effects. The HDAC inhibitors have an anti-rheumatic mechanism involving the development of seizures in rheumatoid arthritis synovial fibroblasts, by showing protective effects on bone and cartilage against their destruction.

TNFα is involved in the occurrence of RA, a fact supported by treatments with anti-TNF-α factors. A present study indicates that GA crucially decreased the extent of TNF-α (Fukae et al., 2005). It is expected that regular intake of GA increases serum butyrate quantity. Butyrate reduces the TNF level and decreases the number of degenerating events in rheumatoid arthritis patients (Segain et al., 2000). The latter will also improve the duration and life standard of rheumatoid arthritis patients. Gum Arabic is used as a nutraceutical to provide dietary supplements to RA patients. It also has health-promoting and disease-preventing activity. It consists of high molecular weight polysaccharides and their calcium, magnesium, and potassium salts, which yield arabinose, galactose, rhamnose, and glucuronic acid upon hydrolysis (Kamal et al., 2018).

2.3.4 BOSWELLIA SERRATA

- **Synonym:** Indian olibanum, salaiguggul and sallaki
- **Biological Source:** *Boswellia seratta*, is a moderate to large-sized branching tree, that grows in the dry mountainous region of India.
- **Family:** Burseraceae
- **Genus:** Boswelia

Boswellia serrata is one of the oleo gum resins. The oleo gum exudate contains 30–60% oils resin and 5-10% essential oils. These oils are soluble in organic solvents and are along with polysaccharides. The gummy portion of *Boswellia serrata* includes monoterpenes, diterpenes, triterpenes, tetracyclic triterpenic acids, and four major pentacyclic triterpenic acids (El-Khadem et al., 1972; Pardhy et al., 1978; Pardhy et al., 1992). Waxy gum abstract of B. serrata has been used in traditional medicine for many years. As an anti-inflammatory agent (Gupta et al., 1992), the gum resin extract of Boswellia serrata has application in the Ayurvedic system of remedy to manage abundant disorders like rheumatism, obesity, and many other diseases (Kirtikar et al., 1918; Chatterjee et al., 1984). Clinical studies have examined *Boswellia serrata* extracts as an osteoarthritis treatment as well as joint function treatments with it showing a slight improvement in both pain and function compared with a placebo treatment. The extract contains resins, amino acids, phenols, terpenes, polysaccharides, and β-Boswellic acid, from which beta-Boswellic acid is a major active anti-inflammatory component (Sailer et al., 1996; Sailer, Subramanian et al., 1996) (Figure 2.4).

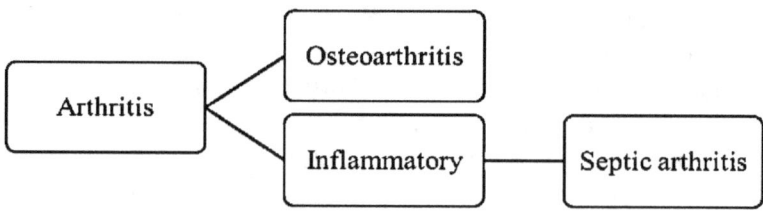

FIGURE 2.4 Synthesis of Boswellic acid.

The non-heme iron-containing enzyme in a person is encoded by the ALOX5 gene, which is the arachidonate 5-lipoxygenase enzyme, also known as ALOX5, 5-lipoxygenase, or 5-LOX. 5-lipoxygenase (5-LOX) is an enzyme that catalyzes the oxygenation of monounsaturated fatty acids like arachidonic acid. Boswellic acid could inhibit 5-lipoxygenase, particularly with anti-inflammatory and anti-arthritic effects (Cicero et al., 2007; Da Costa et al., 2017).

According to research findings, pain, stiffness, and joint function start to improve after a month of taking *Boswellia serrata* and its extract. Some researchers have administered 100–250 mg of *Boswellia serrata* and its extract for secondary outcome analysis in randomized controlled trials (RCTs) involving continuous intervention with *Boswellia* and its extract (minimum 100–250 mg).

2.3.5 CASHEW GUM

- **Synonym:** Anacardium Gum
- **Biological Source:** *Anacardium Occidentale* L. trees were used to collect the cashew Gum
- **Family:** Anacardiaceae

Rheumatoid Arthritis is one of the common constituents of persistent inflammatory joint disorders that affect the standard of living of millions of individuals around the world. *Anacardium Occidentale* L., *Anacardiaceae*, is a plant with appreciable medicinal value and economic nature. It is typically described as a cashew tree and is native to Africa, India, and northeastern Brazil (Smolen et al., 2016).

The Cashew gum is obtained from this plant's bark. The plant's bark contains epithelial cells that produce yellow to brown exudate when attacked by pathogens or mechanical injuries, as a form of protection (Eddy et al., 2019). This gum extract has been typically used in water-soluble compositions, even as an anti-asthmatic and anti-diabetic agent (Lima et al., 2006). A salient feature revealed by some reviews was the lack of 4-o-methyl glucuronic acid units in Indian cashew gum, thus reducing its inherent polyanionic charge requiring modification.

Cashew gum consists of a heteropolysaccharide compound, containing as its main chemical components Galactose (61%), Glucose (8%), Arabinose (14%), Rhamnose (7%), Glucuronic acid (5%), and other sugar residues (<2%) (Silva et al., 2010). It is considered a heteropolysaccharide with a molar mass of 1.5×10^4. The gum has a higher quantity of Galactose compared to other monosaccharides.

Some non-clinical studies have shown the anti-inflammatory effects of cashew gum in various experimental *in vivo* and *in vitro* models, with these activities attributed to the presence of polysaccharides. Cashew gum extract, after the removal of the polysaccharides to obtain a polysaccharide-free extract, was characterized, allowing for the determination of the proportional concentrations of several anacardic acids. Anacardic acids are compounds that contain salicylic acid along with a C-15 or C-17 alkyl side chain, exhibiting a broad spectrum of biological activities (Hemshekhar et al., 2011). A preclinical study conducted in various animal models of irritation and inflammation shows the reduced inflammation activity of anacardic acids (Gomes-Júnior et al., 2020).

Cashews are particularly rich in heart-healthy monounsaturated fatty acids (MUFAs). These MUFAs are healthy fats that replace less healthy fats with unsaturated fats, providing health benefits. Scientific studies suggest that MUFAs can help reduce inflammation and, therefore, are beneficial in the treatment of chronic diseases.

2.3.6 GUGGULU (C. WIGHTII)

➢ **Synonym:** *Commiphora wightii*, Gugal, gugul either mukul myrrh tree

- **Biological Source:** The bark of *Commiphora wightii* is obtained from guggulu which is an olea-gum resin the plant is generally described as a guggul tree.
- **Family:** Burseraceae
- **Genus:** Commiphora

Guggulu comprises Oleo-gum resin that comes as an exudate about the trunk and branches of *Commiphora wightii*. The guggul tree is found in the regions of Mother India, Pakistan, and Bangladesh. Inside India, it is spotted in Rajasthan, Gujarat, Assam and Karnataka.

The tree produces a yellowing gum resin inside a small channel detected all around its bay. These shrubs are drained by giving a slit on the bark. The fresh guggulu is viscid and golden colored. It occurs as a pale yellow to brown-colored mass that has an aromatic odor and bitter astringent taste (Ayurvedic Pharmacopoeia of India et al., 2007; Ayurvedic Pharmacopoeia of India et al., 2001).

Guggulu consists of Monoterpenoids, Sesquiterpenoids, Diterpenoids (α-camphorene, tocembrene-A, and other cembrenoids), Triterpenoids (myrrhanone derivatives), Steroids (Guggulsterol), flavonoids, Guggultetrols, Lignans, Sugars, and other unidentified components.

Guggulu has been used for many years to treat various disorders like arthritis, inflammation, gout, rheumatism, and obesity. Guggulu contains numerous medicinal and curative properties (Urizar et al., 2003).

Anti-inflammatory and antiarthritic results of guggulu have been observed in various scientific studies (Francis et al., 2004; Kimura et al., 2001). Guggulu should be decontaminated prior to administration so that it can take care of adverse effects and show enhancements in therapeutic effects and medicinal properties. Mice exposed to adjuvant-induced air pouch granulomas showed an anti-inflammatory response to methanol extracts containing 50% aqueous methanol. Lipopolysaccharide-stimulated mouse peritoneal macrophages were prevented from producing nitric oxide by a methanolic extract (Kimura et al., 2001). The anti-inflammatory effect is induced by Freund's adjuvant. It prevents the full development of primary injury in adjuvant arthritis and also decreases the severity of lesions. The efficacy of guggulu extract in osteoarthritis (OA) models has also been evidenced by a few animal studies (Arora et al., 1972).

In Lucknow, the Institute of Central Drug Research has been involved in synthetic, therapeutical, and analytical studies on guggulu (Satyavati et al., 1988). Gugulipid, an ethyl acetate extract of the oleoresin, has been marketed in India as a hypolipidemia representative. It contains Z-guggulsterone and E-guggulsterone; these compounds are in charge of the lipid-lowering action of the guggulu (de Morais et al., 2007; Sahni et al., 2005). Researchers have conducted several analytical tests to verify guggulu and gugulipid's lipid-lowering properties. Pharmacodynamic studies have been observed for the lipid-lowering activity of guggulu (Nityanand et al., 1989; Verma et al., 2002). Guggulu can suppress hepatic steroid production, which eventually improves the breakdown of plasma LDL cholesterol. Recently, researchers found that guggulsterone E and Z are highly efficacious antagonists of the Farnesoid X receptor, a nuclear hormone receptor that is activated by bile acids, thus permitting increased cholesterol catabolism and excretion from the body (Wu, Xia et al., 1988; Urizar et al., 2002).

2.4 CONCLUSION

Most researchers have investigated and reported *in vivo* findings regarding gums used as an anti-inflammatory in the treatment of arthritis. In that, Gum Arabic decreased TNFα and ESR. It also decreases SJC, TJC, VAS, and DAS, and improves patients' clinical symptoms and signs. Boswellia and its extract might be a rare drug for patients with OA. *In vitro* and *in vivo* studies demonstrate that the standardized constitution of Boswellia serrata gum resin extract, serratrin, reduces pain through the combined inhibition of cyclooxygenase and 5-lipoxygenase pathways. The Guggulu plant consists of many biologically active components involving terpenoids, steroids, flavonoids, guggultetrols, lignans, sugars, and amino acids. The resin of *Commiphora wightii* guggulu has emerged as a good source of traditional medicines for the treatment of inflammation and arthritis. The interest of researchers has thus shifted toward finding newer and cheaper gums, and one such discovery was Cashew gum. The important reason for this increasing attentiveness in the practice of CG was observed due to its rheological and physicochemical properties which have been found to be similar to Gum Arabic. Consequently, it may be summarized that while much improvement has been made by the untiring efforts of researchers worldwide, there are still numerous challenges that must be overcome.

KEYWORDS

- anti-osteoarthritis
- biodegradable
- distal interphalangeal
- gum Arabic
- metacarpophalangeal
- noncorrosive blocker
- nutraceuticals
- proximal interphalangeal
- rheumatoid arthritis

REFERENCES

Arora, R. B., Taneja, V., Sharma, R. C., & Gupta, S. K. (1972). Anti-inflammatory studies on a crystalline steroid isolated from Commiphora mukul. *Indian Journal of Medical Research*, *60*(6), 929–931.

Chamarthy, S. P., & Pinal, R. (2008). Plasticizer concentration and the performance of a diffusion-controlled polymeric drug delivery system. *Colloids and Surfaces A: Physicochemical and Engineering Aspects*, *331*, 2530.

Chatterjee, G., & Pal, S. (1984). Anti-inflammatory agents from Indian medicinal plants. *Indian Drugs*, *21*, 431.

Chaudhari, K., Rizvi, S., & Syed, B. A. (2016). Rheumatoid arthritis: Current and future trends. *Nature Reviews Drug Discovery*, *15*(5), 305–306.

Chauhan, B., Kumar, G., Kalam, N., & Ansari, S. H. (2013). Current concepts and prospects of herbal nutraceutical: A review. *International Journal of Pharmaceutical Sciences Review and Research*, *4*(1), 1–3.

Cicero, A. F., & Laghi, L. (2007). Activity and potential role of licofelone in the management of osteoarthritis. *Clinical Interventions in Aging*, *2*(1), 73–79.

da Costa, B. R., Reichenbach, S., Keller, N., et al. (2017). Effectiveness of non-steroidal anti-inflammatory drugs for the treatment of pain in knee and hip osteoarthritis: A network meta-analysis. *The Lancet*, *390*(10090), e21–e33.

Davison, R. L. (1980). *Handbook of Water-Soluble Gums and Resins*. New York: McGraw Hill Book Company. v. 1, pp. 1–657. ISBN: 9780070154711.

De Morais, S. M., Facundo, V. A., Bertini, L. M., et al. (2007). Chemical composition and larvicidal activity of essential oils from Piper species. *Biochemical Systematics and Ecology*, *35*(10), 670–675.

Eddy, N., Udofia, I., Okey, E., Odiongenyi, A., & Udofia, P. (2019). Physicochemical, spectroscopic, and rheological characterization of Anacardium occidentale gum exudates. *Advances in Dental Research*, *19*, 1–15.

El-Khadem, H., El-Shafei, Z. M., Elsekeify, M. A., & Abdel Rahman, M. M. (1972). Derivatives of boswellic acids. *Planta Medica*, *22*, 157–159.

Fox, C. Q., & Ahmed, S. S. (2002). *Physician Assistant's Clinical Review Cards*. Philadelphia: F. A. Davis Company. 222 pages, ISBN: 9780803605398.

Francis, J. A., Raja, S. N., & Nair, M. G. (2004). Bioactive terpenoids and guggul steroids from Commiphora mukul gum resin of potential anti-inflammatory interest. *Chemistry & Biodiversity*, *1*(11), 1842–1853.

Fukae, J., Amasaki, Y., Yamashita, Y., et al. (2005). Butyrate suppresses tumor necrosis factor production by regulating specific messenger RNA degradation mediated through a cis-acting AU-rich element. *Arthritis & Rheumatology*, *52*(9), 2697–2707.

Gay, R. D., Clarke, A. W., Elgundi, Z., Domagala, T., Simpson, R. J., Le, N. B., et al. (2010). Anti-TNFα domain antibody construct CEP-37247: Full antibody functionality at half the size. *MAbs*, *2*(6), 625–638.

Girish, J. K., Dhiren, S. P., Vipul, D. P., & Vineet, J. C. (2009). Gums and mucilages: Versatile excipients for pharmaceutical formulations. *Asian Journal of Pharmaceutical Sciences*, *4*, 309–313.

Gomes-Júnior, A. L., Islam, T. M., Nicolau, L. A. D., de Souza, L. K. M., Araújo, T. S. L., Lopes de Oliveira, G. A., de Melo, N. K., da Silva, L. L., Medeiros, J. R., Mubarak, M. S., & Melo-Cavalcante, A. A. C. (2020). Anti-inflammatory, antinociceptive, and antioxidant properties of anacardic acid in experimental models. *ACS Omega*, *5*, 19506–19515.

Gupta, O. P., Sharma, N., & Chand, D. (1992). A sensitive and relevant model for evaluating anti-inflammatory activity—Papaya latex-induced rat paw inflammation. *Journal of Pharmacological and Toxicological Methods*, *28*, 15–19.

Hemshekhar, M., Sebastin, S. M., Kemparaju, K., & Girish, K. S. (2011). Emerging roles of anacardic acid and its derivatives: A pharmacological overview. *Basic & Clinical Pharmacology & Toxicology*, *110*, 122–132. https://doi.org/10.1111/j.1742-7843.2011.00833.x.

Hoxha, M. A. (2018). A systemic review on the role of eicosanoid pathways in rheumatoid arthritis. *Advances in Medical Sciences*, *63*(1), 22–29.

Kamal, E., Kaddam, L. A., Dahawi, M., Osman, M., Salih, M. A., Alagib, A., & Saeed, A. (2018). Gum Arabic fibers decreased inflammatory markers and disease severity score among rheumatoid arthritis patients, Phase II trial. *International Journal of Rheumatology*, *2018*, 1–6.

Kathleen, C., & Stephen, D. (2013). Nutraceuticals: What are they and do they work? Kentucky Equine Research, Inc., *7*(4), 1–50.

Kimura, M., Yoshikawa, S., Kobayashi, S., et al. (2001). New triterpenes, myrrhanol A and myrrhanone A, from guggul-gum resins, and their potent anti-inflammatory effect on adjuvant-induced air-pouch granuloma of mice. *Bioorganic & Medicinal Chemistry Letters*, *11*(8), 985–989.

Kirtikar, K. R., & Basu, B. D. (1918). *Indian Medicinal Plants*. Plates Vol. 1. Panini Office, Bhuvaneswari Ashram, India. Vol. 2, pp. 798.

Kulkarni, G. T., Gowthamarajan, K., Dhobe, R. R., Yohanan, F., & Suresh, B. (2005). Development of controlled release spheroids using natural polysaccharide as release modifier. *Drug Delivery*, *12*(4), 201–206.

Kvale, D., & Brandtzaeg, P. (1995). Constitutive and cytokine-induced expression of HLA molecules, secretory component, and intercellular adhesion molecule-1 is modulated by butyrate in the colonic epithelial cell line HT-29. *Gut*, *36*(5), 737–742.

Lee, J. E., Kim, I. J., Cho, M. S., & Lee, J. (2017). A case of rheumatoid vasculitis involving hepatic artery in early rheumatoid arthritis. *Journal of Korean Medical Science, 32*(7), 1207–1210.

Lima, J. L. S., Furtado, D. A., Pereira, J. P. G., Baracuhy, J. G. V., & Xavier, H. S. (2006). Plantas medicinais de uso comum no Nordeste do Brasil. Universidade Federal de Campina Grande, E-book. Campina Grande 1.1.

Luhrs, H., Gerke, T., Schauber, J., et al. (2001). Cytokine-activated degradation of inhibitory B protein is inhibited by the short-chain fatty acid butyrate. *International Journal of Colorectal Disease, 16*(4), 195–201.

Mahajan, B., Taneja, S. C., Sethi, V. K., & Dhar, K. L. (1995). Two triterpenoids from Boswellia serrata gum resin. *Phytochemistry, 39*, 453–455.

Matsumoto, N., Riley, S., Fraser, D., et al. (2006). Butyrate modulates TGF-β1 generation and function: Potential renal benefit for Acacia(Sen) SUPERGUM (gum Arabic)? *Kidney International, 69*(2), 257–265.

McGonagle, D., Hermann, K. G., & Tan, A. L. (2015). Differentiation between osteoarthritis and psoriatic arthritis: Implications for pathogenesis and treatment in the biologic therapy era. *Rheumatology (Oxford), 54*(1), 29–38.

McInnes, I. B., & Schett, G. (2011). The pathogenesis of rheumatoid arthritis. *New England Journal of Medicine, 365*(23), 2205–2219.

Mohammad Sadegh Amiri, Vahideh Mohammad Zadeh, Mohammad Ehsan Taghavizadeh Yazdi, Mahmood Barani, Abbas Rahdar, & George Z. Kyzas. (2021). Plant-based gums and mucilage's applications in pharmacology and nanomedicine: A review. *Molecules, 26*(6), 1770–1793.

Naga Vamsi Krishna, L., Kulkarni, P. K., Dixit, M., Lavanya, D., & Prudhvi Kanth Raavi, P. K. (2011). Brief introduction of natural gums, mucilage's and their applications in novel drug delivery systems—A review. *International Journal of Drug Formulation and Research, 2*(6), 55.

Nithyashree, R. S., & Deveswaran, R. (2020). A comprehensive review on rheumatoid arthritis. *Journal of Pharmaceutical Research International, 32*(12), 18–32.

Nityanand, S., Srivastava, J. S., & Asthana, O. P. (1989). Clinical trials with Gugu lipid—a new hypolipidemic agent. *The Journal of the Association of Physicians of India, 37*(5), 323–328.

Olaiya, C. O., Soetan, K. O., & Esan, A. (2016). The role of nutraceuticals, functional foods, and value-added food products in the prevention and treatment of chronic diseases. *African Journal of Food Science, 10*(10), 185–193.

Pandey, R., & Khuller, G. K. (2004). Polymer-based drug delivery systems for mycobacterial infections. *Current Drug Delivery, 1*, 195–201.

Pardhy, R. S., & Bhattacharyya, S. C. (1978). Tetracyclic triterpene acids from the resin of Boswellia serrata Roxb. *Indian Journal of Chemistry, 16B*, 174–175.

Pardhy, R. S., & Bhattacharyya, S. C. (1978). β-Boswellic acid, acetyl-β-Boswellia acid, acetyl-11-keto-β-Boswellia acid, and 11-keto-β-Boswellia acid, four pentacyclic triterpenic acids from the resin of Boswellia serrata Roxb. *Indian Journal of Chemistry, 16B*, 176–178.

Pelletier, J. P., Martel-Pelletier, J., & Abramson, S. B. (2001). Osteoarthritis, an inflammatory disease: Potential implication for the selection of new therapeutic targets. *Arthritis & Rheumatism, 44*, 1237–1247.

Picerno, V., Ferro, F., Adinolfi, A., Valentini, E., Tani, C., & Alunno, A. (2015). One year in review: The pathogenesis of rheumatoid arthritis. *Clinical and Experimental Rheumatology, 33*(4), 551–558.

Piyarulli, D., & Koolaee, R. M. (2016). A 22-Year-Old Female with Joint Pain. In D. Piyarulli & R. M. Koolaee (Eds.), *Medicine Morning Report: Beyond the Pearls* (pp. 65–77). Cambridge: Elsevier.

Praveshkumar, N., Nirdeshkumar, & Omer, T. (2016). Nutraceuticals: Critical supplement for building a healthy India. *World Journal of Pharmacy and Pharmaceutical Sciences, 5*(3), 579–594.

Rajasekaran, A., Sivagnanam, G., & Xavier, R. (2008). Nutraceuticals as therapeutic agents: A review. *Research Journal of Pharmacy and Technology, 1*(4), 328–340.

Sahni, S., Hepfinger, C. A., & Sauer, K. A. (2005). Guggulipid use in hyperlipidemia: Case report and review of the literature. *American Journal of Health-System Pharmacy, 62*(16), 1690–1692.

Sailer, E. R., Subramanian, L. R., Rall, B., Hoernlein, R. F., Ammon, H. P. T., & Safayhi, H. (1996). Acetyl-11-keto-β-Boswellic Acid (AKBA): Structure requirements for binding and 5-lipoxygenase inhibitory activity. *British Journal of Pharmacology, 117*(4), 615–618.

Sailer, E.-R., Hoernlein, R. F., Ammon, H. P. T., & Safayhi, H. (1996). Structure-activity relationships of the nonredox-type non-competitive leukotriene biosynthesis inhibitor acetyl-11-keto-β-boswellic acid. *Phytomedicine, 3*(1), 73–74.

Satyavati, G. V. (1988). Gum guggul (*Commiphora mukul*)—The success story of an ancient insight leading to a modern discovery. *Indian Journal of Medical Research, 87*(4), 327–335.

Segain, J. P., Galmiche, J. P., Raingeard de la Blétière, D., et al. (2000). Butyrate inhibits inflammatory responses through NF-κB inhibition: implications for Crohn's disease. *Gut, 47*(3), 397–403.

Silva, T. M., Santiago, P. O., Purcena, L. L. A., & Fernandes, K. F. (2010). Study of the cashew gum polysaccharide for the horseradish peroxidase immobilization: Structural characteristics, stability, and recovery. *Materials Science and Engineering: C, 30*, 526–530.

Smith, F., & Montgomery, R. (1959). *The Chemistry of Plant Gums and Mucilages and Some Related Polysaccharides*. New York: Reinhold Publishing Corp. 627 pages.

Smolen, J. S., Aletaha, D., & McInnes, I. B. (2016). Rheumatoid arthritis. *Lancet, 388*, 2023–2038.

The Ayurvedic Pharmacopoeia of India (Formulations). (2007). Department of Indian Systems of Medicine and Homeopathy, Ministry of Health and Family Welfare, Government of India, New Delhi, India (1st ed.).

The Ayurvedic Pharmacopoeia of India. (2001). Department of Indian Systems of Medicine and Homeopathy, Ministry of Health and Family Welfare, Government of India, New Delhi, India (1st ed.).

Urizar, N. L., & Moore, D. D. (2003). Gugu lipid: A natural cholesterol-lowering agent. *Annual Review of Nutrition, 23*, 303–313.

Urizar, N. L., Liverman, A. B., Dodds, D. T., et al. (2002). A natural product that lowers cholesterol as an antagonist ligand for FXR. *Science, 296*(5573), 1703–1706.

Verma, S. K., & Bordia, A. (2002). Effect of Commiphora mukul (gum guggul) in patients of hyperlipidemia with special reference to HDL-cholesterol. *Indian Journal of Molecular Endocrinology, 16*(7), 1590–1597.

Whistler, R. L. (1996). Drug-release retarding polymers are the key performers. In *Industrial Gums* (2nd ed.). Academic Press, London, UK.

Wu, J., Xia, C., Meier, J., Li, S., Hu, X., & Lala, D. S. (2002). The hypolipidemic natural product guggulsterone acts as an antagonist of the bile acid receptor. *Molecular Endocrinology*, *16*(7), 1590–1597.

Zatz, J. L., & Kushla, G. P. (1989). Oral aqueous suspensions and gels. In M. M. Reiger & G. S. Banker (Eds.), *Pharmaceutical Dosage Forms: Disperse Systems* (Vol. 2, pp. 164–405). New York, NY: Marcel Dekker.

CHAPTER 3

ROLE OF NUTRACEUTICALS IN THE PREVENTION AND TREATMENT OF ARTHRITIS

PANKAJ KUMAR[1] and ROHIT[2]

[1]*Professor, Department of Pharmacology, Adesh Institute of Pharmacy and Biomedical Science, Adesh University, Bathinda, Punjab, India*

[2]*Department of Pharmacy Practice, ISF College of Pharmacy, Moga, Punjab, India*

ABSTRACT

Swollen, painful, and stiff joints on both sides of the body are the result of rheumatoid arthritis, a chronic inflammatory illness. Between the ages of 30 and 50 is when you'll see it most often. An autoimmune disorder, roughly speaking. To put it simply, "nutraceuticals" are any food or food component that has both nutritional value and medicinal properties. Not only does this unique quality help people stay healthy, but it also plays a role in warding off and treating certain diseases. As both qualitative and quantitative decision-making elements have progressed, so has the need for these items. The outcome is a multibillion-dollar business devoted to nutraceuticals all over the globe. The use of nutraceuticals is essential in the treatment of chronic inflammatory diseases like rheumatoid arthritis. The production of pro-inflammatory cytokines like IL-1β and IL-6 may be suppressed and reactive oxygen species reduced with the use of nutraceuticals. Both conventional nonsteroidal anti-inflammatory drugs and anti-inflammatory nutraceuticals work by targeting the same underlying molecular mechanism.

3.1 INTRODUCTION

The synovial tissue of joints, cartilage, bone, and, less often, extra-articular locations, becomes inflamed due to the inflammatory illness rheumatoid arthritis (RA) (Scutellari & Orzincolo, 1998). Increased oxidative damage and inflammation characterize this chronic inflammatory illness (Tak et al., 2000). Rheumatoid arthritis affects around 5 out of every 1,000 people worldwide. Two to three times as Maq: any women as men are afflicted, and it may strike at any moment. The painful swelling of joints in the hands and feet is a hallmark of rheumatoid arthritis (Shrivastava & Pandey, 2013). Edema is most common in the hands and feet, particularly the wrists, metacarpophalangeal joints, metatarsophalangeal joints, and proximal interphalangeal joints. As a result, you may have morning stiffness that lasts for at least 30 minutes and up to several hours. Synovitis and effusion often cause a "soft" (as opposed to "hard;" boney) swelling in the joint, which differentiates it from osteoarthritis (Bird et al., 1985).

In cases of psoriatic arthritis affecting the fingers, the swelling is fusiform rather than generalized throughout the whole digit ("sausage digit"). Extra-articular symptoms may emerge if rheumatoid arthritis is not managed properly. Rheumatoid nodules are by far the most typical manifestation of this condition (hard subcutaneous lumps around bony prominences such as the elbow) (Cushnaghan & McDowell, 1999). Rheumatoid vasculitis, a necrotizing inflammation of small or medium-sized arteries, is a more dangerous symptom. It most often affects the skin and vasa nervorum, but may also affect arteries in other organs (Genta et al., 2006). Multiple comorbidities have been linked to increased symptoms for those with rheumatoid arthritis. Inflammation is a hallmark of RA, and cardiovascular disease is the major cause of death in people with the condition (Carmona et al., 2007). Heart disease is more strongly linked to disease activity in RA patients than to traditional cardiovascular risk factors (Corrales et al., 2015). Rheumatoid arthritis alters a person's capacity for physical and occupational tasks and has a negative impact on their quality of life. Without proper treatment, in 10 years 80% of patients would have misaligned joints, rendering 40% of them permanently unable from employment (Kaplan et al., 1993). Daily activities are impacted by rheumatoid arthritis in every way. In the long term, poorly managed disease, the development of joint degeneration, which is permanent in rheumatoid arthritis, leads to disability.

Obesity, starvation, and weight loss have all been noted as symptoms of rheumatoid arthritis, according to published research. Possible explanations for this variety include differences in disease progression, hereditary variables, and therapeutic approach (Chapple et al., 2017) (Figure 3.1).

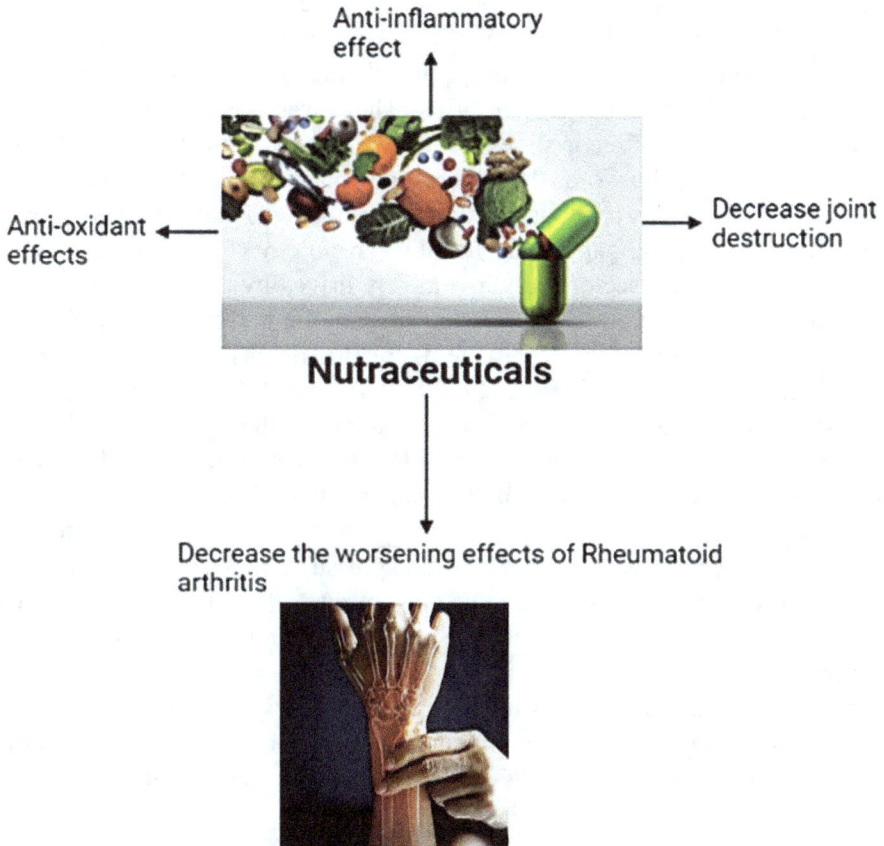

FIGURE 3.1 Nutraceuticals' role in rheumatoid arthritis.

The nutritional condition of Egyptian patients with rheumatoid arthritis was evaluated using anthropometric measures and food intake, and the results showed that 75% of the patients were either overweight or obese, while 14% were malnourished (Al-Okbi, 2014). Rheumatoid arthritis, and by extension other inflammatory disorders, has a poorly understood pathogenesis, and there is no evidence that dietary nutritional variables influence this pathogenesis. In people with rheumatoid arthritis, malnutrition seems to be very frequent. Loss of lean tissues, which contain the majority of the body's proteins, may account for the prevalence of malabsorption, anorexia, and weight loss in rheumatoid arthritis patients (Kalantar-Zadeh et al., 2003). Protein intake and low blood albumin levels pointed to a significant protein deficit in associated rheumatic illnesses. Patients with rheumatoid arthritis had lower than optimal intakes of Fe, Zn, and niacin, and they also consumed fewer calories than advised (Stone et al., 1997). Obesity (Jarouliya & Keservani, 2019a), vitamin deficiencies, and inadequate dietary consumption are all factors that have been linked to a higher risk of rheumatoid arthritis. There was no correlation between weight gain and a decline in illness severity. The word "nutraceutical" comes from a merging of the words "nutrition" and "pharmaceutical." What we call "nutraceuticals" refers to foods and dietary components that have a significant role in regulating and supporting healthy physiology (Pandey et al., 2010). Global nutraceutical sector growth is mostly driven by current demographic and health trends. Nutraceuticals may be anything from dietary fiber to probiotics to polyunsaturated fatty acids to antioxidants to various herbal or natural foods (Keservani et al., 2017, 2020). An example of a nutraceutical is "a food (or part of a meal) that gives medical or health benefits, including the prevention or treatment of sickness" (Kalra, 2003). Nutraceuticals have been shown to be effective in preventing a broad variety of diseases and conditions, including arthritis, the common cold, cough, sleep disorders, gastrointestinal problems, cancer, osteoporosis, high blood pressure, high cholesterol, chronic pain, depression, and diabetes. Dietary sources of nutraceuticals include polyunsaturated fatty acids, probiotics, prebiotics, and dietary fiber. Chronic inflammatory diseases may benefit from nutraceuticals derived from foods high in antioxidants and anti-inflammatory bioactive components such as phenolic compounds, polyunsaturated fatty acids, phytosterols, tocopherols, and carotenoids (Andlauer & Fürst, 2002; Keservani et al., 2010a, b, 2017, 2020; Arya et al., 2022).

3.2 RHEUMATOID ARTHRITIS

Chronic inflammatory polyarthritis of both big and small joints is a hallmark of RA, an autoimmune disease that causes symmetrical joint damage over time. Between the ages of 30 and 50 is when it usually first becomes noticeable (Arvikar et al., 2017). There are about 25 males and 54 females affected for every 100,000 persons in the United States, making it the most prevalent form of inflammatory arthritis. This condition accounts for 250,000 hospitalizations and 9 million doctor visits annually (Rindfleisch & Muller, 2005). Rheumatoid arthritis may be more common in the Western hemisphere than in Asia, according to studies. Although the exact cause of rheumatoid arthritis is unknown, researchers believe a combination of hereditary and environmental factors has a role. The severity of an illness is strongly influenced by one's genetic makeup (Bogdanos et al., 2012). Joint inflammation is caused by an underlying condition, such as an autoimmune response or a viral infection. Joint damage and systemic ramifications are caused by a coordinated effort between several immune cell types and their cytokines, proteinases, and growth factors. Rheumatoid arthritis is exacerbated by several cytokines that exploit broken signal transduction pathways. Aberrant fibroblast-like synoviocytes (FLS) proliferation is caused by the inadequate regulation of many signaling pathways at the local inflammatory site, the joint. The pathophysiology of RA involves many signaling networks, including the Mitogen-activated protein kinase (MAPK) signaling system, the nuclear factor-kappa B (NF-κB) route, the PI3K/AKT signaling pathway, and the JAK/STAT signaling circuit (Morel & Berenbaum, 2004).

3.2.1 MAPK SIGNALING PATHWAY

Neurotransmitters, hormones, inflammatory substances, stress conditions, viruses, and growth factors are only some of the stimuli that might activate the MAPK signaling pathway. The cell surface relays extracellular signals to the central core of the downstream effector (Sujitha & Rasool, 2017). Numerous cellular responses are regulated by the mitogen-activated protein kinase (MAPK) signaling pathway, which includes cell proliferation, differentiation, and death. Phosphorylation by MKK3/MKK6 and perhaps by MKK4 is the first step in activating p38 MAPK, which is then activated by the MAPKKKs. Recent research has shown that MKK3 and MKK6 are involved in p38 MAPK activation in rheumatoid synovial fibroblasts in response to cytokine stimulation, indicating that blocking either one alone is insufficient. MLK, Tpl2 (tumor progression locus-2), TGF-activated protein kinase (TAK)-1, and apoptosis signal-regulating kinase (ASK)-1 are all members of the MAPKKK superfamily (Schett et al., 2008). With the help of p21-activated kinases, tiny GTP-binding proteins like Rac and Cdc42 activate MAPKKKs (PAKs). In inflammation, the most crucial activation process occurs when inflammatory mediators like TNF- and IL-1 bind to their extracellular membrane receptors and recruit intracellular adaptor molecules. Transcription factors ATF-2, CHOP (C/EBP), and MAPK-interacting serine/threonine kinase (MNK), as well as kinases such as MAPK-activated protein kinase (MAPKAPK)-2, mitogen- and stress-activated protein kinase (MSK)-1, and p38-regulated/activated protein kinase (PRAK) (Hammaker et al., 2003). Inflammatory cells such as macrophages, mast cells, and natural killer cells are abundant in the RA synovium. MAPKs play a crucial part in the signaling cascade downstream of IL-1, IL-17, and TNF receptors, and they also control the production of pro-inflammatory cytokines in damaged joint tissue. Matrix metalloproteinase-mediated degradation of cartilage is a primary mechanism through which JNK MAPKs contribute to the development of RA (MMP) (Malemud, 2013). The downstream JNK signaling pathway is activated by TNF-α and interleukin-1, and it promotes extracellular matrix disintegration by controlling MMP production in chondrocytes and FLS. While investigating potential inhibitors of proinflammatory cytokines, which human monocytes activate by reacting to bacterial LPS, researchers stumbled onto the p38 MAPK. The fact that p38 inhibitors may dampen the production of IL-17 while also inhibiting TNF-α, IL-1, MMP-1, MMP-3, IL-6, and IL-8 shows that the p38 MAPK pathway's main job is to regulate IL-17 signal transduction. MMPs are crucial to the progression of damage because they may destroy all components of the extracellular matrix (Shen et al., 2022). MMPs may be broken down into five categories: Interstitial collagens (types I, II, and III) are degraded by collagenases (MMP-1, 8, 13, 2), gelatinases (MMP-2, -9), and metalloproteinases (MMP-6, 7). Matrix metalloproteinases (MMP) 3, 10, and 11 break down matrix proteins other than collagen. Membrane-type MMPs (MMP-14, -15, -16, -17, -24, 25), and a varied group including MMP-7, -11, -12, -20, and MMP-23 (Giannelli et al., 2004). The proteolytic enzymes stromelysins and matrilysins have been linked to the breakdown of noncollagen matrix components in both rheumatoid arthritis and osteoarthritis. MMP-3 (stromelysin-1) activity may be related to proteoglycan loss, and stromelysins have a wide selectivity for molecules including fibronectin, elastin, laminin, and aggrecan. Although clinical trials have not yet identified p38 kinase inhibitors that are effective, this target has been identified as a potential one for the treatment of RA in preclinical studies. Trials for the p38 MAPK inhibitor VX-702 have shown modest therapeutic effectiveness associated with transient reductions in inflammatory markers, but the drug may not have a substantial and long-lasting inhibitory effect on the chronic inflammation seen in rheumatoid arthritis (Schett et al., 2008). Important in this signaling are nutraceuticals, which may inhibit a large number of signaling pathways and thereby lower inflammation. MMP overexpression is inhibited by anti-inflammatory nutraceutical components such as olive (Olea europaea), and curcumin (Vyas et al., 2010; Kesharwani et al., 2015, 2018; Mishra et al., 2019; Singh et al., 2013a, b, 2015, 2016; Upadhyaya et al., 2009; Kesharwani & Misra, 2011), turmeric, phenolic compounds, phytosterols, tocopherols, and polyunsaturated fatty acids, which in turn slows the development of rheumatoid arthritis.

Curcumin reduces joint inflammation in rheumatoid arthritis by inhibiting the production of adhesion molecules called integrins 3 and 7. Furthermore, it inhibits the synthesis of inflammatory cytokines. It is a powerful anti-inflammatory supplement that blocks the enzyme lipoxygenase in addition to the cyclooxygenase-2 enzyme. *In vitro* and *in vivo* studies show that it reduces inflammation of both the acute and chronic varieties (Pourhabibi-Zarandi et al., 2021).

3.2.2 NF-KB SIGNALING PATHWAY

The NF-κB signaling system may be activated by a variety of stimuli, such as pathogen-related molecular patterns from microbes, endogenous damage-associated molecular patterns recognized by patterns such as toll-like receptors (TLRs), and environmental stimulation. Synovial tissue from people with rheumatoid arthritis has been demonstrated to exhibit a higher level of nuclear factor kappa B (NF-κB) (Barrow, 2021). Accelerating the development of rheumatoid arthritis, highly active NF-κB may stimulate the production of pro-inflammatory cytokines such as TNF-alpha, IL-1β, and IL-6. Rheumatoid arthritis is exacerbated by a positive feedback loop caused by the production of pro-inflammatory cytokines, which regulate NF-κB activation (Han et al., 1998). Abnormal FLS apoptosis is caused by the overactivation of NF-κB in rheumatoid arthritis. Synovial hyperplasia in rheumatoid arthritis is primarily caused by aberrant apoptosis in FLS, which occurs in the context of the inflammatory milieu of the synovium. Medicinal and edible plants including soybean, garlic, ginger, and tea are the primary sources of phytochemicals found in nutraceuticals.

Rheumatoid arthritis development may be slowed by ingesting carotenoids, flavonoids, sulfur-containing substances, and other phenolic compounds. They may prevent the release of inflammatory cytokines (Mohanty et al., 2020).

3.2.3 JAK/STAT SIGNALING PATHWAY

The JAK/STAT pathway is a crucial mechanism for signaling cytokines. It has a role in immunological modulation as well as cell division, differentiation, and death. Studies have revealed that blocking the activity of the enzyme Janus kinase (JAK) might have a profound effect on autoimmune illnesses like rheumatoid arthritis (STAT & EGF, 2005). The primary pathogenic alteration in rheumatoid arthritis is synovitis (Malemud, 2018). Certain transcription factors and signal transduction pathways are linked to the inflammatory reactions seen in the synovium of rheumatoid arthritis patients, including the activation of cytokines and adhesion molecules. Interaction with pro-inflammatory cytokines results in JAK phosphorylation and subsequent STAT protein activation. Researchers have found a correlation between STAT gene transcription and the severity of joint damage in rheumatoid arthritis. Inhibitors of Janus kinase (JAK) are a novel family of small drugs that disrupt intracellular signaling and contribute significantly to the management of rheumatoid arthritis (STAT & EGF, 2005). Due to the diversity of compounds with the capacity to suppress JAK/STAT signaling, nutraceuticals play an essential role in this scenario. Curcumin, a key ingredient in many nutraceuticals, has been shown to block the activation of the inflammatory pathway JAKS/STATs. The JAK/STAT signaling system is one of the molecular mechanisms that mediate the inflammatory response. There is evidence that blocking the STAT signaling pathway reduces the production and release of inflammatory cytokines, therefore ameliorating the symptoms of inflammatory disorders (Ciobanu et al., 2020) (Figure 3.2).

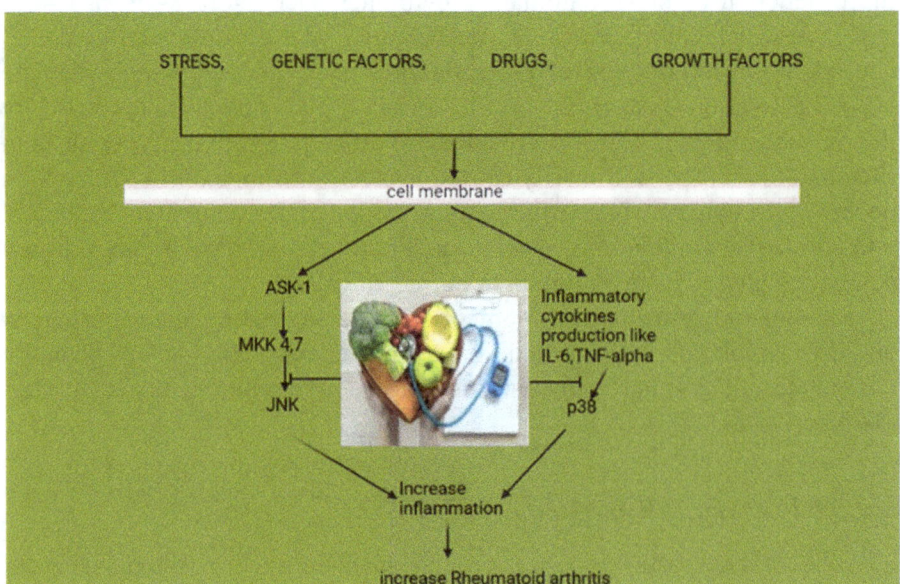

FIGURE 3.2 Role of various inflammatory pathways in the progression of rheumatoid arthritis.

3.3 NUTRACEUTICAL'S ROLE IN RHEUMATOID ARTHRITIS

Bioactive foods, or nutraceuticals, are nutritional supplements with anti-cancer and anti-heart-disease effects beyond those of the foods themselves (Albini et al., 2019). Recently, the utilization of nutraceuticals and bioactive foods derived from natural sources has been recognized as a viable treatment option for a wide variety of diseases, including inflammatory disorders and cardiovascular issues. The nutritional advantages of vitamins (Singh et al., 2019a), minerals, and nutraceuticals, as well as those of food and dietary supplements, are important in maintaining good health and warding off illness. Nutraceuticals have grabbed the attention of scientists not just because of the nutritional benefits they provide, but also because of the incredible safety and powerful biological activity they exhibit (Mannucci et al., 2021).

High demand may be attributed to the fact that nutraceuticals are effective in improving health, prolonging cell life, and promoting overall well-being without the harmful side effects that are often associated with conventional medicine. Nutraceuticals are preferred over conventional medicines because they provide better therapeutic results with fewer adverse effects. Various biological processes, such as antioxidant protection activation, signal transduction pathway activation, gene expression related to cell survival, cell proliferation, differentiation, and mitochondrial integrity preservation, have been shown to be a part of the mechanical behavior of nutraceuticals (Curtis et al., 2004). These characteristics seem to be crucial for the security of many conditions associated with aging or chronic use. Scientific research confirms that a diet rich in fruits and vegetables is vital for optimal health. Lycopene and beta-carotene shield the skin from the harmful effects of ultraviolet radiation; lutein and zeaxanthin promote cardiovascular health; and lycopene is also used to treat prostate cancer (Salami et al., 2013). Nutraceuticals, due to their anti-inflammatory properties, are widely employed in the treatment of rheumatoid arthritis (Figure 3.3).

Exaggerated levels of oxidative stress and inflammatory indicators are characteristic of rheumatoid arthritis, a chronic inflammatory illness (Mannucci et al., 2021). In light of the rapid reactions and/or unpleasant side effects of the synthetic medications now used in its therapy, research into other, less risky therapeutic options is ongoing. Polyunsaturated fatty acids, phytosterols, tocopherols, and phenolic compounds are all examples of natural anti-inflammatory chemicals present in the diet. Pro-inflammatory cytokines like IL-1β and IL-6 may be suppressed by nutraceuticals as well. Both nonsteroidal anti-inflammatory medications and anti-inflammatory nutraceuticals work by targeting the same molecular mechanism (Simioni et al., 2018).

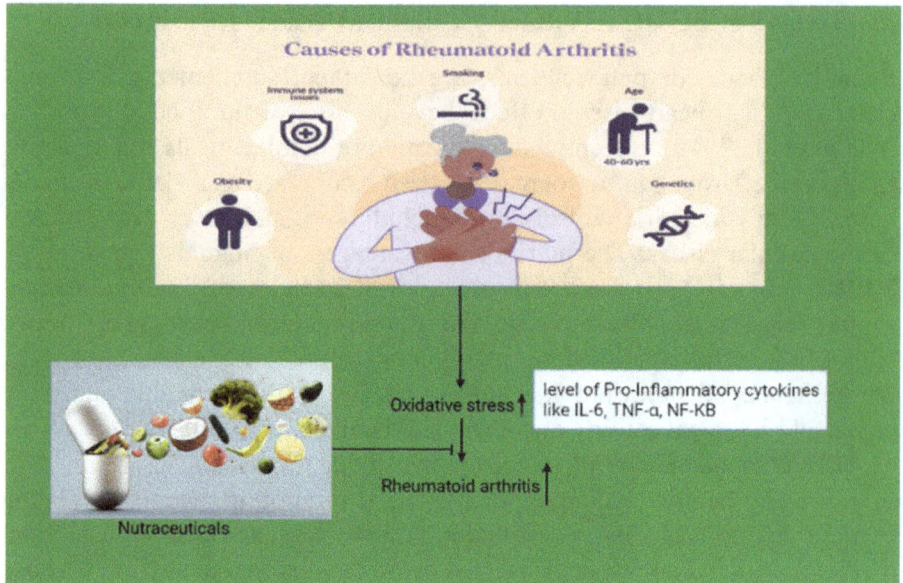

FIGURE 3.3 Role of nutraceuticals in the inhibition of oxidative stress.

By activating NF-kappa B, producing and upregulating proinflammatory cytokines, and producing reactive oxygen species, nutraceuticals have the potential to suppress inflammatory metastatic processes. Therefore, they are useful in treating rheumatoid arthritis. Differences in the mechanism of action between steroidal and non-steroidal anti-inflammatory drugs exist. The eicosanoid metabolic pathways that steroidal anti-inflammatory drugs disrupt, and maybe stimulate the production of many lipocortin-like proteins, are essential to their efficacy (Cui et al., 2004; Jarouliya & Keservani, 2019b; Singh et al., 2017b). By reducing phospholipase A2 activity, lipocortins reduce the amount of AA available, which in turn inhibits the production of cyclooxygenase and lipoxygenase (Vane & Botting, 1987). In addition to reducing inflammation-related vasodilation, steroidal anti-inflammatory drugs also inhibit cellular and fluid egress from the vascular space to inflammatory sites, dampen inflammatory cell activities, and postpone leukocyte recruitment into damaged regions (Serhan & Savill, 2005). As a result, immune system activity is dampened. T-lymphocytes in the immune system become less responsive to IL-1β and IL-18, two activating cytokines. Prostaglandin production and/or action suppression seems to be associated with nonsteroidal anti-inflammatory drugs; on the other hand (Laveti et al., 2013). Most of them work by blocking the enzyme cyclooxygenase, which is essential for the production of harmful cyclic endoperoxides from arachidonic acid. The strong antioxidant content of nutraceuticals means they may help with conditions like rheumatoid arthritis. Some examples of these are vitamin E, carotenoids, phenolic compounds, phytosterols, probiotics, prebiotics, omega-3 fatty acids, and symbiotics (Gordon & Kubomura, 2003).

3.3.1 VITAMIN E

Antioxidant supplementation techniques for rheumatoid arthritis prevention and therapy have been explored. Vitamin E (α, β, γ, and δ-tocopherol and α, β, γ, and δ-tocotrienol) is a strong antioxidant that has been shown to be useful in rheumatoid arthritis (Al-Okbi, 2014). Some oils and foods may naturally contain vitamin E. Nuts, seeds, vegetable oils, greens, and fortified cereals are only a few of the nutritional sources of alpha-tocopherol (Rizvi et al., 2014). While fat oxidation occurs, vitamin E acts as a powerful antioxidant, preventing the creation of reactive oxygen species molecules and the development of free radical events. Compared to alpha-tocopherol alone, tocopherols significantly reduce lipid peroxidation in human erythrocytes (Singh et al., 2005). It preserves polyunsaturated fatty acids in membrane phospholipids and plasma lipoproteins by scavenging peroxyl radicals. In addition to oxidizing other lipids, Tocopheroxyl radicals can also: (1) combine with another Tocopheroxyl radical to form non-reactive tocopherol dimers; (2) be reduced to tocopherol by other antioxidants; (3) combine with another Tocopheroxyl radical to form non-reactive tocopherol quinones; or (4) be reduced to tocopherol by other antioxidants (Noguchi et al., 2002). One possible mechanism by which vitamin E exerts its anti-inflammatory effects is by blocking the arachidonic acid pathway, the source of proinflammatory lipid mediators including prostaglandins and leukotrienes. (Nanda et al., 2007) While α-tocopherol is well known for its antioxidant properties, it may also have other bioactivities. Pro-oxidants include α-tocopherol and ascorbic acid. Overexpression of several so-called "pro-inflammatory" genes, such as tumor necrosis factor, has been related to the transcription factor nuclear factor κB (NF-κB), which α-tocopherol has been shown to inhibit.

3.3.2 OMEGA-3-FATTY ACIDS

Many studies have looked at the potential benefits of polyunsaturated fatty acids for the treatment of rheumatoid arthritis. There is a difference in the metabolic processing of PUFAs between those found in animal diets and those found in plant foods (Kasprzyk et al.). Patients with rheumatoid arthritis who were assigned to the intervention group and who consumed a diet rich in polyunsaturated fatty acids and low in saturated fatty acids while also taking eicosapentaenoic acid (EPA) at a dose of 1.8 g daily experienced a decrease in the number of painful joints and morning stiffness (Tidow-Kebritchi & Mobarhan, 2001). Higher consumption of long-chain n-3 PUFAs (>0.21 g/day) was related to a 35% reduced risk of acquiring rheumatoid arthritis in a prospective trial of 205 women with rheumatoid arthritis (multivariable-adjusted relative risk (RR) 0.65; 95% CI: 0.48 to 0.90) (Tański et al., 2022). Some studies suggest that taking omega-3 PUFA supplements may help reduce rheumatoid arthritis symptoms, the number of painful joints, the severity of morning stiffness, and the need for nonsteroidal anti-inflammatory drugs (NSAIDs) (Efthimiou & Kukar, 2010). The World Health Organization and North American dietary guidelines propose that lipids make up 20%–35% of daily calorie intake (DEI). This number is now between 35% and 40% in France. The consumption of omega-3 fatty acids is one of these suggestions. The precursor of EPA and DHA, linolenic acid (ALA), should account for 0.5%–1% of DEI (about 0.8–1 g/day). However, recommendations for dietary EPA and DHA of at least 0.25 g/day were also advised, perhaps as a result of the poor ALA bioconversion to EPA and DHA (Lanchais et al., 2020). Supplementation delivered above 1 g/day and commonly reached 2–4 g/day in clinical studies for cardiovascular disease and rheumatoid arthritis (Di Stasi et al., 2004). Fish oil omega-3 supplementation in a rheumatoid arthritis animal model resulted in lower plasma levels of interleukins 6, 10, and 12, tumor necrosis factor-alpha, prostaglandin PGE2, and thromboxane TXB2. In patients with inflammatory arthritis, taking 2.4 g/day of EPA and DHA decreased pain and inflammation and elevated plasmatic concentrations of resolvins and resolvin E2 in synovial fluid.

3.3.3 PROBIOTICS

To put it simply, probiotics are healthy bacteria that may be beneficial to your health if consumed in sufficient quantities. Some of the metabolic products created by the probiotic community include short-chain fatty acids (SCFAs) and vitamins, both of which are used as fuel by enterocytes. It's no surprise that these substances may modulate intestinal immunity and gut microbiota to keep things in balance in the digestive tract. (Jäger et al., 2019) Randomized controlled studies are looking at the efficacy of probiotic bacteria such as *Lactobacillus rhamnosus*, *Lactobacillus casei*, *Bacillus coagulans*,

Lactobacillus reuteri, *Lactobacillus acidophilus*, and *Bifidobacterium bifidum* in treating rheumatoid arthritis. (Fijan, 2014) Evidence suggests that probiotic bacteria may modulate the host's innate and adaptive immune systems and have therapeutic value for a variety of chronic inflammatory illnesses. Bacteria like lactic acid bacteria (LAB) and bifidobacteria get the most attention, although yeasts and bacilli have also been employed as probiotics. Blood levels of proinflammatory cytokines (TNF-a, IL-6, and IL-12) and levels of regulatory cytokine (IL-10) were shown to be much lower in L. casei than in rheumatoid arthritis patients in recent studies. (Saez-Lara et al., 2015). Patients with RA may use these probiotics with confidence since they have been demonstrated to be safe and helpful. Blood levels of cytokines such as IL-1, IL-6, IL-10, IL-12p70, and TNF-α were reduced in rheumatoid arthritis patients who took the Lactobacillus probiotics *L. rhamnosus* GR-1 and *L. reuteri* RC-14 together (Bungau et al., 2021). Further research indicated that L. casei, a probiotic, reduced IL-12 and TNF-α levels and joint inflammation in individuals with rheumatoid arthritis (Vaghef-Mehrabany et al., 2014).

3.3.4 PRE-BIOTICS

Prebiotics and symbiotics have been shown to increase mineral absorption, namely calcium and magnesium. The increased production of short-chain fatty acids by bacteria, which is aided by an increased substrate supply, increases mineral solubility; the promotion of enterocyte proliferation by bacterial fermentation products, primarily lactate and butyrate, increases the absorption surface; the expression of calcium-binding proteins improves gut health; and the breakdown of mineral complexin increases mineral solubility. (Scholz-Ahrens et al., 2007) Prebiotics are a kind of food that improves the health of the host by selectively promoting the production and/or activity of particular members of the gut microbiota. They are typically made up of oligosaccharides that are not digested by the host. (Lim et al., 2005) Currently, inulin and galacto-oligosaccharides are the only two naturally occurring dietary components found in plants as storage carbohydrates that meet all the requirements for prebiotic categorization. (Gibson et al., 2017) In the upper gastrointestinal tract, the host lacks the enzymatic ability to break down fiber carbohydrates (including cellulose, pectin, gums, beta-glucan, and lignin). Once in the colon, however, it is expected that these chemicals are preferentially processed by resident bacteria into SCFAs, especially acetate, propionate, butyrate, and lactate. Most bacteria in the intestines are anaerobes that survive on fermentation rather than oxygen.

The evolution of several enzymes and transport proteins suggests that the gut bacteria may digest dietary fiber. Researchers believe that SCFAs are responsible for fiber's anti-inflammatory effects. For a long time, people have understood that SCFAs are good for the digestive tract. It is probable that a decrease in anaerobic bacteria is responsible for the decreased amounts of "good" microbiota and SCFAs in patients with IBD. However, it has been shown that SCFA supplementation is useful and effective in the treatment of colitis and other inflammatory bowel illnesses. Among SCFAs, butyrate has been investigated the most. Colonic epithelial cells rely on butyrate for energy, and this nutrient has effects on cell proliferation and barrier function while also reducing oxidative DNA damage (Tedelind et al., 2007). A combination of prebiotics and beneficial bacteria (probiotics) that can convert the prebiotics into usable energy is one way to boost the health of the host. Symbiotics are synergistic mixtures of probiotic and prebiotic bacteria. The potential health advantages of prebiotics, probiotics, and symbiotics are now the subject of investigation in a variety of circumstances, and this is backed by the safety and convenience of using these substances. (Hasan et al., 2019) The advantages of intestinal homeostasis, which may be induced by the management of the gut microbiota, extend well beyond the digestive system. Obesity, arthritis, diabetes, cancer, asthma, alcoholic liver disease, and cardiovascular disease are only a few of the chronic disorders where the host-microbe interaction is being studied for prebiotic and probiotic effects (Carding et al., 2015).

3.4 FLAVONOIDS AND RHEUMATOID ARTHRITIS

Natural sources of flavonoids (Keservani & Sharma, 2014; Keservani et al., 2016a, b) include many different types of plants and fungi. Flavonoids' involvement in inflammatory diseases, including atherosclerosis and rheumatoid arthritis, may be attributed to their antioxidant, antibacterial, and anti-inflammatory capabilities (Yu et al., 2016). It is unclear how exactly flavonoids help in the treatment of rheumatoid arthritis. Natural polyphenolic compounds are used to treat and/or manage metabolic, cardiovascular, neurological, and cancer illnesses in humans (Rengasamy et al., 2019). Inflammatory mediators, including nitric oxide (NO) and reactive oxygen species (ROS), are downregulated, and inflammatory enzyme activities like COXs and iNOS are modulated by flavonoids, demonstrating their role in the inflammatory response (Leyva-López et al., 2016). Flavonoids' effect is due in part to their ability to inhibit both the manufacture and expression of cytokines, as well as the activity of transcription factors including nuclear factor-light chain-enhancer of activated B cells (NF-kB) and activating protein-1 (AP-1). They commonly form complexes with reactive species, which halt reactions before any damage is done to the cell. Proinflammatory interferons, such as cytokines, are generated as a byproduct of inflammatory processes initiated by oxidative metabolism's overproduction of reactive oxygen species. Significant factors in the onset of inflammatory processes that lead to a variety of chronic illnesses include the activation of nuclear factor kappa B/active protein-1 (NF-kB/AP-1) and the creation of tumor necrosis factor-alpha (TNF-α) (Baltazar). Flavonoids such as genkwanin, hydroxy genkwanin, luteolin, and apigenin make up the bulk of D. genkwa. We investigated if these flavonoids may help with rheumatoid arthritis by testing their anti-inflammatory and immune-regulatory effects (Ali et al., 2017).

When faced with an invader or irritant, the immune system reacts with inflammation. Large amounts of NO are produced by iNOS during the inflammatory phase. NF-κB is a transcription factor that regulates immunological and inflammatory responses (Wang et al., 2019). It affects immunological and inflammatory responses, cell proliferation, and cell death by controlling the manufacture of proinflammatory cytokines and growth factors (Hotchkiss & Nicholson, 2006). In the treatment of rheumatoid arthritis, the NF-κB pathway is crucial because inducible nitric oxide synthase (iNOS) and cyclooxygenase-2 (COX-2) are essential proteins in the NF-kappaB signal transduction pathway. Inflammatory illnesses like RA may benefit from flavonoids because of their ability to inhibit NF-κB signaling (Roman-Blas & Jimenez, 2006).

KEYWORDS

- cyclooxygenase-2
- **mitogen-activated protein kinase**
- **necrosis factor-alpha**
- **nitric oxide synthase**
- **nuclear factor-kappa B**
- **rheumatoid arthritis**
- **short-chain fatty acids**
- **toll-like receptors**

REFERENCES

Albini, A., Bassani, B., Baci, D., Dallaglio, K., Gallazzi, M., Corradino, P., Bruno, A., & Noonan, D. M. (2019). Nutraceuticals and cancer. *Current Medicinal Chemistry*, *26*(6), 973–987.

Ali, F., Rahul, Naz, F., Jyoti, S., & Siddique, Y. H. (2017). Health functionality of apigenin: A review. *International Journal of Food Properties*, *20*(11), 1197–1238.

Al-Okbi, S. Y. (2014). Nutraceuticals of anti-inflammatory activity as a complementary therapy for rheumatoid arthritis. *Toxicology and Industrial Health*, *30*(8), 738–749.

Andlauer, W., & Fürst, P. (2002). Nutraceuticals: A piece of history, present status, and outlook. *Food Research International*, *35*(2–3), 171–176.

Arvikar, S. L., Crowley, J. T., Sulka, K. B., & Steere, A. C. (2017). Autoimmune arthritides, rheumatoid arthritis, psoriatic arthritis, or peripheral spondylarthritis following Lyme disease. *Arthritis & Rheumatology*, *69*(1), 194–202.

Arya, R. K. K., Sati, D., Bisht, D., & Keservani, R. K. (2022). Nanotechnology-Based Bacterial Immunotherapy. In Kesharwani, R. K., Keservani, R. K., & Sharma, A. K. (Eds.), *Nutraceuticals and Functional Foods in Immunomodulators* (pp. 3–19). Springer, Singapore. https://doi.org/10.1007/978-981-19-2507-8_1.

Baltazar, M. T., Dinis-Oliveira, R. J., Guilhermino, L., Bastos Mde, L., Duarte, J. A., & Carvalho, F. (2013). New formulation of paraquat with lysine acetylsalicylate with low mammalian toxicity and effective herbicidal activity. *Pest Manag Sci. 69*(4), 553–8. doi: 10.1002/ps.3412. Epub 2012 Oct 29. PMID: 23109273.

Barrow, M. (2021). An overview of the NF-kB mechanism of pathophysiology in rheumatoid arthritis, investigation of the NF-kB ligand RANKL, and related nutritional interventions. *Autoimmunity Reviews*, *20*(3), 102741.

Bird, H., Gallez, P. L., & Hill, J. (1985). The nursing process and rheumatology nursing. In *Combined Care of the Rheumatic Patient*, pp. 71–129. Springer.

Bogdanos, D. P., Smyk, D. S., Rigopoulou, E. I., Mytilinaiou, M. G., Heneghan, M. A., Selmi, C., & Gershwin, M. E. (2012). Twin studies in autoimmune disease: Genetics, gender and environment. *Journal of Autoimmunity*, *38*(2–3), J156–J169.

Bungau, S. G., Behl, T., Singh, A., Sehgal, A., Singh, S., Chigurupati, S., Vijayabalan, S., Das, S., & Palanimuthu, V. R. (2021). Targeting probiotics in rheumatoid arthritis. *Nutrients*, *13*(10), 3376.

Carding, S., Verbeke, K., Vipond, D. T., Corfe, B. M., & Owen, L. J. (2015). Dysbiosis of the gut microbiota in disease. *Microbial Ecology in Health and Disease*, *26*(1), 26191.

Carmona, L., Descalzo, M. A., Perez-Pampin, E., Ruiz-Montesinos, D., Erra, A., Cobo, T., & Gómez-Reino, J. J. (2007). All-cause and cause-specific mortality in rheumatoid arthritis are not greater than expected when treated with tumor necrosis factor antagonists. *Annals of the Rheumatic Diseases*, *66*(7), 880–885.

Chapple, I. L., Bouchard, P., Cagetti, M. G., Campus, G., Carra, M. C., Cocco, F., Nibali, L., Hujoel, P., Laine, M. L., & Lingström, P. (2017). Interaction of lifestyle, behavior or systemic diseases with dental caries and periodontal diseases: Consensus report of group 2 of the joint EFP/ORCA workshop on the boundaries between caries and periodontal diseases. *Journal of Clinical Periodontology*, *44*(S18), S39–S51.

Ciobanu, D. A., Poenariu, I. S., Crînguș, L.-I., Vreju, F. A., Turcu-Stiolica, A., Tica, A. A., Padureanu, V., Dumitrascu, R. M., Banicioiu-Covei, S., & Dinescu, S. C. (2020). JAK/

STAT pathway in pathology of rheumatoid arthritis. *Experimental and Therapeutic Medicine*, *20*(4), 3498–3503.

Corrales, A., Dessein, P. H., Tsang, L., Pina, T., Blanco, R., Gonzalez-Juanatey, C., Llorca, J., & Gonzalez-Gay, M. A. (2015). Carotid artery plaque in women with rheumatoid arthritis and low estimated cardiovascular disease risk: A cross-sectional study. *Arthritis Research & Therapy*, *17*(1), 1–8.

Cui, K., Luo, X., Xu, K., & Murthy, M. V. (2004). Role of oxidative stress in neurodegeneration: Recent developments in assay methods for oxidative stress and nutraceutical antioxidants. *Progress in Neuro-Psychopharmacology and Biological Psychiatry*, *28*(5), 771–799.

Curtis, C. L., Harwood, J. L., Dent, C. M., & Caterson, B. (2004). Biological basis for the benefit of nutraceutical supplementation in arthritis. *Drug Discovery Today*, *9*(4), 165–172.

Cushnaghan, J., & McDowell, J. (1999). Rheumatological conditions. In *Drug Therapy in Rheumatology Nursing* (pp. 1–20). Gateshead: Whurr Publishers.

Di Stasi, D., Bernasconi, R., Marchioli, R., Marfisi, R. M., Rossi, G., Tognoni, G., & Tacconi, M. T. (2004). Early modifications of fatty acid composition in plasma phospholipids, platelets, and mononucleates of healthy volunteers after low doses of n-3 polyunsaturated fatty acids. *European Journal of Clinical Pharmacology*, *60*(3), 183–190.

Efthimiou, P., & Kukar, M. (2010). Complementary and alternative medicine use in rheumatoid arthritis: Proposed mechanism of action and efficacy of commonly used modalities. *Rheumatology International*, *30*(5), 571–586.

Fijan, S. (2014). Microorganisms with claimed probiotic properties: An overview of recent literature. *International Journal of Environmental Research and Public Health*, *11*(5), 4745–4767.

Genta, M. S., Genta, R. M., & Gabay, C. (2006). Systemic rheumatoid vasculitis: A review. *Seminars in Arthritis and Rheumatism*, *36*(2), 88–98.

Giannelli, G., Erriquez, R., Iannone, F., Marinosci, F., Lapadula, G., & Antonaci, S. (2004). MMP-2, MMP-9, TIMP-1, and TIMP-2 levels in patients with rheumatoid arthritis and psoriatic arthritis. *Clinical and Experimental Rheumatology*, *22*(3), 335–338.

Gibson, G. R., Hutkins, R., Sanders, M. E., Prescott, S. L., Reimer, R. A., Salminen, S. J., Scott, K., Stanton, C., Swanson, K. S., & Cani, P. D. (2017). Expert consensus document: The International Scientific Association for Probiotics and Prebiotics (ISAPP) consensus statement on the definition and scope of prebiotics. *Nature Reviews Gastroenterology & Hepatology*, *14*(8), 491–502.

Gordon, D. T., & Kubomura, K. (2003). Beverages as delivery systems for nutraceuticals. In *Beverage Quality and Safety* (pp. 15–72).

Hammaker, D., Sweeney, S., & Firestein, G. (2003). Signal transduction networks in rheumatoid arthritis. *Annals of the Rheumatic Diseases*, *62*(suppl 2), ii86–ii89.

Han, Z., Boyle, D., Manning, A., & Firestein, G. (1998). AP-1 and NF-kB regulation in rheumatoid arthritis and murine collagen-induced arthritis. *Autoimmunity*, *28*(4), 197–208.

Hasan, M. T., Jang, W. J., Lee, J. M., Lee, B. J., Hur, S. W., Gu Lim, S., Kim, K. W., Han, H. S., & Kong, I. S. (2019). Effects of immunostimulants, prebiotics, probiotics, symbiotic, and potentially immunoreactive feed additives on olive flounder (*Paralichthys olivaceus*): A review. *Reviews in Fisheries Science & Aquaculture*, *27*(3), 417–437.

Hotchkiss, R. S., & Nicholson, D. W. (2006). Apoptosis and caspases regulate death and inflammation in sepsis. *Nature Reviews Immunology*, *6*(11), 813–822.

Jäger, R., Mohr, A. E., Carpenter, K. C., Kerksick, C. M., Purpura, M., Moussa, A., Townsend, J. R., Lamprecht, M., West, N. P., & Black, K. (2019). International Society of Sports

Nutrition position stand: Probiotics. *Journal of the International Society of Sports Nutrition*, *16*(1), 62.

Jarouliya, U., & Keservani, R. K. (2019a). Pathways leading to child obesity. In D. Bagchi (Ed.), *Global Perspectives on Childhood Obesity: Current Status, Consequences and Prevention* (2nd ed., pp. 137–146). Academic Press, Elsevier. ISBN: 9780128128404.

Jarouliya, U., & Keservani, R. K. (2019b). Protein functions as a cell surface and nuclear receptor in human diseases. In S. Bharti & D. K. Mahapatra (Eds.), *Medicinal Chemistry with Pharmaceutical Product Development* (pp. 1–32). Apple Academic Press, CRC Press, Taylor & Francis Group. ISBN: 9781771887106.

Kalantar-Zadeh, K., Ikizler, T. A., Block, G., Avram, M. M., & Kopple, J. D. (2003). Malnutrition-inflammation complex syndrome in dialysis patients: Causes and consequences. *American Journal of Kidney Diseases*, *42*(5), 864–881.

Kalra, E. K. (2003). Nutraceutical definition and introduction. *AAPS Pharmsci.*, *5*(3), 27–28.

Kaplan, R. M., Anderson, J. P., & Ganiats, T. G. (1993). The quality of well-being scale: Rationale for a single quality of life index. In S. R. Walker & R. M. Rosser (Eds.), *Quality of Life Assessment: Key Issues in the 1990s* (pp. 65–94). Springer.

Kasprzyk, N., Poniewierski, P., Kostiukow, A., & Samborski, W. (2022) The role of diet in rheumatoid arthritis therapy: A review of the literature. *Journal of Health Study and Medicine*, *1*, 19–32.

Keservani, R. K., & Sharma, A. K. (2014). Flavonoids: Emerging trends and potential health benefits. *Journal of Chinese Pharmaceutical Sciences*, *23*(12), 815–824.

Keservani, R. K., Kesharwani, R. K., Vyas, N., Jain, S., Raghuvanshi, R., & Sharma, A. K. (2010). Nutraceutical and functional food as future food: A review. *Der Pharmacia Lettre*, *2*(1), 106–116.

Keservani, R. K., Sharma, A. K., & Kesharwani, R. K. (2016a). Nutraceutical and functional foods for cardiovascular health. In *Food Process Engineering* (pp. 291–312). Apple Academic Press, CRC Press. ISBN: 9781771884020.

Keservani, R. K., Sharma, A. K., & Kesharwani, R. K. (2016b). Medicinal effect of nutraceutical fruits for cognition and brain health. *Scientifica*, 2016, Article ID 3109254, 10 pages. https://doi.org/10.1155/2016/3109254.

Keservani, R. K., Sharma, A. K., & Kesharwani, R. K. (2017). An overview and therapeutic applications of nutraceutical and functional foods. In *Recent Advances in Drug Delivery Technology* (pp. 160–201). ISBN: 9781522507543.

Keservani, R. K., Sharma, A. K., & Kesharwani, R. K. (Eds.). (2020). *Nutraceuticals and Dietary Supplements: Applications in Health Improvement and Disease Management*, Apple Academic Press, CRC Press. pp. 1–344. ISBN: 9781771888738.

Keservani, R.K., Kesharwani, R.K., Sharma, A.K., Vyas, N., & Chadoker, A. (2010). Nutritional Supplements: An Overview. *International Journal of Current Pharmaceutical Review and Research*, *1*(1), 59–75.

Kesharwani, R. K., & Misra, K. (2011). Prediction of the binding site for curcuminoids at human topoisomerase II α protein; an in-silico approach. *Current Science*, *100*(7), 1060–1065.

Kesharwani, R. K., Singh, D. B., Singh, D. V., & Misra, K. (2018). Computational study of curcumin analogs by targeting DNA topoisomerase II: A structure-based drug designing approach. *Network Modeling Analysis in Health Informatics and Bioinformatics*, *7*(1), 1–7.

Kesharwani, R. K., Srivastava, V., Singh, P., Rizvi, S. I., Adeppa, K., & Misra, K. (2015). A novel approach for overcoming drug resistance in breast cancer chemotherapy by targeting new synthetic curcumin analogs against aldehyde dehydrogenase 1 (ALDH1A1) and glycogen synthase kinase-3β (GSK-3β). *Applied Biochemistry and Biotechnology, 176*(7), 1996–2017.

Lanchais, K., Capel, F., & Tournadre, A. (2020). Could omega-3 fatty acids preserve muscle health in rheumatoid arthritis? *Nutrients, 12*(1), 223.

Laveti, D., Kumar, M., Hemalatha, R., Sistla, R., Naidu, V. G. M., Talla, V., Verma, V., Kaur, N., & Nagpal, R. (2013). Anti-inflammatory treatments for chronic diseases: A review. *Inflammation & Allergy-Drug Targets, 12*(5), 349–361.

Leyva-López, N., Gutierrez-Grijalva, E. P., Ambriz-Perez, D. L., & Heredia, J. B. (2016). Flavonoids as cytokine modulators: A possible therapy for inflammation-related diseases. *International Journal of Molecular Sciences, 17*(6), 921.

Lim, C. C., Ferguson, L. R., & Tannock, G. W. (2005). Dietary fibers as "prebiotics": Implications for colorectal cancer. *Molecular Nutrition & Food Research, 49*(6), 609–619.

Malemud, C. J. (2013). Intracellular signaling pathways in rheumatoid arthritis. *Journal of Clinical & Cellular Immunology, 4*(4), 160.

Malemud, C. J. (2018). The role of the JAK/STAT signal pathway in rheumatoid arthritis. *Therapeutic Advances in Musculoskeletal Disease, 10*(5–6), 117–127.

Mannucci, C., Casciaro, M., Sorbara, E. E., Calapai, F., Di Salvo, E., Pioggia, G., Navarra, M., Calapai, G., & Gangemi, S. (2021). Nutraceuticals against oxidative stress in autoimmune disorders. *Antioxidants, 10*(2), 261.

Mishra, H., Kesharwani, R. K., Singh, D. B., Tripathi, S., Dubey, S. K., & Misra, K. (2019). Computational simulation of inhibitory effects of curcumin, retinoic acid, and their conjugates on GSK-3 beta. *Network Modeling Analysis in Health Informatics and Bioinformatics, 8*(1), 3.

Mohanty, S., Pal, A., & Si, S. C. (2020). Flavonoid as nutraceuticals: A therapeutic approach to rheumatoid arthritis. *Research Journal of Pharmacy and Technology, 13*(2), 991–998.

Morel, J., & Berenbaum, F. (2004). Signal transduction pathways: New targets for treating rheumatoid arthritis. *Joint Bone Spine, 71*(6), 503–510.

Nanda, B., Nataraju, A., Rajesh, R., Rangappa, K., Shekar, M., & Vishwanath, B. S. (2007). PLA2 mediated arachidonate free radicals: PLA2 inhibition and neutralization of free radicals by anti-oxidants-a new role as an anti-inflammatory molecule. *Current Topics in Medicinal Chemistry, 7*(8), 765–777.

Noguchi, N., Yamashita, H., Hamahara, J., Nakamura, A., Kühn, H., & Niki, E. (2002). The specificity of lipoxygenase-catalyzed lipid peroxidation and the effects of radical-scavenging antioxidants. *Biological Chemistry, 383*(3–4), 619–626.

Pandey, M., Verma, R. K., & Saraf, S. A. (2010). Nutraceuticals: New era of medicine and health. *Asian Journal of Pharmaceutical and Clinical Research, 3*(1), 11–15.

Pourhabibi-Zarandi, F., Shojaei-Zarghani, S., & Rafraf, M. (2021). Curcumin and rheumatoid arthritis: A systematic review of the literature. *International Journal of Clinical Practice, 75*(2), e14280.

Rengasamy, K. R., Khan, H., Gowrishankar, S., Lagoa, R. J., Mahomoodally, F. M., Khan, Z., Suroowan, S., Tewari, D., Zengin, G., & Hassan, S. T. (2019). The role of flavonoids in autoimmune diseases: Therapeutic updates. *Pharmacology & Therapeutics, 194*, 107–131.

Rindfleisch, A. J., & Muller, D. (2005). Diagnosis and management of rheumatoid arthritis. *American Family Physician, 72*(6), 1037–1047.

Rizvi, S., Raza, S. T., Ahmed, F., Ahmad, A., Abbas, S., & Mahdi, F. (2014). The role of vitamin E in human health and some diseases. *Sultan Qaboos University Medical Journal, 14*(2), e157–e165.

Roman-Blas, J. A., & Jimenez, S. A. (2006). NF-κB is a potential therapeutic target in osteoarthritis and rheumatoid arthritis. *Osteoarthritis and Cartilage, 14*(8), 839–848.

Saez-Lara, M. J., Gomez-Llorente, C., Plaza-Diaz, J., & Gil, A. (2015). The role of probiotic lactic acid bacteria and bifidobacteria in the prevention and treatment of inflammatory bowel disease and other related diseases: A systematic review of randomized human clinical trials. *BioMed Research International, 2015*, Article ID 505878.

Salami, A., Seydi, E., & Pourahmad, J. (2013). Use of nutraceuticals for prevention and treatment of cancer. *Iranian Journal of Pharmaceutical Research: IJPR, 12*(2), 219–229.

Schett, G., Zwerina, J., & Firestein, G. (2008). The p38 mitogen-activated protein kinase (MAPK) pathway in rheumatoid arthritis. *Annals of the Rheumatic Diseases, 67*(7), 909–916.

Scholz-Ahrens, K. E., Ade, P., Marten, B., Weber, P., Timm, W., Açil, Y., Glüer, C. C., & Schrezenmeir, J. (2007). Prebiotics, probiotics, and symbiotics affect mineral absorption, bone mineral content, and bone structure. *The Journal of Nutrition, 137*(3 Suppl 2), 838S–846S.

Scutellari, P. N., & Orzincolo, C. (1998). Rheumatoid arthritis: Sequences. *European Journal of Radiology, 27*(Suppl 1), S31–S38.

Serhan, C. N., & Savill, J. (2005). Resolution of inflammation: The beginning programs the end. *Nature Immunology, 6*(12), 1191–1197.

Shen, Y., Teng, L., Qu, Y., Liu, J., Zhu, X., Chen, S., Yang, L., Huang, Y., Song, Q., & Fu, Q. (2022). Anti-proliferation and anti-inflammation effects of corilagin in rheumatoid arthritis by downregulating NF-κB and MAPK signaling pathways. *Journal of Ethnopharmacology, 284*, 114791.

Shrivastava, A. K., & Pandey, A. (2013). Inflammation and rheumatoid arthritis. *Journal of Physiology and Biochemistry, 69*(2), 335–347.

Simioni, C., Zauli, G., Martelli, A. M., Vitale, M., Sacchetti, G., Gonelli, A., & Neri, L. M. (2018). Oxidative stress: Role of physical exercise and antioxidant nutraceuticals in adulthood and aging. *Oncotarget, 9*(24), 17181–17198.

Singh, D. B., Gupta, M. K., Kesharwani, R. K., & Misra, K. (2013a). Comparative docking and ADMET study of some curcumin derivatives and herbal congeners targeting β-amyloid. *Network Modeling Analysis in Health Informatics and Bioinformatics, 2*(1), 13–27.

Singh, D. V., Agarwal, S., Kesharwani, R. K., & Misra, K. (2013b). 3D QSAR and pharmacophore study of curcuminoids and curcumin analogs: Interaction with thioredoxin reductase. *Interdisciplinary Sciences: Computational Life Sciences, 5*(4), 286–295.

Singh, P., Kesharwani, R. K., & Keservani, R. K. (2017a). Antioxidants and vitamins: Roles in cellular function and metabolism. In *Sustained Energy for Enhanced Human Functions and Activity* (pp. 385–407). Academic Press. ISBN: 9780128054130.

Singh, P., Kesharwani, R. K., & Keservani, R. K. (2017b). Protein, carbohydrates, and fats: Energy metabolism. In *Sustained Energy for Enhanced Human Functions and Activity* (pp. 103–115). Academic Press. ISBN: 9780128054130.

Singh, P., Kesharwani, R. K., Misra, K., & Rizvi, S. I. (2015). The modulation of erythrocyte Na+/K+-ATPase activity by curcumin. *Journal of Advanced Research, 6*(6), 1023–1030.

Singh, P., Kesharwani, R. K., Misra, K., & Rizvi, S. I. (2016). Modulation of erythrocyte plasma membrane redox system activity by curcumin. *Biochemistry Research International, 2016*, Article ID 702039.

Singh, U., Devaraj, S., & Jialal, I. (2005). Vitamin E, oxidative stress, and inflammation. *Annual Review of Nutrition, 25*, 151–174.

Stat, C. J. K., & Egf, P. (2005). The Jak-STAT pathway in rheumatoid arthritis. *The Journal of Rheumatology, 32*(9), 1650–1653.

Stone, J., Doube, A., Dudson, D., & Wallace, J. (1997). Inadequate calcium, folic acid, vitamin E, zinc, and selenium intake in rheumatoid arthritis patients: Results of a dietary survey. *Seminars in Arthritis and Rheumatism, 27*(3), 180–185.

Sujitha, S., & Rasool, M. (2017). MicroRNAs and bioactive compounds on TLR/MAPK signaling in rheumatoid arthritis. *Clinica Chimica Acta, 473*, 106–115.

Tak, P. P., Zvaifler, N. J., Green, D. R., & Firestein, G. S. (2000). Rheumatoid arthritis and p53: How oxidative stress might alter the course of inflammatory diseases. *Immunology Today, 21*(2), 78–82.

Tański, W., Świątoniowska-Lonc, N., Tabin, M., & Jankowska-Polańska, B. (2022). The relationship between fatty acids and the development, course, and treatment of rheumatoid arthritis. *Nutrients, 14*(5), 1030.

Tedelind, S., Westberg, F., Kjerrulf, M., & Vidal, A. (2007). Anti-inflammatory properties of the short-chain fatty acids acetate and propionate: A study with relevance to inflammatory bowel disease. *World Journal of Gastroenterology: WJG, 13*(20), 2826–2832.

Tidow-Kebritchi, S., & Mobarhan, S. (2001). Effects of diets containing fish oil and vitamin E on rheumatoid arthritis. *Nutrition Reviews, 59*(10), 335–338.

Upadhyaya, J., Kesharwani, R. K., & Misra, K. (2009). Metabolism, pharmacokinetics, and bioavailability of ascorbic acid; synergistic effect with tocopherols and curcumin. *Journal of Computational Intelligence in Bioinformatics, 2*(1), 77–84.

Vaghef-Mehrabany, E., Alipour, B., Homayouni-Rad, A., Sharif, S. K., Asghari-Jafarabadi, M., & Zavvari, S. (2014). Probiotic supplementation improves inflammatory status in patients with rheumatoid arthritis. *Nutrition, 30*(4), 430–435.

Vane, J. R., & Botting, R. M. (1987). Inflammation and the mechanism of action of anti-inflammatory drugs. *The FASEB Journal, 1*(2), 89–96.

Vyas, N., Keservani, R. K., Nayak, A., Jain, S., & Singhal, M. (2010). Effect of Tamarindus indica and Curcuma longa on stress-induced alopecia. *Pharmacology online, 1*, 377–384.

Wang, H. M.-D., Fu, L., Cheng, C. C., Gao, R., Lin, M. Y., Su, H. L., Belinda, N. E., Nguyen, T. H., Lin, W.-H., & Lee, P. C. (2019). Inhibition of LPS-induced oxidative damages and potential anti-inflammatory effects of *Phyllanthus emblica* extract via down-regulating NF-κB, COX-2, and iNOS in RAW 264.7 cells. *Antioxidants, 8*(9), 270.

Yu, J., Bi, X., Yu, B., & Chen, D. (2016). Isoflavones: Anti-inflammatory benefit and possible caveats. *Nutrients, 8*(6), 361.

CHAPTER 4

ARTHRITIS DISEASE AND OMEGA POLYUNSATURATED FATTY ACIDS

AARTI TIWARI,[1] SATYA PRAKASH SINGH,[1] AJAY KUMAR SHUKLA,[1] VIMAL KUMAR YADAV,[1] VISHNU PRASAD YADAV,[1] SHAILENDRA KUMAR,[2] MANISH KUMAR,[3] and VIJAY KUMAR YADAV[4]

[1]*Institute of Pharmacy, Dr. Ram Manohar Lohia Avadh University, Ayodhya, Uttar Pradesh, India*

[2]*Institute of Microbiology, Dr. Ram Manohar Lohia Avadh University, Ayodhya, Uttar Pradesh, India*

[3]*Department of Pharmacy, Madhav University, Pindwara, Rajasthan, India*

[4]*Dr. Bhimrao Ambedkar University, Chhalesar Campus, Agra, Uttar Pradesh, India*

ABSTRACT

Omega-3 fatty acids (OMG-FA) are a type of healthy fats that are important for our bodies. They are called "essential" because our bodies can't make them on their own, so we need to get them from the food we eat. These OMG-FA are helpful for our brains and eyes. They play a role in the development and functioning of our neurological system and the retina in our eyes. They also provide some protection against heart disease and stroke. Omega-3s may also have an effect on our immune system. They can help control inflammation in our bodies by acting as building blocks for certain substances that regulate inflammation. This means they can limit or modify the body's response to inflammation. In studies done on animals with arthritis,

OMG-3-FA was found to avoid or diminish the symptoms of arthritis. This suggests that they might be helpful in treating rheumatoid arthritis, a type of arthritis that causes swollen and painful joints. In clinical studies involving people with arthritis, OMG-3-FA was shown to have a positive effect on the disease and diminish swollen and painful joints. It is helpful to lower disease activity. The OMG-3-FA has many health benefits. They are important for our brain, eyes, and heart. They also have the potential to reduce inflammation and improve symptoms of arthritis.

4.1 INTRODUCTION

OMG-3-FA is well-known for its numerous therapeutic effects on health management and treatment of diseases. OMG-3-FA has been found to be very effective in protecting against cardiovascular disease and arthritis (Kromhout et al., 1985). OMG-3-FA can be used for the treatment and management of myocardial infarction, etc. (Holub et al., 2004) because it has an anti-arrhythmic action (Galano et al., 2018). It can reduce inflammation (Innes et al., 2018; Calder et al., 2017). Therefore, inflammatory bowel disease can be effectively treated with OMG-3-FA, according to research (Ungaro et al., 2017). OMG-3-FA has also been effective in the treatment of multiple sclerosis (Pantzaris et al., 2013; Harbige et al., 2007). OMG-3-FA has immunomodulatory properties (Riccio et al., 2011; Calder et al., 2019; Rajaei et al., 2015). In this chapter, the effect of OMG-3-FA-related information and its therapeutic roles on rheumatoid arthritis (RA) disease are covered and discussed.

Fatty acids are of two types: first, monounsaturated; and second, polyunsaturated (Din et al., 2004). Saturated fatty acids are solid when it's not excessively hot or cold, like in a regular room, whereas unsaturated fatty acids are often liquid. This is the primary physical difference between the two types of fatty acids. So, if you have fat like butter or lard, which is solid at room temperature, it is likely to contain more saturated fats. On the other hand, oils like olive oil or vegetable oil, which are in a liquid state at room temperature, tend to have more unsaturated fats (Jarouliya & Keservani, 2019). There are two varieties of polyunsaturated FA: OMG-3-PUFA and OMG-6 PUFA. Vegetable oils are a common source of OMG-3-FA. OMG-3-FA occurs naturally in three different forms: linolenic acid, which is found in vegetable oils; eicosapentaenoic acid; and docosahexaenoic acid, which is typically derived from marine sources. Linoleic acid (LA) is a base material for the biosynthesis of various fatty acids. LA is an originator of the OMG-6 series of FA and α-linolenic acid. Both fatty acids are the precursors of the OMG-3 series of FA, and they are considered essential fatty acids because mammals cannot biosynthesize them. The name of fatty acids depends on the position of double unsaturated bonds. These double bonds are present between carbon atoms. Omega-3-FA has its first double bond at the 3-carbon molecule from the CH_3 methyl or n or ω end of the molecule, but Omega-6-FA has the first double bond at the 6-carbon molecule from the CH_3 methyl or n or ω end of the fatty acid molecule (Wall et al., 2010). Omega-6 LA, a type of fatty acid also known as linolenic acid, is found in several plants. Arachidonic acid is a different fatty acid that our bodies can use to create linoleic acid. Eicosapentaenoic acid and docosahexaenoic acid are two more fatty acids that can be altered and transformed from linolenic acid. People tend to consume more Omega-6-FA than Omega-3-FA in Western nations. Their diet typically has an Omega-6 to Omega-3 FA ratio of roughly 20 to 30 (Simopoulos et al., 2003; Kang et al., 2003).

4.2 MECHANISM OF ACTION

OMEGA-3 fatty acids (OMEGA-3-FA) are precursors of the synthesis of anti-inflammatory protective biomolecules. Therefore, OMEGA-3-FA has significant anti-inflammatory action. OMEGA-3-FA is synthesized from OMEGA-6 and OMEGA-3 fatty acids. Arachidonic acid and eicosapentaenoic acid are transformed into eicosanoids by the enzymes cyclo-oxygenase and lipoxygenase. Bioactive molecules formed from OMEGA-3 fatty acids are anti-inflammatory and prevent platelet aggregation activity, while arachidonic acid is pro-inflammatory and pro-aggregatory. Therefore, we can say that the beneficial effects of OMEGA-3-FA relate to them as well as to their metabolites, including maresins, protectins, and resolvins. Clinically, resolution is where the majority of OMEGA-3 metabolites are discovered. It is separated into two classes: class D resolvins, which are made from docosahexaenoic acid, and class E resolvins, which are made from eicosapentaenoic acid (Serhan et al., 2006; Serhan et al., 2000; Hong et al., 2003). Both metabolites of OMEGA-3 fatty acids (OMEGA-3-FA) participate with OMEGA-6 acid metabolites to enhance the resolution of the inflammatory cycle (Neuhofer et al., 2013; Watson et al., 2019). This metabolite plays an important role in reducing inflammation and regulating autoimmunity action.

Polyunsaturated fatty acids, like n-3 and n-6 FAs, have different effects on our bodies. The amount of these fats we eat is important for how they affect us. It's been noticed that as n-3 intake has decreased recently, chronic inflammation has become more severe. These fats can change certain genes and cause inflammation in the gut, leading to inflammatory bowel diseases. Scientists have been studying this for many years. In this chapter, we will discuss the role of polyunsaturated fatty acids and how they affect digestion, focusing on their connection to inflammation (Watson et al., 2019). The general mechanism and roles of omega-3 fatty acids are exposed in Figures 4.1 and 4.2, respectively.

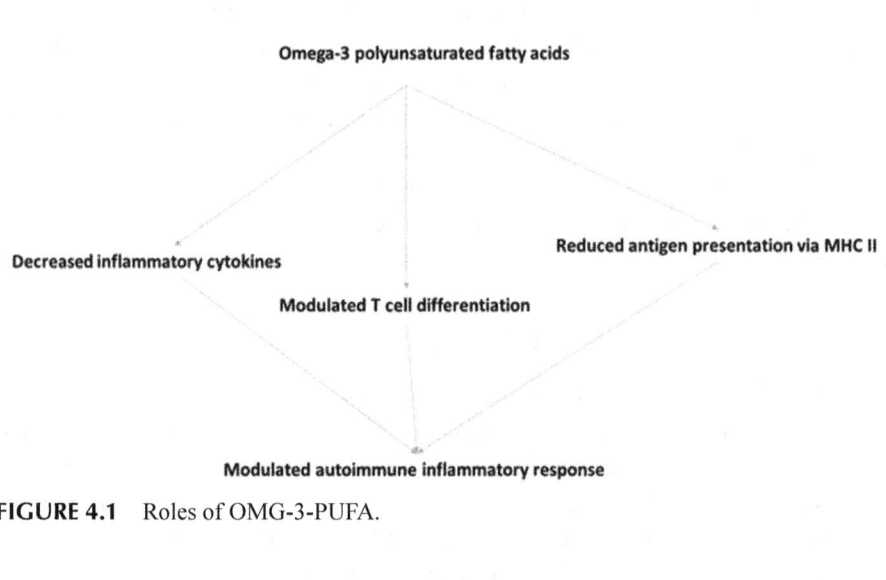

FIGURE 4.1 Roles of OMG-3-PUFA.

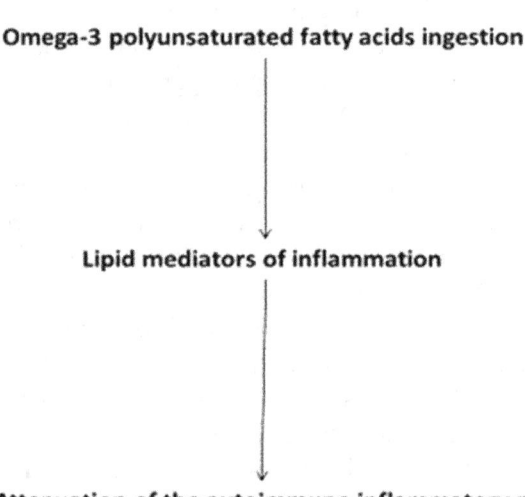

FIGURE 4.2 Biological response and OMG-3-PUFA.

OMG-3-FA is a type of supplement that might affect the release of certain chemicals in our body that cause inflammation. In a study involving people with rheumatoid arthritis, scientists found that when these individuals took fish oil regularly, it helped reduce the amount of a specific substance called plasma interleukin-1β (IL-1β) which is known to promote inflammation (Espersen et al., 1992). According to clinical studies, fish oil supplementation also caused endotoxin-stimulated monocyte cells' levels of substances including tumor necrosis factor-alpha (TNF-α), interleukin-1 (IL-1), and interleukin-6 (IL-6) to decline (Caughey et al., 1996) respectively. Docosahexaenoic acid, eicosapentaenoic acid, and the number of CD4+ T cells were all reduced by fish oil intake. CD4+ T cells generate interferon-γ (IFN-γ) and interleukin-17 (IL-17) (Ye et al., 2012). Eicosapentaenoic acid and docosahexaenoic acid have been discovered to inhibit the production of cytokines including TNF-α, IL-1, and IL-6, which are well-known pro-inflammatory mediators (Novak et al., 2003; Babcock et al., 2002; Zhao et al., 2004; Trebble et al., 2003). Clinical researchers have found that Omega-3 fatty acids (OMG-3-FA) and their metabolites significantly reduce inflammation (Kang et al., 2004; Wei et al., 2010). OMG-3-FA reduces the inflammation-causing action of cytokines and the inflammation-causing factor in RA disease. Eicosapentaenoic acid and docosahexaenoic acid have been demonstrated to reduce the development of human T cells and the generation of IL-2 in clinical investigations (Pompos et al., 2002; Bi et al., 2017). The dietary OMG-3-FA is very effective for maintaining the balance between TH1 and TH2 ratios in RA and autoimmune encephalitis disease (Mizota et al., 2009; Sierra et al., 2006). Clinical results revealed that OMG-3-FA regulates the proliferation and differentiation of T cells.

Researchers have found in lab studies that a substance called Omega-3 fatty acids (OMG-3-FA) can lower the production of a specific protein called major histocompatibility complex (MHC) II. This protein is important for presenting antigens, which are molecules that trigger an immune response. It was also found that this effect of OMG-3-FA on MHC II was seen in both mice and humans, confirming the results from the lab studies (Khair-El-Din et al., 1995; Hughes et al., 1997). The above-mentioned data showed that Omega-3 fatty acids (OM-3-FA) reduce the inflammatory action of cytokines, modulate T-cell differentiation, and reduce antigen presentation via MHC II. Consequently, it enhances the inflammatory autoimmune response (Leslie et al., 1985; Ierna et al., 2010) (Figure 4.1). Omega-3 polyunsaturated fatty acids (OMG-3-PUFA) chiefly include eicosapentaenoic acid (EPA) and docosahexaenoic acid (DHA). Both PUFAs are obtained from fish oil, and alpha-linolenic acid (ALA) from plant sources (Volker et al., 2010; Woo et al., 2015; Adkins et al., 2019).

OMG-3 (n-3) PUFAs result in a reduction in the mRNA levels of numerous proteins that are known to be crucial in the pathophysiology of OA. They offer a mechanistic explanation of the health benefits of consuming OMG-3-PUFAs, at least in part. The complex symptoms of many ailments may be eliminated by the OMFA diet. OMG-3-PUFAs may be especially beneficial as dietary supplements for people with joint pain illnesses because of the limited efficacy of EPA.

The addition of a high-fat diet and even a small amount of OMG-3-FA eliminates the harmful effects of dietary weight loss on osteoarthritis, "said Farshid Guilak, co-author of a study in rats and now published in the Annals of the Rheumatic Diseases. "Although OMG-3-FA did not reverse the osteoarthritis caused by injury," Guilak continues, "they significantly reduce bone density compared with OMG-6 or saturated fatty foods (Nicholas et al., 2014)."

4.3 FAT CATEGORIES

Carbon, hydrogen, and oxygen make up fatty acids as constituent elements. Due to the chemical makeup of these substances, they do not dissolve in water. Fatty acids come in a variety of forms, including saturated, monounsaturated, and polyunsaturated varieties. These categories have various characteristics. At room temperature, saturated fats, such as the fat in butter and animal meats, are solid. Olive oil is an example of a monounsaturated fat that is liquid at room temperature but solidifies when placed in the refrigerator. Oils from grains and seeds contain polyunsaturated fats that remain liquid at room temperature as well as in the refrigerator.

The two types of polyunsaturated fatty acids (PUFAs) are omega-3 and omega-6. They are given names based on where the fatty acid's carbon double bond is found. Counting the carbon atoms starting at the methyl (omega) end of the chemical yields the location of this bond. While omega-6 PUFAs have it at the 6-carbon position, omega-3 PUFAs have it at the 3-carbon position. Oleic acid, an omega-9 lipid, is found in olive oil, with its single double bond at the ninth carbon in the chain. PUFAs that are necessary fatty acids include linolenic acid (LA) and alpha-linolenic acid (ALA). This means that because our bodies are unable to create them, we must obtain them through diet. To stay healthy, it's crucial to have these fatty acids in our meals (Harper et al., 2001; Roche et al., 1999).

4.4 DIETARY COMPOSITION OF PUFA

OMEGA-6-FA is more common in the modern Western diet than OMEGA-3-FA. OMEGA-6 to OMEGA-3-FA ratios are typically 4 to 1. However, this ratio has greatly increased over time, often exceeding 25 to 1. This is primarily due to the usage of partially hydrogenated FA, which is added to snacks and processed convenience meals to extend their shelf lives. PUFAs are the main source of OMEGA-6-FA in our diet. Other sources of PUFAs include beef, poultry, nuts, grains, vegetables, and seed oils. OMEGA-6-FA is a component of arachidonic acid, a compound that plays a role in inducing inflammatory reactions in our bodies. The prevalence of chronic inflammatory disorders that we observe today is rising in part due to the modern dietary practices we have adopted (Rakel et al., 2003).

4.5 PHARMACOLOGIC ACTIONS OF OMGA-3-FAUFA

which stands for polyunsaturated fatty acids, is an important substance that we get from our diet. Two examples of UFA are EPA and DHA, which are types of OMG-3-FA. These OMG-3-FA play a crucial role in our body by serving as building blocks for eicosanoids. Eicosanoids are molecules that have various effects on our body, such as reducing inflammation, preventing blood clotting, and widening blood vessels. Our body can also produce eicosanoids from a different type of OMG-3-FA called ALA, but this conversion process is not very efficient. The reason for this is that ALA and another type of fatty acid called OMG-6-FA compete for the same enzyme, called delta-6 desaturase, which is needed for the conversion. This enzyme controls how OMG-6 and OMG-3-FA are transformed into their respective eicosanoids. When we consume more OMG-6-FA, especially a specific type called arachidonic acid, it leads to the production of eicosanoids that can promote inflammation, blood clotting, and the release of substances like tumor necrosis factor-alpha (TNF-alpha), thromboxane A2, prostaglandin E2, and leukotriene B4. These effects can be harmful to our bodies and cause problems. So, it's important to have a good balance of omega-3 and omega-6 fatty acids in our diet. By consuming enough omega-3 fatty acids like EPA and DHA, we can support the production of eicosanoids that have positive effects on our body and help maintain our health (Gerster et al., 1998). Fish oil contains a substance called EPA, which was discovered by EPA researchers. EPA works by blocking the process of arachidonic acid metabolism. This leads to the production of fewer substances in the body that can cause blood clotting and inflammation. These substances are called eicosanoids and they are made from omega-3 fatty acids. Eicosanoids have the ability to cause inflammation in our cells, but the ones derived from EPA are much less powerful compared to those derived from omega-6 fatty acids (Alexander et al., 1998).

OMEGA-3-PUFA is a crucial nutrient that is present in some forms of fat. Omega-3-PUFAs come in a variety of forms, such as alpha-linolenic acid (ALA), stearidonic acid (SDA), eicosapentaenoic acid (EPA), docosapentaenoic acid (DPA), and docosahexaenoic acid (DHA). To comprehend how these fatty acids affect human health, they have been the subject of numerous studies. OMEGA-3-PUFAs come in a variety of dietary sources and have diverse structural variations. Fatty acids are also metabolized by our body. The impact of OMEGA-3-PUFAs on a range of health issues, including heart disease, diabetes, cancer, Alzheimer's disease, dementia, depression, vision, mood swings, and the health of expectant women and children, has been studied by researchers. OMEGA-3-PUFAs have been linked in numerous studies to favorable health effects, although there are still some debates and divergent views. The efficiency and overall advantages of these fatty acids have drawn criticism from some studies. Clarifying these debates and providing more accurate information regarding the health impacts of OMEGA-3 PUFA are priorities for future research.

4.6 PATHOPHYSIOLOGY OF EICOSANOID IMMUNOMODULATORY FUNCTIONS IN RHEUMATOID ARTHRITIS AND CARDIOVASCULAR DISEASE

Arachidonic acid-derived eicosanoids like TNF-alpha and interleukin-1 beta (IL-1 beta) are substances that play a big role in causing tissue damage and pain. These substances have been found in the fluid and tissues of joints affected by rheumatoid arthritis, as well as in the lesions of people with atherosclerosis (a condition where arteries become clogged). However, they have not been observed in healthy blood vessels (Fontana et al., 1992; Di Giovine et al., 1988). In clinical research, scientists have found that certain substances in our bodies called cytokines play a role in causing swelling and damage in different parts of our body. These cytokines can make the lining of our joints grow too much, cause immune cells to gather in these areas, and break down the protective layer of our cartilage. They can also affect blood vessels that have fatty deposits, causing them to become swollen and damaged. Inflammatory cytokines like TNF-alpha and growth factors from platelets are particularly responsible for these effects. These growth factors make cells in the inner and outer layers of blood vessels multiply, which leads to the growth of plaques and makes them larger (Arend et al., 1995; Barath et al., 1990).

When there is inflammation, the body produces a chemical called C-reactive protein (CRP). CRP levels rise in the body of a person who has rheumatoid arthritis (RA) while the condition is active. Furthermore, CRP has a role in the development of atherosclerosis, a condition in which artery plaque builds up. Numerous studies have shown that higher levels of CRP are associated with an increased risk of cardiovascular events, including heart attacks and strokes. Ridker et al. in 2000 described numerous methods by which this occurs. The level of CRP in the body is directly related to the levels of a substance called interleukin-6. This substance promotes the sticking of white blood cells to the walls of blood vessels (Wolbink et al., 1996). CRP helps macrophages produce tissue factors. These factors are important for blood clotting and are found in plaques that build up in blood vessels (Cermak et al., 1993). In the treatment of rheumatoid arthritis (RA), some medications, like corticosteroids, can contribute to the development of these plaques. Even though corticosteroids are used in low doses, they can still have a negative impact on cholesterol levels in the blood. However, some research studies have not found a clear link between the use of steroids in RA and an increased risk of cardiovascular death (Wallberg-Jonsson et al., 1997; Stern et al., 1973).

Methotrexate and sulfasalazine are two medications that can cause the development of atherogenesis, which is the formation of fatty plaques in blood vessels. This happens because these drugs affect the body's ability to process folate, leading to increased levels of homocysteine, a substance that can contribute to the development of atherosclerosis. When homocysteine levels are high, it increases the risk of developing a condition called atherothrombosis, which involves the formation of blood clots in the arteries. Methotrexate and sulfasalazine can directly harm the cells that line the blood vessels (called endothelial cells), and they also promote the oxidation of LDL cholesterol, which can further damage the arteries. Additionally, these drugs can make the blood more prone to clotting. However, there is a way to reduce the risk associated with these medications. By ensuring an adequate intake of folate through a balanced diet or folate supplements, the harmful effects of methotrexate can be minimized. Folate helps counteract the negative impact of these drugs on homocysteine levels and therefore lowers the risk of atherogenesis and atherothrombosis (Welch et al., 1998).

4.7 DIETARY STUDIES

According to a study in clinical medicine, taking fish oil supplements in the form of tiny capsules can lessen the body's synthesis of several molecules that promote inflammation. These chemicals are known as TNF-alpha and IL-1 beta in mononuclear cells. However, taking a lot of medicines every day can be expensive and come with potential difficulties and adverse effects for individuals. Additionally, two different diets were contrasted in the study. One group of subjects consumed flaxseed, which has a low concentration of omega-6 polyunsaturated fatty acids (PUFAs) but is a good source of omega-3 fatty acids. The other group followed a diet that included sunflower products, which are a common source of omega-6 PUFAs. Examples of sunflower products are sunflower oil, spreads, and dressings. The researchers found that the group following the flaxseed diet had a significant decrease in the production of TNF-alpha, IL-1 beta, thromboxane B2, and prostaglandin E2. These substances are all involved in causing inflammation. On the other hand, the group following the sunflower diet did not show as much effectiveness in reducing the production of these inflammatory substances. These clinical studies showed that increasing the intake of OMG-3 fatty acids, whether from fish oil (specifically EPA) or its precursor called ALA and at the same time reducing the intake of OMG-6 PUFAs through dietary restrictions can significantly lower the levels of these inflammatory substances in our body (Caughey et al., 1996). OMG-6-FA is a special fat that our bodies need but can't make on their own. We have to get them from the food we eat. They work together with another type of fat called OMG-3s to help our brains work well, and they're important for our bodies to grow and develop properly. These fats, also known as OMG-6s, help our skin and hair grow, keep our bones healthy, control how our bodies use energy, and make sure our reproductive system functions normally.

To eat healthy, it's important to limit your intake of bad fats and focus on consuming more good fats. This means choosing foods like fruits, vegetables, whole grains, and lean proteins while minimizing the consumption of processed and fried foods. Two important types of fats are Omega-3 and Omega-6 fatty acids. Omega-3 fats are good because they can help reduce inflammation in our bodies, which is a normal response when we get hurt or sick. On the other hand, some Omega-6 fats can actually make inflammation worse. If we have too much of these Omega-6 fats, it may increase the chances of having regional pain syndrome, which is a condition that causes chronic pain in certain parts of the body. Unfortunately, the typical American diet has a lot more omega-6 fats compared to Omega-3 fats. In fact, it can have 14 to 25 times more Omega-6 fats! This imbalance is not good for our health because it can make inflammation problems worse. To stay healthy, it's important to have a diet that has a good balance of Omega-3 and Omega-6 fatty acids.

OMG-6 fatty acids come in a variety of forms, but not all of them lead to inflammation in our systems. The majority of OMG-6 fatty acids that humans consume come from vegetable oils like linoleic acid (LA), which are found in meals. Alpha-linolenic acid (ALA), an OMG-3 fatty acid, and linoleic acid should not be confused. Gamma-linolenic acid (GLA), which is produced by our bodies from linoleic acid, is ingested. Arachidonic acid (AA) can then be produced from GLA. Evening primrose oil (EPO), borage oil, and black currant seed oil are examples of plant-based oils that contain GLA, an OMG-6 fatty acid.

4.8 CLINICAL STUDIES

In some medical research, scientists have discovered that people who eat baked or broiled fish (except tuna) with omega-3 fatty acids more than two times a week have a lower chance of getting rheumatoid arthritis (RA). They also found that those who already have RA may have milder symptoms if they eat this type of fish regularly. These findings are supported by a report from clinical studies (Shapiro et al., 1996).

A new study was conducted on 50 patients with rheumatoid arthritis (RA). The study lasted for 15 weeks and it was designed in a way that some patients received a fake treatment (placebo) while others were given omega-6 fatty acids as part of their diet. The study was also conducted in a way that neither the patients nor the researchers knew who was receiving the real treatment or the placebo (double-blind), and the assignment of treatments was random. The researchers found that omega-6 fatty acids had a significant impact on the patients' RA-related problems when taken regularly. These problems included stiffness, inflammation, and pain. The researchers evaluated the activity of arthritis and used a Health Assessment Questionnaire score to measure the patient's condition. However, the positive results were not seen in patients who took omega-6 fatty acids for only 15 days. Therefore, the researchers concluded that RA patients need to regularly consume omega-6 fatty acids through their diet or in the form of fish oil. Having a regular diet that includes omega-6 fatty acids or taking supplements can help decrease the symptoms associated with RA, reduce the risk of disease, alleviate pain, and decrease inflammation.

Multiple studies have shown that taking fish oil supplements can be very helpful for people with rheumatoid arthritis (RA). These studies, known as clinical meta-analyzes, have analyzed the findings from various research papers, including those by Kremer et al. in 1987; Cleland et al. in 1988; and Geusens et al. in 1994. The meta-analyzes researchers discovered that taking fish oil supplements significantly improves RA-related joint issues and morning stiffness. In their research, they took into account a variety of disease-related characteristics, including age, gender, rheumatoid factor status, length of the disease, and medication use. In comparison to other treatments like nonsteroidal anti-inflammatory medicines (NSAIDs) and slow-acting antirheumatic drugs (SAARDs), the findings of their investigation showed that consuming OMG-3-FA from fish oil is more beneficial in lowering sensitive joints and the length of morning stiffness. In other words, the level of relief in painful joints and morning stiffness was not as great in patients who remained taking NSAIDs and SAARDs as it was in patients who received OMG-3-FA from fish oil (Fortin et al., 1995).

4.9 DRUG/DIET TREATMENT COMBINATIONS FOR RA

Using a combination of drugs and a special diet can be a highly effective treatment for patients with rheumatoid arthritis (RA). The combination of anti-rheumatoid drugs and an omega-3 and omega-6 fatty acids (OMFA) diet has been found to greatly reduce the production of a substance called eicosanoid, which plays a role in inflammation. By combining the drugs and the diet, the therapeutic effect is increased, leading to better results for patients. Clinical researchers have been studying the effects of giving patients both the drug and the specific dietary regimen. The diet regimen includes a specific ratio of omega-6 fatty acids (LA) to omega-3 fatty acids (ALA), which is 4:1. This particular ratio has been found to be very effective for treating RA. In addition, the researchers found that when patients took a combination of the dietary omega-3 fatty acid EPA and the drug auranofin, it significantly reduced the production of another substance called LTB4, which is involved in inflammation (Lau et al., 1993; James et al., 1992).

It is important to study the possibility of using a lower dose of a dietary supplement to effectively treat rheumatoid arthritis (RA). This study is crucial for RA patients because the pharmaceutical company conducting the research has found that the supplement can be effective for patients who regularly take medication. All clinical studies can be short-term or long-term, and these studies have shown that many patients with RA have a chronic and progressive disease despite treatment. RA patients often need to change their medications because they either don't work well or cause side effects. According to a study by Prashker et al., the side effects of RA medications make up about 60% of the total cost of treating RA patients in the United States (Pincus et al., 1992; Prashker et al., 1995).

Researchers have discovered that taking LA/ALA (alpha-lipoic acid/alpha-linolenic acid) and fish oil together in a 4:1 ratio for a long period of time can lead to increased loss or breakdown of antioxidants in the body. This can cause more complications in the body. Therefore, it is important to take antioxidants along with dietary supplements of OMFA (OMG-3 fatty acids). A study from 1996 showed that consuming fish oil should be accompanied by vitamins E and C. This helps ensure a balanced diet and prevents the negative effects of free radicals, which can worsen cardiovascular problems (Darlington et al., 2001).

4.10 DOSAGE

EPA and DHA content determines the varied dosages of fish oil supplements that are available. The average amount of EPA and DHA in a fish oil capsule is 0.18 grams (180 milligrams) and 0.12 grams (120 milligrams), respectively. EPA and DHA concentrations in wild fish are often higher than those in farmed fish, according to research (Darlington et al., 2001; Bender et al., 1998).

4.11 HARMFUL EFFECTS

A special kind of oil called omega-3 fatty acids (OMFA) can help reduce allergic reactions to products that contain fish. It can also reduce the negative effects that nuts can have on some people. When people have allergies, they may experience symptoms like feeling sick, burping more, having heartburn, feeling uncomfortable in the stomach, or having a fishy taste in their mouth. These symptoms can be reduced if people take fish oil supplements with their meals, starting with a small amount and gradually increasing the dose. The FDA, which is responsible for ensuring the safety of medicines, has given guidelines about omega-3 fatty acids and has confirmed that fish supplements are safe to use. The EPA and the Department of Health and Human Services have cautioned against eating some species of fish like sharks, swordfish, king mackerel, and tilefish if you are a pregnant woman, a breastfeeding mother, or a young child. These large sea creatures may contain dangerous amounts of methylmercury, a hazardous chemical. If you're using a medicine that prevents blood from clotting, such as antiplatelet or anticoagulant pills, it's crucial to be careful because fish and fish-based products can make blood take longer to clot. These fish-derived products can make bleeding take longer to stop (Buckley et al., 2004). If you take fish oil for many months, it can lead to a lack of vitamin E and lower levels of antioxidants in your body. But you can prevent this by eating fresh fruits and vegetables, which are rich in vitamin E and vitamin C. When fish oils are packaged as capsules, they are often mixed with vitamin E (in the form of d-alpha-tocopherol) and sometimes with vitamin C to prevent damage to the oils. To make sure you have enough of these vitamins, it is recommended to take 400 IU (International Units) of vitamin E, 200 mg of vitamin C, and 200 mcg (micrograms) of selenium each day (Darlington et al., 2001).

4.12 STORAGE PRECAUTIONS

OMEGA-3 fatty acid supplements are important, but you need to be careful about how you store them. These supplements can get damaged when they are exposed to sunlight or high temperatures. So, it's essential to store them in the right container, keep them in a cool place, and protect them from sunlight to make sure they last longer. Some OMEGA-3-FA supplements even need to be refrigerated once you open them.

4.13 RECOMMENDATIONS

According to studies done by doctors and researchers, it has been found that if you have rheumatoid arthritis (RA) or cardiovascular problems and you want to get better results from your treatment, it's important to take OMEGA-3-FA oils and supplements for a period of 60 days. These oils and supplements have been shown to reduce the symptoms and issues associated with RA and cardiovascular problems. It's crucial to remember that consuming OMEGA-3-FA supplements and oils may potentially cause your body's level of antioxidants to decline. Antioxidants are chemicals that aid in defending your body from harm brought on by dangerous compounds. It is advised to routinely eat fruits high in antioxidants in order to maintain a healthy balance of antioxidants in your body. The researchers also recommended that patients adhere to a diet that supports heart and joint health. This entails choosing wholesome foods that are good for your heart and joints. By adhering to these recommendations, you can enhance your general health and support the therapeutic effects of OMEGA-3-FA oils and supplements.

4.14 CONCLUSION

Higher omega-3 to omega-6 fatty acid ratios in the diet reduce the generation of TNF-alpha, IL-1 beta, inflammation, and a number of other RA disease-related symptoms. Omega-3 to omega-6-FA diets offer a more supportive environment for the management and effective treatment of RA. Dietary supplements like DHA and EPA in fish oil or fatty fish meals are also available. These serve as a direct supply of omega-3-FA, which has a key function in decreasing medicine use, adverse effect profiles, and mortality among individuals with RA and cardiovascular disease. Omega-3-FA pills and oils have drawbacks such as short shelf life, medication interactions, and unfavorable storage conditions. Omega-3-FA oils and supplements speed up bleeding, thus anyone who takes them should take extra precautions while taking anticoagulants. According to clinical studies, omega-3-FA exerts its anti-inflammatory effects by reducing the production of proinflammatory mediators like cytokines and by inducing the synthesis of eicosanoids. Clinical studies have found that fish oil supplements work well and are safe as nutraceuticals. There are various healing properties in fish oil. It may supplement current RA therapy plans. However, there is still work to be done on studies with longer-term trials and larger patient cohorts. This kind of extensive research can offer useful insights into the advantages of taking fish oil supplements for RA and other conditions. N-3 PUFAs' effects on synovial histology, radiographic progression, their contribution to the development of early arthritis, and their interaction with biologics are still being studied.

KEYWORDS

- arthritis
- biologics
- eicosanoids
- linoleic acid
- omega-3 fatty acids
- rheumatoid arthritis
- tumor necrosis factor-alpha

REFERENCES

Adkins, Y., Soulika, A. M., Mackey, B., & Kelley, D. S. (2019). Docosahexaenoic acid (22:6n-3) ameliorated the onset and severity of experimental autoimmune encephalomyelitis in mice. *Lipids, 54*(1), 13–23.

Alexander, J. W. (1998). Immunonutrition: The role of omega-3 fatty acids. *Nutrition, 14*, 627–633.

Arend, W. P., & Dayer, J. M. (1995). Inhibition of the production and effects of interleukin-1 and tumor necrosis factor-alpha in rheumatoid arthritis. *Arthritis Rheum., 38*(2), 151–160.

Babcock, T. A., Novak, T., Ong, E., Jho, D. H., Helton, W. S., & Espat, N. J. (2002). Modulation of lipopolysaccharide-stimulated macrophage tumor necrosis factor-alpha production by omega-3 fatty acid is associated with differential cyclooxygenase-2 protein expression and is independent of interleukin-10. *J. Surg. Res., 107*(1), 135–139.

Barath, P., et al. (1990). Tumor necrosis factor gene expression in human vascular intimal smooth muscle cells determined by in situ hybridization. *Am. J. Pathol., 137*(3), 503–509.

Bender, N. K., et al. (1998). Effects of marine fish oils on the anticoagulation status of patients receiving chronic warfarin therapy. *J. Thromb. Thrombolysis, 5*, 257–261.

Bi, X., Li, F., Liu, S., Jin, Y., Zhang, X., Yang, T., et al. (2017). ω-3 polyunsaturated fatty acids ameliorate type 1 diabetes and autoimmunity. *J. Clin. Invest., 127*(5), 1757–1771.

Bowen, K. J., Harris, W. S., & Kris-Etherton, P. M. (2016). Omega-3 fatty acids and cardiovascular disease: Are there benefits? *Curr. Treat Options Cardiovasc. Med., 18*, 69.

Buckley, M. S., et al. (2004). Fish oil interaction with warfarin. *Ann. Pharmacother., 38*(1), 50–52.

Calder, P. C. (2017). Omega-3 fatty acids and inflammatory processes: From molecules to man. *Biochem. Soc. Trans., 45*(5), 1105–1115.

Calder, P. C. (2019). Intravenous lipid emulsions to deliver bioactive omega-3 fatty acids for improved patient outcomes. *Mar Drugs, 17*(5), 274.

Caughey, G. E., et al. (1996). The effect on human tumor necrosis factor-alpha and interleukin 1 beta production of diets enriched in n-3 fatty acids from vegetable oil or fish oil. *Am. J. Clin. Nutr., 63*(1), 116–122.

Cermak, J., et al. (1993). C-reactive protein induces human peripheral blood monocytes to synthesize tissue factors. *Blood, 82*(2), 513–520.

Cleland, L. G., et al. (1988). Clinical and biochemical effects of dietary fish oil supplements in rheumatoid arthritis. *J. Rheumatol., 15*(9), 1471–1475.

Covington, M. B. (2004). Omega-3 fatty acids. *Am. Fam. Physician., 70*, 133–140.

Darlington, L. G., & Stone, T. W. (2001). Antioxidants and fatty acids in the amelioration of rheumatoid arthritis and related disorders. *Br. J. Nutr., 85*, 251–269.

Dawczynski, C., Schubert, R., Hein, G., Müller, A., Eidner, T., Vogelsang, H., & Jahreis, G. (2009). Long-term moderate intervention with n-3 long-chain PUFA-supplemented dairy products: Effects on pathophysiological biomarkers in patients with rheumatoid arthritis. *Br. J. Nutr., 101*(11), 1517–1526.

Di Giovine, F. S., et al. (1988). Tumor necrosis factor in synovial exudates. *Ann. Rheum. Dis., 47*(10), 768–772.

Din, J. N., Newby, D. E., & Flapan, A. D. (2004). Omega 3 fatty acids and cardiovascular disease–fishing for a natural treatment. *BMJ, 328*(7430), 30–35.

Endres, S., et al. (1989). The effect of dietary supplementation with n-3 polyunsaturated fatty acids on the synthesis of interleukin-1 and tumor necrosis factor by mononuclear cells. *New England Journal of Medicine, 320*, 265–271.

Espersen, G. T., Grunnet, N., Lervang, H. H., Nielsen, G. L., Thomsen, B. S., Faarvang, K. L., et al. (1992). Decreased interleukin-1 beta levels in plasma from rheumatoid arthritis patients after dietary supplementation with n-3 polyunsaturated fatty acids. *Clinical Rheumatology, 11*(3), 393–395.

Fontana, A., et al. (1982). Interleukin 1 activity in the synovial fluid of patients with rheumatoid arthritis. *Rheumatology International, 2*, 49–53.

Fortin, P. R., et al. (1995). Validation of a meta-analysis: The effects of fish oil in rheumatoid arthritis. *Journal of Clinical Epidemiology, 48*, 1379–1390.

Galano, J. M., Roy, J., Durand, T., Lee, J., Le Guennec, J. Y., Oger, C., et al. (2018). Biological activities of non-enzymatic oxygenated metabolites of polyunsaturated fatty acids (NEO-PUFAs) derived from EPA and DHA: New anti-arrhythmic compounds? *Molecular Aspects of Medicine, 64*, 161–168.

Gerster, H. (1998). Can adults adequately convert alpha-linolenic acid (18:3n-3) to eicosapentaenoic acid (20:5n-3) and docosahexaenoic acid (22:6n-3)? *International Journal of Vitamin and Nutrition Research, 68*, 159–173.

Geusens, P., et al. (1994). Long-term effect of omega-3 fatty acid supplementation in active rheumatoid arthritis. A 12-month, double-blind controlled study. *Arthritis & Rheumatism, 37*, 824–829.

Gui, H., Tong, Q., Qu, W., Mao, C. M., & Dai, S. M. (2015). The endocannabinoid system and its therapeutic implications in rheumatoid arthritis. *International Immunopharmacology, 26*, 86–91.

Harbige, L. S., & Sharief, M. K. (2007). Polyunsaturated fatty acids in the pathogenesis and treatment of multiple sclerosis. *British Journal of Nutrition, 98*(Suppl 1), S46–S53.

Harper, C. R., & Jacobson, T. A. (2001). The facts of life: The role of omega-3 fatty acids in the prevention of coronary heart disease. *Archives of Internal Medicine, 161*, 2185–2192.

Holub, D. J., & Holub, B. J. (2004). Omega-3 fatty acids from fish oils and cardiovascular disease. *Molecular and Cellular Biochemistry, 263*(1–2), 217–225.

Hong, S., Gronert, K., Devchand, P. R., Moussignac, R. L., & Serhan, C. N. (2003). Novel docosatrienes and 17S-resolvins generated from docosahexaenoic acid in murine brain, human blood, and glial cells. Autacoids in anti-inflammation. *Journal of Biological Chemistry, 278*(17), 14677–14687.

Horrobin, D. F. (1987). Low prevalence of coronary heart disease (CHD), psoriasis, asthma, and rheumatoid arthritis in Eskimos: Are they caused by high dietary intake of eicosatetraenoic acid (EPA), a genetic variation of essential fatty acid (EFA) metabolism or a combination of both? *Medical Hypotheses, 22*, 421–428.

Hughes, D. A., & Pinder, A. C. (1997). N-3 polyunsaturated fatty acids modulate the expression of functionally associated molecules on human monocytes and inhibit antigen-presentation in vitro. *Clinical and Experimental Immunology, 110*(3), 516–523.

Ierna, M., Kerr, A., Scales, H., Berge, K., & Griinari, M. (2010). Supplementation of diet with krill oil protects against experimental rheumatoid arthritis. *BMC Musculoskeletal Disorders, 11*, 136.

Innes, J. K., & Calder, P. C. (2018). Omega-6 fatty acids and inflammation. *Prostaglandins, Leukotrienes, and Essential Fatty Acids, 132*, 41–48.

James, M. J., et al. (1992). Inhibition of human neutrophil leukotriene B4 synthesis by a combination of auranofin and eicosatetraenoic acid. *Biochemical Pharmacology, 43*, 695–700.

Jarouliya, U., & Keservani, Raj K. (2019). Protein functions as a cell surface and nuclear receptor in human diseases. In S. Bharti & D. K. Mahapatra (Eds.), *Medicinal Chemistry with Pharmaceutical Product Development* (pp. 1–32). Apple Academic Press, CRC Press, Taylor & Francis Group.

Kang, J. X. (2003). The importance of omega-6/omega-3 fatty acid ratio in cell function. The gene transfer of omega-3 fatty acid desaturase. *World Review of Nutrition and Dietetics, 92*, 23–36.

Kang, J. X., Wang, J., Wu, L., & Kang, Z. B. (2004). Transgenic mice: fat-1 mice convert n-6 to n-3 fatty acids. *Nature, 427*(6974), 504.

Khair-el-Din, T. A., Sicher, S. C., Vazquez, M. A., Wright, W. J., & Lu, C. Y. (1995). Docosahexaenoic acid, a major constituent of fetal serum and fish oil diets, inhibits IFN gamma-induced IA expression by murine macrophages in vitro. *Journal of Immunology, 154*(3), 1296–1306.

Kremer, J. M., et al. (1987). Fish-oil fatty acid supplementation in active rheumatoid arthritis. A double-blinded, controlled, crossover study. *Annals of Internal Medicine, 106*, 497–503.

Kromhout, D., Bosschieter, E. B., & de Lezenne Coulander, C. (1985). The inverse relation between fish consumption and 20-year mortality from coronary heart disease. *New England Journal of Medicine, 312*(19), 1205–1209.

Lands, W. E. (1992). Biochemistry and physiology of n-3 fatty acids. *The FASEB Journal, 6*, 2530–2536.

Lau, C. S., et al. (1993). Effects of fish oil supplementation on non-steroidal anti-inflammatory drug requirements in patients with mild rheumatoid arthritis—A double-blind, placebo-controlled study. *British Journal of Rheumatology, 32*, 982–989.

Leslie, C. A., Gonnerman, W. A., Ullman, M. D., Hayes, K. C., Franzblau, C., & Cathcart, E. S. (1985). Dietary fish oil modulates macrophage fatty acids and decreases arthritis susceptibility in mice. *Journal of Experimental Medicine, 162*(4), 1336–1349.

Leslie, M. A., Cohen, D. J., Liddle, D. M., Robinson, L. E., & Ma, D. W. (2015). A review of the effect of omega-3 polyunsaturated fatty acids on blood triacylglycerol levels in normolipidemic and borderline hyperlipidemic individuals. *Lipids in Health and Disease, 14*, 53.

Lowin, T., Apitz, M., Anders, S., & Straub, R. H. (2015). Anti-inflammatory effects of N-acylethanolamines in rheumatoid arthritis synovial cells are mediated by TRPV1 and TRPA1 in a CO_{x-2}-dependent manner. *Arthritis Research & Therapy, 17*, 321.

Meydani, M., et al. (1991). Effect of long-term fish oil supplementation on vitamin E status and lipid peroxidation in women. *Journal of Nutrition, 121*, 484–491.

Mizota, T., Fujita-Kambara, C., Matsuya, N., Hamasaki, S., Fukudome, T., Goto, H., et al. (2009). Effect of dietary fatty acid composition on Th_1/Th_2 polarization in lymphocytes. *JPEN Journal of Parenteral and Enteral Nutrition, 33*(4), 390–396.

Neuhofer, A., Zeyda, M., Mascher, D., Itariu, B. K., Murano, I., Leitner, L., et al. (2013). Impaired local production of pro-resolving lipid mediators in obesity and 17-HDHA as a potential treatment for obesity-associated inflammation. *Diabetes, 62*(6), 1945–1956.

Nicholas, J. B. (2014). From arthritis to omega PUFAs regulate OA in obesity. *Nature Reviews Rheumatology, 10*, 514.

Novak, T. E., Babcock, T. A., Jho, D. H., Helton, W. S., & Espat, N. J. (2003). NF-kappa B inhibition by omega-3 fatty acids modulates LPS-stimulated macrophage TNF-alpha transcription. *American Journal of Physiology. Lung Cellular and Molecular Physiology, 284*(1), L84–L89.

Ooi, E. M., Watts, G. F., Ng, T. W., & Barrett, P. H. (2015). Effect of dietary fatty acids on human lipoprotein metabolism: A comprehensive update. *Nutrients, 7*, 4416–4425.

Pantzaris, M. C., Loukaides, G. N., Ntzani, E. E., & Patrikios, I. S. (2013). A novel oral nutraceutical formula of omega-3 and omega-6 fatty acids with vitamins (PLP10) in relapsing remitting multiple sclerosis: a randomized, double-blind, placebo-controlled proof-of-concept clinical trial. *BMJ Open, 3*(4), 1–16.

Pincus, T. (1992). The paradox of effective therapies but poor long-term outcomes in rheumatoid arthritis. *Seminars in Arthritis and Rheumatism, 21*(6 Suppl 3), 2–15.

Pompos, L. J., & Fritsche, K. L. (2002). Antigen-driven murine CD4+ T lymphocyte proliferation and interleukin-2 production are diminished by dietary (n–3) polyunsaturated fatty acids. *Journal of Nutrition, 132*(11), 3293–3300.

Prashker, M. J., & Meenan, R. F. (1995). The total costs of drug therapy for rheumatoid arthritis: A model based on costs of drug, monitoring, and toxicity. *Arthritis & Rheumatism, 38*, 318–325.

Rajaei, E., Mowla, K., Ghorbani, A., Bahadoram, S., Bahadoram, M., & Dargahi-Malamir, M. (2015). The Effect of Omega-3 Fatty Acids in Patients with Active Rheumatoid Arthritis Receiving DMARDs Therapy: Double-Blind Randomized Controlled Trial. *Global Journal of Health Science, 8*(7), 18–25.

Rakel, D. (Ed.). (2003). *Integrative Medicine*. St. Louis, MO: Saunders, 668–676. ISBN: 9-781-437-717-938.

Recht, L., et al. (1990). Hand handicap and rheumatoid arthritis in a fish-eating society (the Faroe Islands). *Journal of Internal Medicine, 227*, 49–55.

Riccio, P. (2011). The molecular basis of nutritional intervention in multiple sclerosis: a narrative review. *Complementary Therapies in Medicine, 19*(4), 228–237.

Richardson, D., Pearson, R. G., Kurian, N., Latif, M. L., Garle, M. J., Barrett, D. A., Kendall, D. A., Scammell, B. E., Reeve, A. J., & Chapman, V. (2008). Characterization of the cannabinoid receptor system in synovial tissue and fluid in patients with osteoarthritis and rheumatoid arthritis. *Arthritis Research & Therapy, 10*, R43.

Ridker, P. M., et al. (2000). C-reactive protein and other markers of inflammation in the prediction of cardiovascular disease in women. *New England Journal of Medicine, 342*, 836–843.

Roche, H. M. (1999). Unsaturated fatty acids. *Proceedings of the Nutrition Society, 58*, 397–401.

Rontoyanni, V. G., Sfikakis, P. P., Kitas, G. D., & Protogerou, A. D. (2012). Marine n-3 fatty acids for cardiovascular risk reduction and disease control in rheumatoid arthritis: "kill two birds with one stone"? *Current Pharmaceutical Design, 18*, 1531–1542.

Serhan, C. N., Clish, C. B., Brannon, J., Colgan, S. P., Chiang, N., & Gronert, K. (2000). Novel functional sets of lipid-derived mediators with anti-inflammatory actions generated from omega-3 fatty acids via cyclooxygenase 2-nonsteroidal anti-inflammatory drugs and transcellular processing. *Journal of Experimental Medicine, 192*(8), 1197–1204.

Serhan, C. N., Gotlinger, K., Hong, S., Lu, Y., Siegelman, J., Baer, T., et al. (2006). Anti-inflammatory actions of neuroprotectin D1/protectin D1 and its natural stereoisomers: Assignments of dihydroxy-containing docosatrienes. *Journal of Immunology, 176*(3), 1848–1859.

Shapiro, J. A., et al. (1996). Diet and rheumatoid arthritis in women: A possible protective effect of fish consumption. *Epidemiology, 7*, 256–263.

Sierra, S., Lara-Villoslada, F., Comalada, M., Olivares, M., & Xaus, J. (2006). Dietary fish oil n-3 fatty acids increase regulatory cytokine production and exert anti-inflammatory effects in two murine models of inflammation. *Lipids, 41*(12), 1115–1125.

Simopoulos, A. P. (2003). Importance of the ratio of omega-6/omega-3 essential fatty acids: Evolutionary aspects. *World Review of Nutrition and Dietetics, 92*, 1–22.

Stern, M. P., et al. (1973). Adrenocortical steroid treatment of rheumatic diseases: Effects on lipid metabolism. *Archives of Internal Medicine, 132*, 97–101.

Trebble, T., Arden, N. K., Stroud, M. A., Wootton, S. A., Burdge, G. C., Miles, E. A., et al. (2003). Inhibition of tumor necrosis factor-alpha and interleukin 6 production by mononuclear cells following dietary fish-oil supplementation in healthy men and response to antioxidant co-supplementation. *British Journal of Nutrition, 90*(2), 405–412.

Ungaro, F., Rubbino, F., Danese, S., & D'Alessio, S. (2017). Actors and factors in the resolution of intestinal inflammation: Lipid mediators as a new approach to therapy in inflammatory bowel diseases. *Frontiers in Immunology, 8*, 1331.

Volker, D. H., FitzGerald, P. E., & Garg, M. L. (2000). The eicosapentaenoic to docosahexaenoic acid ratio of diets affects the pathogenesis of arthritis in Lew/SSN rats. *Journal of Nutrition, 130*(3), 559–565.

Volker, D., et al. (2000). Efficacy of fish oil concentrates in the treatment of rheumatoid arthritis. *Journal of Rheumatology, 27*, 2343–2346.

Wall, R., Ross, R. P., Fitzgerald, G. F., & Stanton, C. (2010). Fatty acids from fish: the anti-inflammatory potential of long-chain omega-3 fatty acids. *Nutrition Reviews, 68*(5), 280–289.

Wallberg-Jonsson, S., et al. (1997). Cardiovascular morbidity and mortality in patients with seropositive rheumatoid arthritis in Northern Sweden. *Journal of Rheumatology, 24*, 445–451.

Watson, J. E., Kim, J. S., & Das, A. (2019). An emerging class of omega-3 fatty acid endocannabinoids & their derivatives. *Prostaglandins & Other Lipid Mediators, 143*, 106337.

Wei, D., Li, J., Shen, M., Jia, W., Chen, N., Chen, T., et al. (2010). Cellular production of n-3 PUFAs and reduction of n-6-to-n-3 ratios in the pancreatic beta-cells and islets enhance insulin secretion and confer protection against cytokine-induced cell death. *Diabetes, 59*(2), 471–478.

Welch, G. N., & Loscalzo, J. (1998). Homocysteine and atherothrombosis. *New England Journal of Medicine, 338*, 1042–1050.

Wolbink, G. J., et al. (1996). CRP-mediated activation of complement in vivo: Assessment by measuring circulating complement-C-reactive protein complexes. *Journal of Immunology, 157*, 473–479.

Woo, S. J., Lim, K., Park, S. Y., Jung, M. Y., Lim, H. S., Jeon, M. G., et al. (2015). Endogenous conversion of n-6 to n-3 polyunsaturated fatty acids attenuates K/BxN serum-transfer arthritis in fat-1 mice. *Journal of Nutritional Biochemistry, 26*(7), 713–720.

Yamano, T., Kubo, T., Shiono, Y., Shimamura, K., Orii, M., Tanimoto, T., et al. (2015). Impact of eicosapentaenoic acid treatment on the fibrous cap thickness in patients with coronary atherosclerotic plaque: an optical coherence tomography study. *Journal of Atherosclerosis and Thrombosis, 22*, 52–61.

Ye, P., Li, J., Wang, S., Xie, A., Sun, W., & Xia, J. (2012). Eicosapentaenoic acid disrupts the balance between Tregs and IL-17+ T cells through PPARgamma nuclear receptor activation and protects cardiac allografts. *Journal of Surgical Research, 173*(1), 161–170.

Zhao, Y., Joshi-Barve, S., Barve, S., & Chen, L. H. (2004). Eicosapentaenoic acid prevents LPS-induced TNF-alpha expression by preventing NF-kappaB activation. *Journal of the American College of Nutrition, 23*(1), 71–78.

CHAPTER 5

MICROALGAE AND THEIR USE AS NUTRACEUTICAL IN ARTHRITIS

PANKAJ KUMAR

Professor, Department of Pharmacology, Adesh Institute of Pharmacy and Biomedical Science, Adesh University, Bathinda, Punjab, India

ABSTRACT

This chapter discusses the importance of Microalgae as a Nutraceuticals in Arthritis. The phrase "nutraceuticals" refers to any product, regardless of its nature found in food sources that has additional advantages to one's health in addition to the fundamental amount of healthy food found in food. Some bioactive compounds found in Microalgae have nutritional value for health as well as medicinal importance for the treatment of Arthritis.

5.1 INTRODUCTION

Microalgae are also called microphytes. They are unicellular photosynthetic microorganisms that use the combination of carbon dioxide, water, and sunlight to produce biomass. They are invisible to the human eye and are mostly found in saline or freshwater environments. Microalgae are present in about 75% of algae species (Marcello Nicoletti, 2016). Microalgae are very important in arthritis treatment because they contain many bioactive substances used in arthritis treatment, such as lutein, algal extracts, polysaccharides, polyunsaturated fatty acids, chlorophyll, beta-carotene, phycobiliprotein, sterol, natural dyes, antioxidants, fatty acids, enzymes, polymers, peptides, fucoxanthin, and toxins like taxanthin (Joshi Nilesh Hemantkumar

& Mor Ilza Rahimbhai, 2019; Thurman, 1997). This is why microalgae are a valuable source of nutraceuticals. Recent discoveries suggest that brown algae are a source of a polysaccharide, which is a long-chain sugar molecule. This material, the polysaccharide alginate, is derived from the stems of brown algae, specifically cuvie (Latin: *Laminaria hyperborea*). It is similar to certain extracellular macromolecules found in cartilage. In cell culture studies, this 'alginate' that has been chemically modified reduces oxidative stress, has an anti-inflammatory effect, and inhibits the immune response to cartilage cells, helping combat the causes of arthritis (Anne Kerschenmeyer, 2017; EMPA, 2017).

Nutraceuticals derived from microalgae have been shown to offer anti-inflammatory qualities due to their ability to lower the expression of inflammatory genes and suppress the generation of cytokines that contribute to inflammation (Choo et al., 2020). Docosahexaenoic acid found in microalgae is used in the treatment of rheumatoid arthritis (Dawczynski, 2018).

Nutraceuticals are products that are classified under diet but are also used for medicinal purposes (Keservani et al., 2010a, b, 2017, 2020). Due to the fact that they are derived from foods and food components, they are sometimes referred to as bioceuticals (Vig & Deshmukh, 2022). In the year 2020, the size of the worldwide Nutraceuticals industry was estimated to be $413 billion. Current market research has suggested that the Nutraceutical market will expand worldwide and reach US $650 billion in the following years. The Indian market is expanding at a rate that is equivalent to 21% every single year. In developed countries, many factors, namely unhealthy lifestyles with poor eating habits, high incomes, and the growing number of older people in particular, have a responsibility to promote the growth of the Nutraceutical industry (Sangeeta, 2020).

5.2 ARTHRITIS

Arthritis is the most widespread joint disease, affecting approximately 90% of people over the age of 60 in different ways. Arthritis is characterized by pain, swelling, and stiffness of one or more joints due to inflammation, regardless of the causes. The areas where two bones come together to form a single structure are known as joints. The majority of kinds of arthritis are associated with joint discomfort and swelling. There are more than 100 different forms of arthritis, and each one has its specific therapy, progression, and prognosis. Osteoarthritis, rheumatoid arthritis, arthritis, and psoriatic arthritis are the most common forms of arthritis (Md. Nur Alam et al., 2014). But nowadays this disease is found a lot in the youth as well (Anne Kerschenmeyer, 2017; EMPA, 2017). Chronic inflammation can provide a path to the development of diseases like rheumatoid arthritis (Lee, 2021).

5.2.1 RISK FACTORS OF ARTHRITIS

1. **Age:** The risk of various types of arthritis like osteoarthritis, both rheumatoid arthritis and gout, increases as people get older.
2. **Previous Joint Injury:** Arthritis in a joint is more likely to occur among those who had previously damaged that joint, possibly while participating in a sport.
3. **Family History:** Different kinds of arthritis can be found in family members if their parents or siblings have a history of arthritis.
4. **Genetics:** Rheumatoid arthritis, systemic lupus erythematosus, and ankylosing spondylitis are some forms of arthritis that have been linked to particular genes, increasing the chance of developing the disease.
5. **Obesity:** When you carry around extra weight, your joints, particularly your knees, hips, and spine, bear the brunt of the strain. Individuals who are already obese have a greater likelihood of gaining additional weight.
6. **Sex:** Women have a higher risk of developing rheumatoid arthritis compared to males, although men make up the majority of those who suffer from gout.
7. **Smoking:** Scientists have discovered a link between smoking and arthritis. Smoking increases the risk of developing arthritis.
8. **Stress:** Some researchers believe that stress may be a cause of arthritis.

All the above factors are responsible for developing/causing Arthritis (www.arthritis.ca).

5.2.2 NUTRACEUTICALS IN ARTHRITIS

Nutraceuticals, also known as bioceuticals, are nutrients from food or food products that not only add to the diet but also help prevent or treat diseases and/or disorders. There are more than 470 nutritious and effective food products available for sale with researched health benefits (Bishop, 2012). Anti-inflammatory and antioxidant nutraceuticals may act as complementary medicine for the treatment of arthritis (Sahar Y. Al-Okbi, 2014). Nutraceuticals and herbal supplements (Sharma et al., 2020; Rane et al., 2020a, b, c) have long been used in traditional medicine, and there is ample evidence that nutraceuticals have the potential to play a significant role in the inflammation and destruction of osteoarthritis joints (Nahid Akhtar et al., 2012).

5.2.3 USE OF MICROALGAE IN THE TREATMENT OF ARTHRITIS

5.2.3.1 ARTHROSPIRA (SPIRULINA) PLATENSIS

Arthrospira is a multicellular filamentous, spiral-shaped blue-green microalgae (Mayada Ragab Farag, 2015). *Arthrospira* (Spirulina) platensis (SPI), also known as nutraceutical spirulina. *Spirulina platensis* is widely used as a source of bioactive compounds like carotenoids, protein, vitamins, minerals, polyunsaturated fatty acids, phycobiliprotein, lutein, β-carotene, astaxanthin, and chlorophyll (Izabela Michalak, 2020). Its protein content is about 60–70%. *Spirulina platensis* possesses antioxidative and anti-inflammatory biological activity, so it is used for the treatment of arthritis (Frontasyev, 2009; Farag, 2016). *Spirulina platensis* has promising protective efficacy against collagen-induced arthritis in rats due to its ability to elevate serum albumin and decrease serum cholesterol, alkaline phosphatase and acid phosphatase activities, and lipid peroxidation (Kumar et al., 2009).

5.2.3.2 PHAEODACTYLUM TRICONUTUM

Recent research has pointed to the microalgae *Phaeodactylum tricornutum* as a potentially important source of fucoxanthin. Fucoxanthin (Fx) is a type of carotenoid present in microalgae that has antioxidant, anti-cancer, anti-obesity, and anti-inflammatory qualities, among many other biological benefits. Fucoxanthin is a useful nutraceutical for relieving inflammation by inhibiting NF-κB activation (Lee, 2021). Macroalgae *Laminaria japonica* and *Undaria pinnatifida* are used for the large-scale production of fucoxanthin, but recently *Phaeodactylum tricornutum* has become a major source of fucoxanthin (Kajikawa, 2012).

5.2.3.3 SCHIZOCHYTRIUM SP.

Schizochytrium sp. Patients with rheumatoid arthritis were given an omega-3 supplement from *Shizochytrium* sp. that included docosahexaenoic acid (DHA) and eicosapentaenoic acid (EPA). This supplement targeted arachidonic acid (AA) pathways by competing with AA (an omega-6 PUFA) during the formation of eicosanoids. The DHA/EPA supplement decreased the number of swollen joints, and blood parameters demonstrated that the supplement decreased the AA:DHA/EPA ratio, which resulted in decreased blood serum levels of AA-derived lipid mediators and improved inflammation conditions (Dawczynski, 2017).

5.2.3.4 NANNOCHLOROPSIS OCULATE

Microalgae are responsible for producing a wide range of sterols, and the sterols derived from plants are known as phytosterols. According to Yasukawa et al.'s (1996) research, phytosterols that were isolated from microalgae were discovered to contain anti-inflammatory characteristics. RAW 264.7 cells were shown in research to be susceptible to having an anti-inflammatory impact when the extract from the microalgae *Nannochloropsis oculata* was applied to them (Choo, 2020).

5.2.3.5 CHLORELLA

The microalgae *Chlorella vulgaris* and *Arthrospira platensis* have been tested as nutraceuticals. *Arthrospira platensis* was found to be rich in saturated fatty acids (FA) and FA-rich monounsaturated *Chlorella vulgaris*. Within the polyunsaturated FA (PUFA), the content of n3 PUFA was less than 1% in *Arthrospira* sp. and more than 10% in *Chlorella vulgaris* (Joana Matos, 2020). Chlorella is an excellent source of many different nutrients, such as vitamins, minerals, antioxidants, and omega-3 fats. There is some evidence that the nutraceuticals included in chlorella, such as niacin, fiber, carotenoids, and antioxidants, can assist in lowering cholesterol levels. Consumption of the *C. variabilis* whole tablet revealed anti-inflammatory effects by effectively reducing TNF- and C-reactive protein concentrations in the blood serum of patients. This was demonstrated by the fact that the qualities were seen (Wan Afifudeen, 2022). In adults, moderately elevated C-reactive protein levels of 10.0–100.0 mg/L of blood, which signifies infection or an inflammatory condition such as rheumatoid arthritis (healthline.com). The role of commercially available lycopene (all-trans) from tomatoes in controlling arthritis has been reported. And it is also reported anti-arthritic effect of lycopene (cis and trans) extracted from the algae Chlorella marina (Renju, 2012; Michele Greque de Morais, 2015).

5.2.3.6 DUNALIELLA SALINA

The green algae *Dunaliella salina* is known for its production of carotenoids. Carotenoids have the potential to play an essential role in the maintenance and improvement of health and in preventing human diseases like rheumatoid arthritis (Farouk K. El-Baz, 2021).

5.2.3.7 HAEMATOCOCCUS PLUVIALIS

Haematococcus pluvialis is a type of microalga that is characterized by the ability to accumulate important concentrations of astaxanthin (Macias-Sánchez, 2021). The green microalga *Haematococcus pluvialis* is considered to be the richest source of astaxanthin. It is well known that astaxanthin is the most powerful carotenoid pigment on the entire planet in the category of nutraceuticals. Astaxanthin (3,3'-dihydroxy-β,β'-carotene-4,4'-ketone) is one of the common nutraceuticals belonging to the group of xanthophylls (Amit H. Batghare, 2021). According to preliminary studies, because of its antioxidant and membrane preservation properties, astaxanthin may be beneficial in relieving pain as well as helping people suffering from rheumatoid arthritis to carry out regular tasks. In addition to strengthening our immune system, astaxanthin can also help reduce inflammation. In particular, this pigment works in the form of active oxygen to reduce the amount of protein that can cause inflammatory diseases such as rheumatoid arthritis, heart disease, celiac disease, and diabetes (www.webmd.com).

5.2.3.8 ODONTELLA AURITA

The marine diatom *Odontella aurita* is the only microalga that is a rich source of EPA (26% of the total fatty acids). Lutein and β-cryptoxanthin may reduce the factors involved in inflammation associated with osteoarthritis and arthritis.

5.3 CONCLUSION

This is strong evidence that certain bioactive compounds obtained from microalgae are safe and effective as nutraceuticals in the treatment of arthritis.

KEYWORDS

- anti-inflammatory
- arachidonic acid
- arthritis
- bioactive compound
- docosahexaenoic acid
- eicosapentaenoic acid
- microalgae
- nutraceuticals
- Spirulina platensis

REFERENCES

Afifudeen, W. C. L., Teh, K. Y., & Cha, T. S. (2022). Bioprospecting of microalgae metabolites against cytokine storm syndrome during COVID-19. *Molecular Biology Reports, 49*, 1475–1490.

Akhtar, N., & Haqqi, T. M. (2012). Current nutraceuticals in the management of osteoarthritis: A review. *Therapeutic Advances in Musculoskeletal Disease, 4*(3), 181–207. https://doi.org/10.1177/1759720X11436238.

Alam, M. N., Rahman, M. M., & Khalil, M. I. (2014). Nutraceuticals in arthritis management: A contemporary prospect of dietary phytochemicals. *The Open Nutraceuticals Journal, 7*, 21–27.

Al-Okbi, S. Y. (2014). Nutraceuticals of anti-inflammatory activity as a complementary therapy for rheumatoid arthritis. *Toxicology and Industrial Health, 30*(8), 738–749. https://doi.org/10.1177/0748233712462468.

Batghare, A. H., & Moholkar, V. S. (2021). Production of nutraceutical astaxanthin from waste resources. In *Waste Biorefinery* (pp. 181–205), Elsevier.

Bishop, W. M., & Zubeck, H. M. (2012). Evaluation of Microalgae for use as Nutraceuticals and Nutritional Supplements. *Journal of Nutrition & Food Sciences, 2*, 147. https://doi.org/10.4172/2155-9600.1000147.

Choo, W. T., Teoh, M. L., Phang, S. M., Convey, P., Yap, W. H., Goh, B. H., & Beardall, J. (2020). Microalgae as Potential Anti-Inflammatory Natural Product Against Human Inflammatory Skin Diseases. *Frontiers in Pharmacology, 11*, 1086. https://doi.org/10.3389/fphar.2020.01086.

Dawczynski, C., Dittrich, M., Neumann, T., Goetze, K., Welzel, A., Oelzner, P., Völker, S., Schaible, A. M., Troisi, F., Thomas, L., Pace, S., Koeberle, A., Werz, O., Schlattmann, P., Lorkowski, S., & Jahreis, G. (2018). Docosahexaenoic acid in the treatment of rheumatoid arthritis: a double-blind, placebo-controlled, randomized cross-over study with microalgae vs. sunflower oil. *Clinical Nutrition, 37*, 494–504. https://doi.org/10.1016/j.clnu.2017.02.021.

El-Baz, F. K., Aly, H. F., & Abd-All, H. I. (2020). The ameliorating effect of carotenoid-rich fraction extracted from *Dunaliella salina* microalga against inflammation-associated cardiac dysfunction in obese rats. *Toxicology Reports, 7*, 118–124.

Farag, M. R., Alagawany, M., Abd El-Hack, M. E., & Dhama, K. (2016). Nutritional and healthical aspects of *Spirulina* (*Arthrospira*) for poultry, animals, and humans. *International Journal of Pharmacology, 12*(1), 36–51.

Frontasyeva, M. F., Pavlov, S. S., Aksenova, N. G., Mosulishvili, L. M., Belokobylskii, A. I., Kirkesali, E. I., Ginturi, E. N., & Kuchava, N. E. (2009). Chromium interaction with blue-green microalga *Spirulina platensis*. *Journal of Analytical Chemistry, 64*(7), 746–749.

Joshi, N. H., & Mor, I. R. (2019). Microalgae and its use in nutraceuticals and food supplements. *Microalgae – From Physiology to Application, 1*, 1–11.

Kajikawa, T., et al. (2012). Stereocontrolled total synthesis of fucoxanthin and its polyene chain-modified derivative. *Organic Letters, 14*, 808–811. https://doi.org/10.1021/ol203344c.

Kerschenmeyer, A., Arlov, Ø., Malheiro, V., Steinwachs, M., Rottmar, M., Maniura-Weber, K., Palazzolo, G., & Zenobi-Wong, M. (2017). Anti-oxidant and immune-modulatory properties of sulfated alginate derivatives on human chondrocytes and macrophages. *Biomaterials Science, 5*(9), 1756. https://doi.org/10.1039/c7bm00341b.

Keservani, R. K., Kesharwani, R. K., Sharma, A. K., Vyas, N., & Chadoker, A. (2010b). Nutritional Supplements: An Overview. *International Journal of Current Pharmaceutical Review and Research, 1*(1), 59–75.

Keservani, R. K., Kesharwani, R. K., Vyas, N., Jain, S., Raghuvanshi, R., & Sharma, A. K. (2010a). Nutraceutical and functional food as future food: A review. *Der Pharmacia Lettre, 2*(1), 106–116.

Keservani, R. K., Sharma, A. K., & Kesharwani, R. K. (2017). An overview and therapeutic applications of nutraceutical and functional foods. In *Recent Advances in Drug Delivery Technology* (pp. 160–201). ISBN: 9781522507543.

Keservani, R. K., Sharma, A. K., & Kesharwani, R. K. (Eds.). (2020). *Nutraceuticals and Dietary Supplements: Applications in Health Improvement and Disease Management*, Apple Academic Press, CRC Press. pp. 1–344. ISBN: 9781771888738.

Kumar, N., Singh, S., Patro, N., & Patro, I. (2009). Evaluation of protective efficacy of *Spirulina platensis* against collagen-induced arthritis in rats. *Inflammopharmacology, 17*, 181–190. https://doi.org/10.1007/s10787-009-0004-1.

Lee, A. H., Shin, H. Y., Park, J. H., et al. (2021). Fucoxanthin from microalgae *Phaeodactylum tricornutum* inhibits pro-inflammatory cytokines by regulating both NF-κB and NLRP3 inflammasome activation. *Scientific Reports, 11*, 543. https://doi.org/10.1038/s41598-020-80748-6.

Macias-Sánchez, M. D. (2021). High-pressure extraction of astaxanthin from *Haematococcus pluvialis*. In *Global Perspectives on Astaxanthin*, pp. 355–373, Academic Press.

Matos, J., Cardoso, C. L., Falé, P., Afonso, C. M., & Bandarra, N. M. (2020). Investigation of nutraceutical potential of the microalgae *Chlorella vulgaris* and *Arthrospira platensis*. *Institute of Food Science and Technology, 55*(1), 303–312.

Michalak, I., Mironiuk, M., Godlewska, K., Trynda, J., & Marycz, K. (2020). *Arthrospira (Spirulina) platensis*: An effective biosorbent for nutrients. *Process Biochemistry, 88,* 129–137. https://doi.org/10.1016/j.procbio.2019.10.004.

Mohanty, S., Pal, A., & Si, S. C. (2020). Flavonoid as nutraceuticals: A therapeutic approach to rheumatoid arthritis. *Research Journal of Pharmacy and Technology, 13*(2), 991–998. https://doi.org/10.5958/0974-360X.2020.00184.5.

Morais, M. G. de, da Silva Vaz, B., de Morais, E. G., & Costa, J. A. V. (2015). Biologically active metabolites synthesized by microalgae. *BioMed Research International, 2015,* Article ID 835761, 15 pages. https://doi.org/10.1155/2015/835761.

Nicoletti, M. (2016). Microalgae Nutraceuticals. *Foods, 5*(3), 16. https://doi.org/10.3390/foods5030054.

Rane, B. R., Bharath, M. S., Patil, R. R., Keservani, R. K., & Jain, A. S. (2020b). Novel approaches in nutraceuticals. In R. K. Kesharwani, R. K. Keservani, & A. K. Sharma (Eds.), *Enhancing the Therapeutic Efficacy of Herbal Formulations Through Novel Drug Delivery Systems* (pp. 241–266). IGI Global International Publisher. ISBN: 9781799844532.

Rane, B. R., Patil, A. S., Keservani, R. K., & Jain, A. S. (2020a). Novel approaches in herbal formulation. In R. K. Kesharwani, R. K. Keservani, & A. K. Sharma (Eds.), *Enhancing the Therapeutic Efficacy of Herbal Formulations Through Novel Drug Delivery Systems* (pp. 43–68). IGI Global International Publisher. ISBN: 9781799844532.

Rane, B. R., Tadavi, S. A., & Keservani, R. K. (2020c). Naturopathy. In A. K. Sharma, R. K. Keservani, & S. P. Gautam (Eds.), *Herbal Product Development* (pp. 321–347). Apple Academic Press, CRC Press, Taylor & Francis Group. ISBN: 9781771888776.

Renju, G. L., Kurup, G. M., & Kumari, C. H. S. (2013). Anti-inflammatory activity of lycopene isolated from *Chlorella marina* on Type II Collagen-induced arthritis in Sprague Dawley rats. *Immunopharmacology and Immunotoxicology, 35*(2), 282–291.

Sharma, A. K., Keservani, R. K., & Gautam, S. P. (2020). *Herbal Product Development*. Apple Academic Press, CRC Press, Taylor & Francis Group. ISBN: 9781771888776.

Swiss Federal Laboratories for Materials Science and Technology (EMPA). (2017). Treating arthritis with algae: A new weapon in the fight against arthritis? *Science Daily*. Retrieved from: www.sciencedaily.com/releases/2017/08/170823094110.htm (accessed on 6 June 2024).

Thurman, H. V. (1997). *Introductory Oceanography*. Prentice Hall College. ISBN: 978-0-13-262072-7.

Vig, H., & Deshmukh, R. (2022). Nutraceuticals market by type, form, and sales channel: Global opportunity analysis and industry forecast, 2021–2030. *Nutraceuticals Market*, pp. 325. Retrieved from: https://www.alliedmarketresearch.com/nutraceuticals-market (accessed on 6 June 2024).

Yasukawa, K., Akihisa, T., Kanno, H., Kaminaga, T., Izumida, M., Sakoh, T., et al. (1996). Inhibitory effects of sterols isolated from *Chlorella vulgaris* on 12-O-tetradecanoylphorbol-13-acetate-induced inflammation and tumor promotion in mouse skin. *Biological & Pharmaceutical Bulletin, 19*(4), 573–576. https://doi.org/10.1248/bpb.19.573.

CHAPTER 6

MODERN NUTRACEUTICALS FOR TREATMENT OF OSTEOARTHRITIS

BUI THANH TUNG, TRAN VIET LINH, NGUYEN THUY NGOC, TRINH PHUONG THAO, and NGUYEN DUC THUAN

VNU University of Medicine and Pharmacy, Vietnam National University, Ha Noi, Vietnam

ABSTRACT

Osteoarthritis (OA) is a degenerative joint disease that significantly impacts joint function and quality of life. Nutraceuticals derived from herbs have a long history in traditional medicine, and there is evidence suggesting their potential role in managing OA joint issues. Consequently, healthcare providers are more inclined to suggest preventive measures to slow down and control the progression of pathological conditions. Some medicinal plants, such as *Angelica sinensis, Boswellia serrata, Commiphora mukul,* and *Eucommia ulmoides*, are recognized for their beneficial biological effects and are commonly used in OA treatment. In this review, we aim to understand the main molecular targets involved in joint issues and inflammation, along with the safety, effectiveness, and potential toxicities of nutraceuticals for managing OA. We will summarize various studies demonstrating the use of nutraceuticals to alleviate symptoms in OA patients and as a complementary therapy for OA management. The results indicate that incorporating nutraceuticals in osteoarthritis treatment yields positive outcomes and paves the way for future research.

Nutraceuticals in Arthritis and Psoriasis: Management and Prevention of Diseases.
Meenakshi Jaiswal, Raj K. Keservani, Rajesh K. Kesharwani, and Swati G. Talele (Eds.)
© 2025 Apple Academic Press, Inc. Co-published with CRC Press (Taylor & Francis)

6.1 INTRODUCTION

Osteoarthritis (OA) is the most prevalent chronic variety of arthritis. Additionally, it is also called degenerative joint disease or "wear and tear" arthritis (Adatia et al., 2012). It represents a complex musculoskeletal disorder with multiple genetic, constitutional, and biomechanical risk factors (Chen et al., 2012). Any joint can be plagued by osteoarthritis, but the condition most frequently causes problems in the knees, hips, and small joints of the hands, and it often appears in the elderly (Loeser et al., 2012). Osteoarthritis occurs when the cartilage that cushions the ends of bones in your joints gradually deteriorates and wears down. Compared to the normal joint, an OA joint exhibits different clinical and biochemical phenotypes, including narrowed joint space, degrees of synovial inflammation, thickened fibrotic ligaments, hypertrophy of the joint capsule in the knee, and damaged menisci. In particular, the number of chondrocytes within cartilage decreases because of increased apoptosis, creating a detrimental environment within the joint (He et al., 2020). The severity of osteoarthritis symptoms can vary greatly from person to person, and between different affected joints. Its prominent feature is the progressive destruction of articular cartilage which ends up in impaired joint motion, inflammation of synovium, and resorption of the underlying subchondral bone (Kamble et al., 2021). OA causes severe pain, stiffness, swelling, and even reduced function and disability in some serious cases (Adatia et al., 2012). The symptoms of OA are joint pain, stiffness in the joint, loss of flexibility and reduced range of motion, hurt when pressing on joints, and inflammation... they often happen when moving and activating. Some people often confuse between osteoarthritis (OA) and rheumatoid arthritis (RA). They share identical symptoms but are very different conditions (Neogi, 2013). OA is a degenerative condition, which suggests that it increases in severity over time but RA, on the opposite hand, is an autoimmune disorder (Hunter et al., 2008). Currently, an extremely high rate of OA on the globe poses an enormous public health problem, the disease burden is typically measured in direct and indirect costs, and also in less well-defined intangible costs like pain and reduction of quality of life (Hunter et al., 2014). Osteoarthritis can't be reversed, but a lot of treatments can reduce pain and help to move better such as using medications such as nonsteroidal anti-inflammatory drugs (NSAIDs), functional foods, physiotherapy, exercise, surgical and other procedures. However, when symptoms of OA and inflammation are protracted, the regular use of conventional treatment invariably causes deleterious effects, which with time may negate the beneficial effects, especially the use of the medicine. The prolonged use of NSAIDs might have unwanted effects such as an increased risk of gastrointestinal bleeding, hypertension, congestive heart failure, and renal insufficiency (Saad & Mathew, 2021). Additionally, investigational agents in drugs like the anti-TNF-α when used on a prolonged basis are known to increase the risk of infections and malignancies (Barrera et al., 2002). Besides using drugs, we can have a balanced diet or use supportive foods like "nutraceuticals" and functional foods to reduce OA symptoms. Diet is also important for OA treatment and prevention; some nutritional supplements like glucosamine, chondroitin, and omega-3 fatty acids, for example, might help slow joint damage and improve function.

Nutraceuticals, a term coined by DeFelice in 1989 combining the words 'nutrition' and 'pharmaceutical,' are used to describe any product derived from food sources with additional health benefits beyond the essential nutritional value found in foods. Nutraceutical products can be considered non-specific biological therapies used to promote general health, control symptoms, and prevent the development of diseases. Hippocrates said, "Let food be your medicine and medicine be your food," to emphasize the link between food for health and their specific therapeutic benefits (Witkamp & Norren, 2018). Nutraceuticals are divided into four categories that include dietary supplements, functional food, medicinal food, and pharmaceuticals. In some cases, nutraceuticals are referred to as "functional foods." The main ingredients of nutraceuticals include substances with established nutritional functions, such as vitamins, minerals, amino acids, and fatty acids; nutrients; medicinal plants or botanical products as concentrates or herbal extracts; reagents derived from other sources (Asif & Mohd, 2019). When food is being cooked or prepared using "scientific intelligence" with or without the knowledge of how or why it's being used, then the food is named "functional food." When functional food aids in the prevention and/or treatment of diseases or disorders aside from deficiency conditions like anemia, it is called a "nutraceutical" (Jeffrey K Aronson, 2017). Over the past several years, nutraceuticals have attracted interest because of their potential nutritional, safety, and therapeutic effects (Keservani et al., 2010a, b, 2017, 2020; Goswami et al., 2019). These products could have a role in a plethora of biological processes, including antioxidant defenses, cell proliferation, gene expression, and the safeguarding of mitochondrial integrity (Adetuyi et al., 2022). Nutraceuticals only have limited effects on their biological target and significant differences may be reached over time through a buildup effect during which daily benefits add up, and therefore the time window for intervention is longer in chronic diseases. On the other hand, nutraceuticals could provide a safer alternative because their use is mostly void of adverse effects, although this is not universal (Jeffrey K Aronson, 2017).

Therefore, nutraceuticals may improve health, prevent chronic diseases, postpone the aging process, and successively increase anticipation, or simply support the functions and integrity of the body. Especially, these products have a huge advantage in supporting the prevention of life-threatening diseases or disease progression like OA. Today, many people select to use nutraceuticals as a product to prevent or support the treatment of OA. In this chapter, we are discussing the scientific evidence supporting the efficacy of medicinal plants delivered nutraceuticals such as to summarize their efficacies for OA management.

6.2 MEDICINAL PLANTS FOR TREATMENT OF OSTEOARTHRITIS

For centuries, medicinal plants have been widely used in traditional medicine to treat OA and other chronic diseases, especially in Asia, due to their antioxidant, anti-inflammatory, anti-nociceptive, and immunoregulatory effects (Ansaripour & Dehghan, 2020). In fact, analgesics such as NSAIDs and corticosteroids are commonly used to manage osteoarthritis, but they only alleviate the symptoms without affecting the progression and pathophysiology of osteoarthritis (D'Adamo et al., 2020). Furthermore, NSAIDs have shown many side effects on various organs in long-term treatment, so an alternative approach with fewer side effects, such as treatment with medicinal plants, has been considered (Oppedisano et al., 2021). Below, we will summarize some promising medicinal plant candidates, such as *Angelica sinensis, Boswellia serrata,* and *Eucommia ulmoides*, which have shown efficient results in osteoarthritis treatment.

6.2.1 ANGELICA SINENSIS

Angelica sinensis is one of the most commonly used traditional Chinese medicine (TCM) for the treatment of osteoarthritis(Yang et al., 2019). Chondrocyte apoptosis is important in the progression of osteoarthritis. Traditional Chinese medicine *Angelica sinensis* polysaccharide (ASP) has anti-inflammatory and anti-apoptotic properties in chondrocytes. The previous study showed that ASP significantly reduced sodium nitroprusside (SNP)-induced apoptosis in chondrocytes by activating ERK1/2-dependent autophagy, making ASP a potential therapeutic supplement for OA treatment (Xu et al., 2021). ASP has a wide range of pharmacological effects, including promoting immunity, antitumor, anti-inflammatory, antioxidant, anti-aging, anti-virus, liver protection, and so on. As a natural polysaccharide, ASP has the potential to be used as a drug carrier (Nai et al., 2021). Another study demonstrated that the effects of ASP could reduce oxidative stress in human osteoarthritis chondrocytes. Oxidative stress plays a role in the pathogenesis of osteoarthritis, and ASP protects human chondrocytes from H_2O_2-mediated injury (Zhuang et al., 2018). Moreover, ASP may act as a promising osteoarthritis treatment because it reduces IL-1-induced chondrocyte inflammation and ECM degradation by inhibiting NF-κB activation via the PI3K/AKT pathway (Li et al., 2018).

6.2.2 BOSWELLIA SERRATA

Boswellia serrata (Salai/Salai guggul), is a tree derived from dry mountainous regions of India, Africa, and therefore the Arabian Peninsula, which belongs to the family of *Burseraceae* (Ramesh, 2016). It is commonly used as an herbal remedy in the ancient traditional Indian medicine system (Ayurveda) for the treatment of chronic inflammatory diseases like OA, bronchitis, asthma, and chronic inflammatory bowel diseases (Siddiqui, 2011). *Boswellia serrata* contains chemicals that may reduce swelling and enhance the body's response. Extracts of *Boswellia serrata* such as sap, bark, and other plant parts are taken for therapeutic purposes (Kimmatkar et al., 2003). These extracts contain resin, amino acids, phenols, terpenes, polysaccharides, and β-boswellic acid, which are the most important active anti-inflammatory components. Recently, *Boswellia serrata* is more commonly used in the treatment of osteoarthritis. The potent anti-inflammatory, anti-arthritic, and analgesic activities of the natural resin extract from *Boswellia serrata* are being studied and developed. It is also known as "Indian frankincense" (Abdel-Tawab et al., 2011). The natural resin of *Boswellia serrata* contains monoterpenes, diterpenes, triterpenes, tetracyclic triterpene acids, and pentacyclic triterpene acids, called boswellic acid (Siddiqui, 2011). Boswellic acids are potent anti-inflammatory agents and are specific non-redox inhibitors of 5-Lipoxygenase (5-LOX), which help to preserve the structural integrity of joint cartilage, maintain a healthy immune mediator cascade at a cellular level, and against pain and inflammation by inhibiting leukotriene synthesis (Alluri et al., 2020; Kimmatkar et al., 2003). Clinical studies have shown that *Boswellia serrata* extract not only has anti-inflammatory and anti-arthritis properties but also improves pain and physical function (Yu et al., 2020). A limited number of clinical studies were performed to assess the efficacy, safety, and tolerability of *Boswellia serrata* extract for osteoarthritis and joint function, particularly beneficial effects for osteoarthritis of the knee, including research in eight weeks (Gupta et al., 2011). All patients receiving *Boswellia serrata* extract (BSE) treatment reported a decrease in knee pain, increased knee flexion, and increased walking distance, and therefore the frequency of swelling within the articulatio genus was decreased (Kimmatkar et al., 2003). The anti-inflammatory activity of *Boswellia serrata* resin improves radiological findings like joint space, subarticular sclerosis, synovial effusion, articular erosion, and osteophytes. It soothes the joints and also helps treat levels of synovia, making the whole structure lubricated and simple to rotate or maneuver. It helps preserve the structural integrity of the joint cartilage and maintains a healthy immune mediator cascade at a cellular level (Gupta et al., 2011). The test demonstrated the protection and efficacy of Boswellin®, oral supplementation of BSE containing 30% AKBBA, and other bioactive β-boswellic acids, namely, BBA, KBBA, and ABBA, in newly diagnosed or untreated patients with osteoarthritis of the knee (Majeed et al., 2019). Additionally, another study presents the anti-osteoarthritis efficacy of Serratrin®, a singular composition containing the acidic and nonacidic fractions of *Boswellia serrata* natural resin. It strongly inhibited 5-LOX activity, leukotriene B4, and prostaglandin E2 productions in human blood-derived cells. Also, it reduced TNF-α production and has pain relief efficacy in a rodent model. *Boswellia serrata* natural resin would be a unique candidate for managing pain with a further good thing about cartilage protection in progressive osteoarthritis in humans (Alluri et al., 2020). Overall, using *Boswellia serrata* as a nutraceutical could even be beneficial in developing adjunct preventive and/or therapeutic approaches to the prevention and treatment of osteoarthritis. However, clinical trials showing the advantage of *Boswellia serrata* extract on inflammation and osteoarthritis are continuously researched.

6.2.3 COMMIPHORA MUKUL

Commiphora mukul (Guggul) which belongs to the family of *Burseraceae* is found from northern Africa to central Asia but is most common in northern India (Arora et al., 2013). It is used as a herbal in the ancient traditional

Indian medicine system (Ayurveda) for the treatment of lipid disorders, acne vulgaris, osteoarthritis, obesity, and cancer (Lee et al., 2020). The oleo-gum resin of *Commiphora mukul*, which is a yellowish substance, is found in the balsam canals in the phloem of the large veins of the leaf and the base of the stem (Kunnumakkara et al., 2018). It is a complicated mixture of minerals, terpenes, flavanones, lignans, sterols (guggulsterol-I, -II, -III, -IV, -V), sterones (Z-, E-, M-guggulsterone, and dehydroguggulsterone-M), and essential oils (Kunnumakkara et al., 2018). Phenolics, which are common natural products found in guggul trees, such as hydroxybenzoic acid derivatives (gallic acid, gentisic acid, ellagic acid) and cinnamic acid derivatives (caffeic acid, chlorogenic acid, ferulic acid), possess substantial antioxidant and anti-inflammatory effects (Hazra et al., 2018). In particular, guggulsterone is an important biologically active compound of *Commiphora mukul*. It has been shown to inhibit NF-kB activation and downregulate the expression of inflammatory gene products like COX-2 and MMP-9, which are major players in the development of arthritis (Arora et al., 2013). A study of the effects of *Commiphora mukul* resin on the knee articular cartilage of rats showed to be effective in improving histopathological damage and highlighted its chondroprotective effect *in vivo* (Hadipour-Jahromy et al., 2009). The effect in ameliorating the histopathological lesions was emphasized, and a protective *in vivo* chondroprotective effect was noted (Hadipour-Jahromy et al., 2009). In a clinical trial, *Commiphora mukul* has reduced pain and stiffness, relieving symptoms of osteoarthritis after one month of treatment, and showed further improvement in long-term use in 36 patients with moderate to severe arthritis. After treatment, no side effects were reported during the trial (Ragavi & Surendran, 2018). *Commiphora mukul* appears to be a relatively safe and effective supplement to reduce symptoms of osteoarthritis (Singh et al., 2003).

6.2.4 DIPSACUS ASPER

Dipsacus asper, also called "Xu-duan" in Chinese, is a perennial herb in the Caprifoliaceae family. The Korean Medicine Classification of Efficacy describes *Dipsacus asperoides* as a tonifying and replenishing medicine or a yang-tonifying medicine that is traditionally used as an analgesic and anti-inflammatory agent to treat pain, rheumatoid arthritis, and bone fractures (Gong et al., 2019). Research on traditional Chinese medicine shows that "Xu-duan" ranks second in the list of most commonly used

Chinese single herbs for treating OA (Chen et al., 2014). Since the end of the 1990s, scientists have found anti-inflammatory and anticomplementary qualities in saponins extracted from *Dipsacus asper* root (Hung et al., 2005). It contains many chemical compounds such as iridoid glycosides, triterpenoid saponins, alkaloids, and phenolic compounds, along with a range of biological activities such as anti-inflammatory, antioxidant, anti-complementary, apoptosis-inducing, cytotoxic, inhibition of Aβ-induced cytotoxicity, antinociceptive, cardioprotective, and osteoprotective effects (Li et al., 2020). Akebia saponin D, identified as the main active ingredient of DAE, displays anti-inflammatory and antinociceptive actions in several cellular and animal models (Gong et al., 2019; Shin et al., 2019). Loganin, a popular iridoid glycoside present, decreased cartilage degeneration by attenuating IL-1β-induced apoptosis and restoring the function of rat chondrocytes via regulation of Phosphatidylinositol 3-Kinases (PI3K/Akt) signaling (Yang et al., 2019). *Dipsacus asper* extract was demonstrated to have an anti-inflammatory effect on Collagen-induced arthritis in mice by inactivating the production of anti-CIIIgG2a antibodies and inhibiting the levels of inflammatory mediators and bone destruction (Jung et al., 2012). A study using a rat model of monosodium iodoacetate (MIA)-induced osteoarthritis was held to investigate the effect of DAE via RNA-Seq analysis. The results showed that DAE worked effectively with the rats, it reduced the knee joint diameter well and generally improved the structural and histological features of the knee joint (Chun et al., 2021). In conclusion, *Dipsacus asper* may have therapeutic potential for treating osteoarthritis. There are more and more studies demonstrating the effect of DAE on OA treatment and its pharmacological activities. Yet, they are still insufficient and lack clinical evidence; therefore, more studies are needed, either for theories or clinical trials.

6.2.5 *EUCOMMIA ULMOIDES*

Eucommia ulmoides (EU) is a native rubber tree and a valuable tonic Chinese medicine in China with an extended history, it's also employed in other Asian countries. EU is often called "Du Zhong" and belongs to the family of *Eucommiaceae* (Lee et al., 2005). Almost all parts of the EU like the leaves, stem, bark, and even the staminate flowers are used as medicinal remedies. However, only the bark has been used as medicine and other parts of it cannot be fully utilized. They found about 112 bioactive chemical compounds isolated from the EU, which include lignans, iridoids, phenolics, steroids, and other compounds. In traditional Chinese medicine, EU is employed to supplement the liver and kidneys; strengthen tendons and bones; prevent miscarriage; and support the treatment of impotence, spermatorrhea, forgetfulness, osteoporosis, menopause syndrome, hypertension, etc. (Hussain et al., 2016).

EU has been used as a pain remedy, and the bark of it has been used as a treatment for osteoarthritis (Lu et al., 2013). It is the most frequently prescribed herb, and Duhuo Jisheng decoction is the most typically prescribed Chinese formula for osteoarthritis (Chen et al., 2014). A study provides evidence on the anti-osteoarthritis effects of EU extract and finds that EU may prevent the progression of osteoarthritis by reducing pro-inflammatory cytokines and metalloproteinases (MMPs) production and inhibiting the PI3K/Akt signaling pathway, but it still has plenty of restrictions. These findings suggest that the EU could also be a good ancillary agent for the prevention and therapy of osteoarthritis (Xie et al., 2015). EU can protect against cartilage effect in rats with osteoarthritis, potentially by improving cartilage metabolism, inhibiting apoptosis in chondrocytes, and regulating the degradation of the extracellular matrix of the articular cartilage, thus slowing down joint degeneration. Additionally, they demonstrated EU extract inhibited bone loss and maintained metabolic balance (Lu et al., 2013). Recently, the consequences and mechanisms of Cortex Eucommiae (CE) extract on OA were studied *in vitro*, and these studies showed that CE extracts inhibited inflammatory mediators like inducible nitric oxide synthase (iNOS), COX-2, TNF-α, and interleukin-1β (IL-1β) (Ahn et al., 2019). *In vivo* studies have identified the collagen synthesis-promoting and cartilage-protective effects of CE extract with the underlying mechanisms responsible (Li et al., 2000). Another study deeply analyzed the consequences and possible mechanisms of EUP within the treatment of osteoarthritis. The qPCR assay indicated that EUP significantly inhibited the expression of macrophage inflammation-related genes IL-6, IL-18, IL-1β and promoted the expression of osteogenesis and chondrogenesis-related genes BMP-6, Arg-1, and TGF-β. These detections found that the cartilage regeneration was significantly improved, and micro-CT scanning found that EU polysaccharides were beneficial to subchondral bone reconstruction (Sun et al., 2021). Those studies could investigate the efficacy and safety of EU as a treatment for mild osteoarthritis and also the results of the study will function as a foundation for the development of *Eucommia ulmoides* as a dietary supplement.

6.2.6 PUNICA GRANATUM

Punica granatum L. (pomegranate), one of the oldest known edible fruits, is now widely consumed around the world (Wang et al., 2018). The seed, peel, juice, and leaves of the pomegranate are all high in potential bioactive compounds (Eghbali et al., 2021). The role of this fruit in the prevention and treatment of various malignant pathologies has long been cited in both scientific and non-scientific literature, so it's crucial to figure out how it plays a role in pathophysiological processes (Moga et al., 2021). Pomegranate has been shown to improve clinical features and reduce inflammatory, oxidative stress, and apoptosis markers in osteoarthritis in human, animal, and *in vitro* studies (Mahdavi & Javadivala, 2021). This study is to compare the prophylactic mechanisms of *Punica granatum* L. peel (PGP) to indomethacin in collagenase-induced osteoarthritis rats. The results showed that PGP reduced collagenase-induced osteoarthritis when compared to the indomethacin-treated group by lowering blood ALP ($P < 0.001$) and significantly inhibiting cartilage erosion as seen in histological slides with collagen and proteoglycan content retention (Shivnath et al., 2021). Determine whether isolated rosmarinic acid from the rind of *Punica granatum* has anti-arthritic properties. According to the findings of this study, rosmarinic acid has significant anti-arthritic potential in Wistar rats with FCA-induced arthritis. This study demonstrated the therapeutic role of *Punica granatum* rosmarinic acid in the management of arthritis/rheumatoid arthritis/osteoarthritis and related inflammatory complications with minimal side effects, which was still far from complete mitigation with currently available conventional medicines (Gautam et al., 2019). The effects of pomegranate peel extract (PPE) supplementation on the serum lipid profile and antioxidant status in obese women with knee osteoarthritis are being investigated. Short-term PPE supplementation had beneficial effects on serum total cholesterol and triglyceride levels, as well as antioxidant status, in obese women with knee OA, according to the findings (Haghighian et al., 2021). POMx (70% acetone extract of punicalagin peels) significantly reduced IL-1-induced inducible nitric oxide synthase, cyclooxygenase-2, and matrix metalloproteinase-13 protein expression in primary rat chondrocytes, according to this study (PRCs). Punicalagin can be used as an active ingredient in POMx-based functional foods for knee-related diseases (Lee et al., 2018).

6.2.7 ROSA CANINA

Rosa canina is a well-known herb that has been used extensively in folk medicine. Rosehip, derived from dried *Rosa canina* fruits, was produced by Hyben Vital in Langeland, Denmark (Schwager et al., 2011). The rose is usually considered a symbol of love, beauty, war, religion, and politics. However, there is another side to the rose – as a medicinal plant. Rosehip is famous for its anti-inflammatory and antioxidant effects, especially in patients suffering from osteoarthritis. A clinical study in Germany in 2001 reported that physical symptoms in OA patients improved under rosehip treatment (Cutler, 2003). A wide range of potentially bioactive compounds have been identified in the rose extract. High levels of antioxidants, many polyphenols, and carotenoids, as well as vitamins, especially Vitamin C, have been found (Nybom & Werlemark, 2017). Over the past two decades, the pharmacological effects of *Rosa canina* have been demonstrated by numerous publications. Neutralization of reactive oxygen and nitrogen species (RONS) by antioxidative compounds, together with the reduction of OA-specific inflammatory processes including the reduction of pro-inflammatory cytokines and chemokines, NF-kB signaling, and inhibition of pro-inflammatory enzymes (COX1/2, 5-LOX, and iNOS) results in the inhibition of osteoarthritis. In addition, rosehip is responsible for reducing C-reactive protein levels, reducing chemotaxis and chemiluminescence of PMNs, and also inhibiting pro-inflammatory metalloproteases (Gruenwald et al., 2019). Several studies pointed out that in osteoarthritis joints, pro-inflammatory cytokines and anti-inflammatory cytokines such as IL-1, IFN-γ, IL-6, IL-7, IL-10, and TNF-α were increased (Chen et al., 2014). *In vitro*, rosehip preparations have been found to inhibit the expression of iNOS, IL-1α, and MMP-9, and IL-1β-induced ADAMTS-4, MMP-1, MMP-13, IL-1α, and IL-8 in chondrocytes by the specific galactolipid constituent (Mobasheri, 2012). Moreover, rosehip powder (RHP) and its constituent galactolipid, GLGPG (galactolipid (2S)-1,2-di-O-[(9Z,12Z,15Z)-octadeca-9,12,15-trienoyl]-3-O-β-d-galactopyranosyl glycerol) diminished the production of 2 biomarkers: NO and PGE2, which are both able to activate chondrocyte apoptosis. As a result, RHP and its constituents down-regulate catabolic processes and reduce chemotaxis related to osteoarthritis in order to protect the cartilage (Schwager et al., 2011). Additionally, a few relevant studies point out that natural compounds (flavonoids, polyphenols, etc.) originating from *Rosa canina* may alter the symptoms and evolution of osteoarthritis, inducing patients to experience an effect similar to that of analgesic drugs, steroids, or anti-arthritis drugs (IANCU et al., n.d.). A meta-analysis of RCTs by Christensen, R, and his co-workers in order to estimate RHP's capacity to reduce pain in osteoarthritis treatment showed that patients allocated to rosehip powder would respond to therapy twice as likely as those who used a placebo (Christensen et al., 2008). Not only anti-inflammatory and antioxidants but Ayati et al.'s review also revealed other effects such as anti-obesity, anti-cancer, hepatoprotective, nephroprotective, cardioprotective, anti-aging, etc. Different effects can influence each other, for example, anti-inflammatory effects and anti-obesity. The mechanical strain on joints can decrease through weight loss, and the reduction of OA-induced pain allows patients to take more exercise, which will in turn help reduce obesity (Gruenwald et al., 2019). Overall, these literature studies and clinical trials both indicate that *Rosa canina* is a potential nutraceutical choice for replacing NSAIDs in the treatment of osteoarthritis, and more research about it should be continued.

6.2.8 SCUTELLARIA BAICALENSIS

In recent years, Chinese herbal extracts have become more widely used to treat osteoarthritis (Wang et al., 2020). *Scutellaria baicalensis* Georgi. (Lamiaceae) is a Lamiaceae plant, whose root is the most commonly used medicinal part. China, Russia, Mongolia, North Korea, and Japan are all home to this medicinal plant (Zhao et al., 2019). *Scutellaria baicalensis* has been shown to have anti-inflammatory and antioxidant properties in the past. When mice were given *Scutellaria baicalensis* instead of a vehicle, they saw a statistically significant reduction in the severity of osteoarthritis. In mice, immunohistochemistry revealed a significant decrease in protein expression of transforming growth factor $\beta1$ (TGF-$\beta1$), high-temperature receptor A1 (HTRA1), matrix metalloprotease 13 (MMP-13), and NF-κB, supporting cartilage morphology assessments with a decrease in inflammatory and osteoarthritis biomarkers (Smith et al., 2020). *Scutellaria baicalensis* root extract has been used in the treatment of inflammatory and other diseases (Khan, Haseeb, Ansari, & Haqqi, 2017). Antiviral, anti-tumor, anti-bacterial, antioxidant, anti-inflammatory, hepatoprotective, and neuroprotective activities have been reported for extracts of *Scutellaria baicalensis* and its major chemical constituents. After a week of treatment with 500 mg/d of *Scutellaria baicalensis*, patients with knee osteoarthritis reported fewer physical symptoms (Wang et al., 2018). *Scutellaria baicalensis* active constituents have antiviral and antibacterial properties, making them more promising candidate therapeutics for preventing infection-related cytokine storms than drugs with only antimicrobial or anti-inflammatory properties (Liao et al., 2021).

6.2.9 WITHANIA SOMNIFERA

Withania somnifera, commonly known as ashwagandha or Indian ginseng, is a very revered herb in the Indian Ayurvedic system of medicine (Khan & Shah, 2016; Singh et al., 2011). *Withania somnifera*, which belongs to the family Solanaceae, is commonly found in India's drier regions like in the states of Madhya Pradesh, Punjab, Sindh, and Rajasthan (Arora et al., 2013). Additionally, it is widely distributed in the drier parts of tropical and subtropical zones, ranging from the Canary Islands, South Africa, the Middle East, and Sri Lanka, to China (Dar et al., 2015). The whole plant or its different parts have widely been used since antiquity for its medicinal properties (Dar et al., 2015). Roots of *Withania somnifera* contain a wide variety of nutrients and other phytochemicals (Mirjalili et al., 2009). They have been used in traditional Indian medicine for treating various health ailments like cardiac failure, diabetes, neurological disorders, ulcers, and gout, especially osteoarthritis (Tetali et al., 2021). Withanolides, which are extracted from *Withania somnifera*, are oxygenated ergostane-type steroids (Tetali et al., 2021). Withanolides are employed in the treatment of arthritis and are shown to be potent inhibitors of angiogenesis, inflammation, and oxidative stress (Arora et al., 2013). Aqueous extracts of *Withania somnifera* roots showed a transitory chondroprotective effect on damaged human osteoarthritic cartilage by significant and reproducible inhibition of the gelatinase activity of collagenase, the type-2 enzyme *in vitro* (Ganesan et al., 2011; Sumantran et al., 2007). Crude ethanol extract of *Withania somnifera* significantly suppressed lipopolysaccharide, which induced the assembly of pro-inflammatory cytokines TNF-a, IL-1b, and IL-12p40 in peripheral blood mononuclear cells from normal individuals and synovial fluid mononuclear cells from osteoarthritis patients (Dar et al., 2015). Withanolides inhibit the activation of NF-kB and NF-kB-regulated gene expression, which is evidenced by mouse cell line data in a study (Arora et al., 2013). *Withania somnifera* root significantly reduces the amplification and propagation of the inflammatory response, without causing any gastric damage (Arora et al., 2013). In many recent clinical studies, *Withania somnifera* is also combined with many medicinal plants to increase the effect in the treatment of osteoarthritis. The combined use of five Ayurvedic herbal formulations (*Z. officinale, T. cordifolia, E. officinalis, T. terrestris*, and *W. somnifera*) within the treatment of osteoarthritis is perceived to significantly relieve pain in the majority of patients (Logie & Vanden Berghe, 2020). Arvind Chopra et al. demonstrated the potential efficacy and safety of RA-11, which is a standardized multiplant Ayurvedic drug (*W. somnifera, B. serrata, Z. officinale*, & *C. longa*) in the symptomatic treatment of osteoarthritis knees over 32 weeks of therapy (Chopra et al., 2004).

6.2.10 ZINGIBER OFFICINALE

Zingiber officinale, commonly known as ginger, a member of the *Zingiberaceae* family, is a climbing perennial plant grown in tropical and subtropical regions. For decades, it has been widely used for cooking and treating different diseases, especially in Asia. Characterized in traditional medicine as spicy and hot, Ancient Indians and Chinese believed ginger could be used for the treatment of cough and cold, nausea, rheumatism, gingivitis, toothache, asthma, constipation, diabetes, menstrual cramps, cancer, and many more (Khan et al., 2016). Over 160 different bioactive compounds in ginger have been identified, such as gingerol analogs, diarylheptanoids, and terpene compounds (Zhang et al., 2021). There are two essential active components in ginger: 6-gingerol and 6-shogaol, which are responsible for preventing inflammation and oxidative stress (Mohd Sahardi & Makpol, 2019). According to a randomized double-blind placebo-controlled 3-month clinical trial in elderly subjects with knee osteoarthritis, the authors revealed that ginger supplementation was linked with decreased levels of TNF-α and IL-1β after 3 months (Mozaffari-Khosravi et al., 2016). 6-gingerol's anti-inflammatory activity is shown by decreasing inducible NO synthase and TNF-α expression through the repression of I-κBα phosphorylation, NF-κB nuclear activation, and PKC-α translocation (Rondanelli et al., 2020). 6-shogaol is a dehydrated form of 6-gingerol, representing the main bioactive principle of dried rhizomes of *Zingiber officinale* Roscoe. Numerous studies both *in vitro* and *in vivo* demonstrate the 6-shogaol effect by inhibiting pro-inflammatory factors and mediators such as NF-κB or COX-2, attenuating the levels of iNOS resulting in decreased levels of NO, and attenuating the release of pro-inflammatory cytokines such as interferon, TNF, interleukins, and chemokines (Bischoff-Kont & Furst, 2021). Oxidative stress occurs resulting in the formation of reactive oxygen species (ROS), which contribute to the onset of inflammatory signaling. Ginger's high antioxidant activity has been found in several studies. The Nrf2/HO-1 signaling plays a crucial role in the prevention of inflammation-related oxidative stress. The transcription factor nuclear factor erythroid 2-related factor 2 (Nrf2) dissociates from the Keap1-Nrf2 protein-protein interaction, translocates into the nucleus, and binds to the antioxidant response element (ARE) in oxidative stress. 6-shogaol (10 µM) increased the H_2O_2-triggered ARE activity and nuclear protein levels of Nrf2. Nrf2, in the event of oxidative stress within the inflammatory situation, mediates a response that protects from cell damage and activates the transcription of HO-1 which exhibits a cell-protective impact by removing ROS. Moreover, 6-shogaol in H_2O_2-activated HepG2 cells is revealed by Western blot analysis to significantly increase HO-1 protein levels (Bischoff-Kont & Furst, 2021). The US FDA listed ginger in their generally recognized as safe (GRAS) list. Bartels et al. carried out the research by meta-analysis on selected studies demonstrating the efficacy and safety of ginger for the symptomatic treatment of osteoarthritis. The review revealed clinical benefits of OA like reducing pain and disability in osteoarthritis; on the other hand, it pointed out its disadvantages such as "bad taste" or "causing stomach upset." But none of those could be classified as "serious" in terms of causing lasting harm compared to cardiovascular and other effects caused by NSAIDs. The authors, therefore, believed ginger could be seen as a better treatment option than NSAIDs (Bartels et al., 2015). Another review, summarising nine randomized clinical trials, showed that combinations of ginger supplementation and other botanicals are effective in decreasing knee pain in patients with knee osteoarthritis, although not all of them found significant changes (Rondanelli et al., 2020). Currently, *Zingiber officinale* shows its anti-inflammatory effects and potential to decrease OA pain, but more clinical studies are needed using different doses and durations of treatment to validate the exact dosage and duration of treatment of ginger extract alone or in combination with other drugs for the treatment of osteoarthritis.

6.3 BIOACTIVE COMPOUNDS FOR TREATMENT OF OSTEOARTHRITIS

Recently, with the failure of pharmacological treatments for cartilage disease to achieve full tissue regeneration and the side effects of NSAIDs on various human organs, interest in herbal compounds and herbal medicine with anti-osteoarthritis activities is increasing rapidly (Sharma et al., 2020; Rane et al., 2020a, b, c). Traditional Chinese medicine has been used for tonifying deficiency effects nutraceuticals as alternative medicines to treat osteoarthritis for years and has shown few promising results (Li et al., 2017). Additionally, bioactive compounds extracted from natural plants that contain anti-inflammatory, antioxidant, or cartilage-protective effects have also been widely used as a potential treatment for osteoarthritis (Li & Zhang, 2020). In this review, we are going to introduce some bioactive compounds potentially used as substitutes for NSAIDs in treating osteoarthritis such as Kaempferol, Curcumin, EGCG, Wogonin, etc.

6.3.1 BAICALEIN

Baicalin (BA) is a flavonoid monomer extracted from the *Scutellaria baicalensis* Georgi plant that has been shown to have anti-inflammatory, anti-deformation, and anti-bacterial properties. In IL-1β-treated chondrocytes and DMM-treated mice, BA promotes chondrocyte viability and cell-matrix synthesis via the TGF-β/Smad3 pathway. BA could be used as a treatment for osteoarthritis (Yi et al., 2021). Baicalin protected CHON-001 cells from IL-1β-induced inflammatory injury, possibly through down-regulation of miR-126 and thus deactivation of the NF-κB signaling pathway, according to this study (Yang et al., 2018). In an OA rat model, this study found that baicalin has the potential to prevent osteoarthritis by suppressing NLRP3 inflammasome activation without affecting oxidative stress-related molecules and inhibiting cartilage catabolism enzymes (Bai et al., 2021). Baicalin is a key active ingredient in *Achyranthes bidentata*'s treatment of osteoarthritis. *Achyranthes bidentata* plays a pharmacological role in osteoarthritis via apoptosis, inflammation, and immune regulation, according to functional enrichment analysis (Chen et al., 2020). The combination of Baicalin and miR-106a-5p mimic significantly reduced IL-1β-induced inflammatory injury in CHON-001 cells, suggesting that it could be used as a novel therapeutic strategy for osteoarthritis (Xiang et al., 2021). Baicalin treatment of osteoarthritic chondrocytes resulted in a minor improvement in cartilaginous extracellular matrix homeostasis (Chunhui Chen et al., 2017). Baicalin can significantly reduce articular cartilage loss (OARSI score), suppress synovial inflammation (synovitis score), and ameliorate subchondral bone resorption as measured by micro-CT in validation experiments. Baicalin could have a promising application and therapeutic value in the treatment of osteoarthritis (Yi et al., 2021).

6.3.2 CURCUMIN

Curcumin (1,7-bis(4-hydroxy-3-methoxyphenyl)-1,6-heptadiene-3,5-dione), also called diferuloylmethane, is a natural polyphenol mainly discovered in the root of *Curcuma longa* (also known as Turmeric), a plant related to the ginger family, *Zingiberaceae* (Vyas et al., 2010; Kesharwani et al., 2015, 2018; Mishra et al., 2019; Singh et al., 2013a, b, 2015, 2016; Upadhyaya et al., 2009; Kesharwani & Misra, 2011; Hewlings & Kalman, 2017). Originating from India, usually known as a plant-derived curry spice due to its yellow color and flavor, nowadays turmeric can be found in several parts of the world, from Southeast Asia to China and even Latin America (Kotha & Luthria, 2019). Not only used as a natural coloring agent in various fields including foods, cosmetics, and textiles, curcumin has also been used for centuries to treat biliary digestive disorders, wound healing, anorexia, cough, hepatic disorders, and rheumatic diseases (Chattopadhyay et al., 2004). Previous studies demonstrated that curcumin is a multitarget agent that has a wide range of pharmacological activities, including antifungal, antiviral, antioxidant, anti-inflammatory, anti-diabetic, antimicrobial, antitumor, antihypertensive, immunomodulatory effects, and protection in respiratory disorders, nephron, gastro, hepatic, etc. (Rahmani et al., 2018). At the molecular level, this bioactive compound has been confirmed to exhibit anti-inflammatory activity through the suppression of numerous cell signaling pathways including NF-κB, STAT3, Nrf2, ROS, and COX-2 (Kunnumakkara et al., 2017). NF-κB plays a major role in the signaling pathways involved in the pathogenesis of osteoarthritis and significantly regulates inflammatory mediators associated with osteoarthritis (Chen et al., 2017). In an *in vivo* experiment using an OA-EN model similar to TNF-α, it was shown that curcumin down-modulates the activation of NF-κB and NF-κB-promoted proteins involved in the inflammatory and destructive processes of cartilage while upregulating SOX9, a protein-coding gene that acts during chondrocyte differentiation (Buhrmann et al., 2021). Looking at the protective effect of curcumin on (MIA)-induced OA, Yun Zhang and his colleagues initiated a preclinical study using a rat model randomized into four groups: control group, OA group, OA+PBS group, and OA+curcumin group. The results showed that joint diameter and Mankin's score remarkably reduced with curcumin treatment, and the expression of MyD88, p-IκBα, NF-κB, TNF-α, IL-1β, and IL-6 in knee OA rats could be attenuated as well (Zhang & Zeng, 2019). Additionally, curcumin acts as a chondroprotective agent by inhibiting apoptosis of chondrocytes, inhibiting the release of proteoglycans and metalloproteases, and inhibiting the expression of cyclooxygenase, prostaglandin E-2, and inflammatory cytokines in chondrocytes. Curcumin prevented chondrogenesis from suppression and apoptosis of canine chondrocytes induced by IL-1β, which also similarly happened in human primary chondrocyte cultures, whereby all cellular features of apoptosis were reversed by 15–30-minute curcumin treatment with the intensification of the expression of antiapoptotic proteins such as Bcl-2, Bcl-XL, and TNF receptor-associated factor 1, and suppressing caspase-3 as a factor (Chin, 2016). Moreover, curcumin inhibits oxidative stress and ER stress by suppressing the PERK-eIF2α-ATF4-CHOP pathway through the activation of SIRT1 in TBHP-treated chondrocytes, thereby protecting cartilage from destruction (Feng et al., 2019). The limiting factors of using curcumin as a therapeutic agent, such as low solubility and oral bioavailability of curcumin, can recently be solved by delivering curcumin in liposomes or nanoparticles or polymeric micelles, phospholipid complexes, and microemulsions (Liu et al., 2016). A meta-analysis comparing curcuminoids versus NSAIDs reported that although the effects of curcuminoids on pain were not significantly better than NSAIDs, patients receiving curcuminoids were less likely to withdraw and experience any GI adverse event during the treatment (Bannuru et al., 2018). Another meta-analysis and systematic review found that curcumin and *Curcuma longa* extract are safe and more effective compared to placebo in relieving pain and improving joint function and stiffness. Compared to NSAIDs, curcumin shows a similar effect on joint pain, function, and stiffness (Zeng et al., 2021). In the future, more studies, both preclinical and clinical, may be worthy to find out the entire effect of this promising nutraceutical in the treatment of osteoarthritis.

6.3.3 EGCG

EGCG (Epigallocatechin 3-gallate), a class of natural flavonol, is found mainly in green tea, which is derived from the leaves of *Camellia sinensis* and bestows upon us various health benefits and reduces the risk of diseases (Chakrawarti et al., 2016). EGCG represents approximately 59% of the total catechins, which are the main flavonoids (Keservani & Sharma, 2014;

Keservani et al., 2016a, b) in green tea. EGCG has effective antimicrobial, anti-inflammatory, antioxidative, and anticarcinogenic effects (Chakrawarti et al., 2016). EGCG has been reported to reduce post-traumatic osteoarthritis progression through its potent anti-inflammatory and antioxidative properties (Huang et al., 2021). In *in-vitro* studies, the molecular mechanism of EGCG's efficacy showed that EGCG inhibits IL-1β-induced phosphorylation as well as proteasomal degradation of IκBα to suppress NF-κB nuclear translocation (Ahmed, 2010). Because IL-1β has promoted an imbalance between excessive cartilage destruction and has also been a potent inducer of reactive oxygen species, including nitric oxide and inflammatory mediators such as PGE2, *via* enhanced expression of the enzyme's inducible nitric oxide synthase and COX-2, respectively (Ahmed, 2010). EGCG could protect cartilage and attenuate the degraded cartilage. The chondroprotective effects of EGCG in osteoarthritis are due to EGCG increasing the gene expression of aggrecan and type II collagen, which are extracellular matrix components secreted by chondrocytes in the cartilage (Ahmed, 2010; Huang et al., 2021). Besides, EGCG also decreases the expression of matrix metalloproteinases (MMP-1, MMP-3, MMP-13), which are a group of enzymes that play an important role in tissue remodeling as well as in the destruction of cartilage in arthritic joints due to their ability to degrade a large variety of extracellular matrix components (Ahmed, 2010). In addition, it has been demonstrated that EGCG could mitigate osteoarthritis progression by inhibiting the expression of other proinflammatory genes (tumor necrosis factor-α (TNF-α), transforming growth factor-β2, a disintegrin, and metalloproteinase with thrombospondin motifs (ADAMTS)-5) (Huang et al., 2021). In an animal study, EGCG could ameliorate cartilage degradation and improve the running endurance of guinea pigs (Huang et al., 2021). However, the bioavailability of EGCG is poor and it is unstable under alkaline or neutral conditions. So, it is mostly used either in combination with other components or being modified to improve its efficacy and specificity. The application of nanotechnology to encapsulate EGCG compounds has been formulated to address the bioavailability and delivery issues (Chakrawarti et al., 2016). Zheng Y et al. has demonstrated the enhancement of the anti-inflammatory potential of EGCG in the treatment of osteoarthritis through the fabrication and optimization of casein protein nanoparticles (EGC-NPs) (Zheng et al., 2019). EGCG decorated Au-Ag nano-heterostructures were utilized as NIR-sensitive nano-enzymes for the treatment of osteoarthritis through mitochondrial repair and cartilage protection, which are promising for osteoarthritis treatment (Xu et al., 2022).

6.3.4 KAEMPFEROL

Kaempferol (3, 5, 7, 4′-tetrahydroxy flavone), is a class of natural flavonol, that is found in many fruits and vegetables, like grapes, tomatoes, broccoli, tea, and distributed in numerous medicinal plants genera like Delphinium, Camellia, Berberis, Gingko, (Shields, 2017). Kaempferol and its various glycosides exert a spread of pharmacological effects, including anti-inflammatory, anti-cancer, anti-microbial, anti-diabetic, anti-allergic, analgesic, cardioprotective, and neuroprotective activities (Calderón-Montaño et al., 2011). Numerous preclinical studies have shown that kaempferol and a few glycosides of kaempferol have a large range of pharmacological activities, like antioxidant, cardioprotective, neuroprotective, antidiabetic, antiosteoporotic, estrogenic/antiestrogenic, anxiolytic, analgesic, and antiallergic activities (Saldanha et al., 2019). Besides, Kaempferol acts as a scavenger of free radicals and superoxide radicals similarly to preserves the activity of assorted antioxidant enzymes (Rajendran et al., 2014). Kaempferol has been extensively used as traditional therapy for several inflammatory and chronic diseases thanks to its suppressing the discharge of chemical intermediates (nitric oxide, interferons, interleukins, prostaglandins, TNFs,) (Kim et al., 2015; Shields, 2017). Especially, it has been recognized as a good agent for alleviating the clinical symptoms of osteoarthritis. Many studies provide evidence that kaempferol encompasses a huge potential within the management of osteoarthritis (Jiang et al., 2019). A Western blot study was performed to analyze the possible mechanism of action. It inhibits the interleukin-1β-stimulated NF-κB signaling pathway and significantly inhibits the phosphorylation of IκBα and NF-κBp65 in rat osteoarthritis chondrocytes (Piao et al., 2015). These investigation findings suggest that the protective effects of kaempferol on the experimental rat chondrocytes model of osteoarthritis were by suppressing PGE2 and NO formations, and iNOS and COX-2 activities, so it has strong anti-inflammatory and anti-arthritis effects during this study. Kaempferol prevented apoptosis and also the release of proinflammatory cytokines triggered by LPS. miR-146a (Zhuang et al., 2017). In another rat model of osteoarthritis, the expression of miR-146a and Decorin in cartilage tissues was repressed by kaempferol. Also, the administration of kaempferol, the activated PI3K/AKT/mTOR signaling pathway was enhanced in the osteoarthritis animal model (Jiang et al., 2019). In another study, kaempferol inhibited inflammation and extracellular matrix degradation by modulating the XIST/miR-130a/STAT3 axis in chondrocytes. Kaempferol decreased proinflammatory cytokine production, and extracellular matrix degradation in C28/I2 cells, ameliorated XIST expression, and enhanced miR-130a expression (Xiao et al., 2021). Recently, the upcoming role of kaempferol within the management of bone metabolism disorders including osteoarthritis was explored in MC3T3-E1 cells. During this study, kaempferol increased the expression of osteoblast-activated factors like RUNX-2, osterix, BMP-2, and collagen I as well as autophagy-related factors beclin-1, SQSTM1/p62, and also the conversion of LC3-II from LC3-I. Another study showed the osteogenic potential of kaempferol by directly modulating the cytokeratin-14 (Krt-14) pathway (Majumdar & Somani, 2018). These results suggest that kaempferol had significant anti-inflammatory and anti-arthritis effects. Thus, kaempferol, as a unique therapeutic activity, may prevent, stop, or retard the progression of osteoarthritis. In an osteoarthritis patient's diet, supplementing plenty of kaempferol through vegetables or using herbs also reduces osteoarthritis symptoms. Therefore, kaempferol could be a potential compound in the development of nutraceuticals to support, prevent, and control osteoarthritis.

6.3.5 PUNICALAGIN

Punicalagin, a compound isolated from *Punica granatum*, inhibits inflammation by suppressing the expression of the iNOS and COX-2 genes, as well as the production of NO and PGE2. Punicalagin has a lot of potential against the inflammatory pathway, according to the research (Berköz & Allahverdiyev, 2017). Punicalagin, a common anti-inflammatory polyphenol, inhibits LPS-induced chondrocyte injury and osteoarthritis progression by controlling the Foxo1/Prg4/HIF3α axis (Liu et al., 2021). They created a collagen-induced arthritis (CIA) model in this study and discovered a large number of M1 macrophages and pyroptosis, both of which are important sources of proinflammatory cytokines. In CIA mice, punicalagin reduced joint inflammation, cartilage damage, and systemic bone destruction. They came to the conclusion that punicalagin and genipin treatment of cartilage had implications for the treatment of osteoarthritis (Ge et al., 2022). Punicalagin binds to type II collagen and prevents it from being degraded by MMP-13, while genipin (GNP) is a collagen cross-linking agent. Injection of punicalagin reduced cartilage loss compared to saline-injected controls, according to quantitative histology, and the addition of GNP had no effect. This research backs up the idea that delivering Punicalagin via IA could help to prevent OA-related cartilage erosion (Elder et al., 2021). Punicalagin slows the progression of OA in chondrocytes by inhibiting apoptosis, oxidative stress, and ECM degradation, which is mediated by autophagy activation (Kong et al., 2020).

6.3.6 RESVERATROL

Resveratrol (3,5,4′-trihydroxystilbene) is a stilbenoid, a type of natural polyphenol. Resveratrol is present in numerous fruits, wines, vegetables, peanuts, and root extracts of the weed *Polygonum cuspidatum* but is mostly concentrated in the skin of red grapes (Hussain et al., 2018). Red wine, a type of wine made from the skin of grapes, is a widely consumed beverage with many beneficial effects on humans including cardiovascular, breast cancer, bone homeostasis, renal, visual system, etc. (Weiskirchen & Weiskirchen, 2016). About 90% of ingested resveratrol, after being absorbed by passive diffusion or carrier-mediated transport (Chen et al., 2013), reaches the colon intact and then ferments. Once absorbed through the portal vein, the production enters the liver where they are rapidly metabolized to glucuronides or sulfates and then arrive in the target tissues and cells via the systemic circulation (Gowd et al., 2019). Several pharmacological activities exhibited by resveratrol have been reported, such as antioxidant, anti-aging, anti-inflammatory, anti-cancerous, anti-diabetic, cardioprotective, vasorelaxant, and neuroprotective properties (Shaito et al., 2020). Since 2001, Gao et al. showed that resveratrol could suppress the proliferation of spleen cells induced by ConA, IL-2, or allo-antigens, and more effectively prevent lymphocytes from producing IL-2 and IFN-γ, and macrophages from TNF-α or IL-12 (Gao et al., 2001). The inflammatory response is regulated by diverse signaling pathways, including the AA pathway, NF-κB, MAPK, and AP-1 (Meng et al., 2021). *In vitro*, resveratrol suppresses IL-1β-induced apoptosis in chondrocytes through down-regulation of NF-κB and NF-κB-dependent proinflammatory and matrix-degrading gene products by inhibiting IκBα degradation and proteasome function in human chondrocytes (Shakibaei et al., 2008). Additionally, resveratrol intra-articular injection could remarkably prevent the destruction of osteoarthritis cartilage through the activation of SIRT1 thereby silencing HIF-2α (Li et al., 2015). Furthermore, a study on the role of sirtuin 1 showed that SIRT1, a human protein activated by resveratrol, plays a protective role in human chondrocytes via the NF-κB pathway, reducing the up-regulation of MMP 1, 2, 9, 13, and ADAMTS 5 genes caused by IL-1β. Treatment with resveratrol could inhibit the expression of NF-kB caused by TNF-α as a result of up-regulation of SIRT1 (Deng et al., 2019). Moreover, resveratrol injection delayed cartilage degeneration and promoted chondrocyte autophagy in the destabilization of the DMM-induced osteoarthritis model by regulating the HIF-1α-dependent AMPK and mTOR signaling pathway (Qin et al., 2017). An experiment on osteoarthritis models in rabbits confirmed that intra-articular injections of resveratrol have a chondroprotective activity in reducing cartilage destruction during the onset of the disease (Elmali et al., 2005). Zhou et al., after investigating several functional analyses, literature reviews, and experimental verifications, identified that six genes (CXCL1, HIF-1α, IL-6, MMP3, NOX4, and PTGS2) are involved in the progression of osteoarthritis and can also be used as therapeutic targets for osteoarthritis treatment (Zhou et al., 2021). Resveratrol is recently known as a potential compound for the management of osteoarthritis and other chronic diseases. However, there is still a lack of clinical studies on resveratrol's harmful and long-term outcomes. More clinical trials are recommended to evaluate the dosage and safety of treatment using resveratrol.

6.3.7 SINOMENINE

Sinomenine ($C_{19}H_{23}NO_4$) (Adetuyi et al., 2022) is a monomer alkaloid isolated from the root of *Sinomenium acutum* with immunomodulatory, anti-inflammatory, and potential anti-angiogenic activities. In Chinese medicine, this compound has a long history of treating arthritis, as it can inhibit the proliferation of synovial fibroblasts and lymphocytes. Additionally, sinomenine has been shown to suppress the expression of genes involved in inflammation and apoptosis, such as interleukin-6, a pleiotropic inflammatory cytokine, and JAK3 (Janus kinase 3) (Kok et al., 2005). Sinomenine has been demonstrated to be effective in managing neuralgia and arthritis diseases. Sinomenine is also a unique plant alkaloid because it potently releases histamine in association with the degranulation of tissue mast cells in mammalian tissues, which occurs preferentially within the skin and joint capsules (Yamasaki, 1976). Studies have shown that sinomenine can reduce cartilage degeneration and synovial inflammation in joints by inhibiting the expression of inflammatory factors and chondrocyte apoptosis, thereby delaying the progression of osteoarthritis (Huang et al., 2022). Intra-articular injection of SIN is also an efficient treatment method for acute knee osteoarthritis pain but still has challenges. Sinomenine hydrochloride injection may be a sterilized solution product of SIN, which might be directly injected into the affected area through the joint cavity and exert the pharmacological effect of sinomenine. Sinomenine hydrochloride injection as an external preparation of sinomenine has been used ever more frequently within the clinical treatment of osteoarthritis and it's been researched to be efficacious and safe in the treatment of osteoarthritis (Huang et al., 2022). *In vitro* and *in vivo* studies, the anti-inflammatory effects of SIN on IL-1β-induced inflammatory response were confirmed. SIN activates the Nrf2/HO-1 pathway and blocks the NF-κB pathway, so it can prevent the imbalance of IL-1β-induced inflammation and ECM metabolism. The treatment of SIN could reverse the event of osteoarthritis and protect against the degradation of cartilage and ECM. The *in vitro* and *in vivo* results were consistent, showing that SIN has a protective effect against the progression of osteoarthritis. The role of SIN in alleviating osteoarthritis is explored by activating the Nrf2/HO-1 signaling pathway and blocking the activity of NF-κB in mouse cartilage cells (Wu et al., 2019). Recently, sinomenine tablets and sinomenine hydrochloride injections have been widely used clinically in China due to their potential (Huang et al., 2022). However, there is still a scarcity of relevant evidence-based medical studies on its oral efficacy and safety. Therefore, researchers continue to demonstrate the clinical efficacy and safety in the treatment of osteoarthritis. These studies contribute to a new understanding of SIN and its use in the treatment of osteoarthritis, providing a new research direction for the future. Hence, is it possible to research and develop it as nutraceuticals for preventing symptoms and managing osteoarthritis?

6.3.8 WOGONIN

Wogonin (5,7-dihydroxy-8-methoxyflavone), a natural flavonoid derived from the root extract of *Scutellaria baicalensis*, has been used to treat inflammatory and cancer diseases (Khan, Haseeb, Ansari, & Haqqi, 2017). Wogonin exerts chondroprotective effects through inhibition of molecules involved in oxidative stress, inflammation, and matrix degradation in osteoarthritis chondrocytes and cartilage explants. Wogonin suppressed the expression and production of inflammatory mediators including IL-6, COX-2, PGE2, iNOS, and NO in IL-1β-stimulated osteoarthritis chondrocytes (Khan, Haseeb, Ansari, & Haqqi, 2017). Wogonin suppressed the expression of matrix-degrading proteases. Wogonin showed potent chondroprotective potential by switching the matrix degradation signaling axis from catabolic to anabolic ends (Khan, Haseeb, Ansari, Devarapalli, et al., 2017). Besides, Wogonin also inhibited the expression, production, and activities of matrix-degrading proteases including MMP-3, MMP-9, MMP-13, and ADAMTS-4 in osteoarthritis chondrocytes, and blocked the release of s-GAG and COL2A1 in IL-1β-stimulated osteoarthritis cartilage explants (Khan, Ahmad, et al., 2017). A recent study showed that wogonin inhibited MMP-3 expression in rabbit articular chondrocytes (Park et al., 2015). Wogonin increased the expression of the anabolic cartilage factors COL2A1 and ACAN in chondrocytes while also inhibiting IL-1β-mediated depletion of COL2A1 (Khan, Haseeb, Ansari, Devarapalli, et al., 2017). Wogonin didn't inhibit through the inhibition of MAPKs and NF-κB activation but was mediated through the suppression of c-Fos/AP-1 activity at transcriptional and post-transcriptional levels in osteoarthritis chondrocytes (Khan, Haseeb, Ansari, & Haqqi, 2017). Wogonin-induced oxidative stress through ROS generation and cellular GSH depletion. Therefore, Wogonin regulated the cellular redox leading to the induction of Nrf2/ARE pathways through activation of ROS/ERK/Nrf2/HO-1-SOD2-NQO1-GCLC signaling axis in osteoarthritis chondrocytes (Khan, Haseeb, Ansari, Devarapalli, et al., 2017). Recently, the TFNA/wogonin complex (TWC), which is a mixture of tetrahedral framework nucleic acid (TFNA) and wogonin, could be a potential injectable form of therapy for osteoarthritis. TWC showed potential to effectively alleviate inflammatory reactions *in vitro* and *in vivo* and to prevent the destruction of rat cartilage than TFNA and Wogonin when used independently (Sirong et al., 2020). Wogonin has been examined for its pain-reducing, anti-inflammatory, and chondroprotective effects when applied as a topical cream. The topical application of wogonin significantly slows or abrogates joint damage progression and promotes joint health in mice (Smith et al., 2020). Wogonin represents a novel treatment for the disease of osteoarthritis.

6.4 CONCLUSION

Modern nutraceuticals have an excellent value in the treatment of osteoarthritis. The application of natural methods is a cutting-edge strategy. Nutraceuticals include a diverse range of molecules that can have beneficial effects on various joint structures through a variety of mechanisms. This review focused in particular on the anti-inflammatory and antioxidant properties of compounds that improve cartilage conditions, implying that they should be included in a prevention strategy. Therefore, the development of modern nutraceuticals with better bioavailability or alternative formulations is urgently needed. Research in this field is continuously developing and being applied more and more in osteoarthritis problems.

KEYWORDS

- herbal plants
- metalloproteinases
- nitrogen species
- nutraceuticals
- osteoarthritis
- pomegranate peel extract
- reactive oxygen

REFERENCES

Abdel-Tawab, M., Werz, O., & Schubert-Zsilavecz, M. (2011). Boswellia serrata. *Clinical Pharmacokinetics, 50*(6), 349–369. https://doi.org/10.2165/11586800-000000000-00000.

Adatia, A., Rainsford, K. D., & Kean, W. F. (2012). Osteoarthritis of the knee and hip. Part I: a etiology and pathogenesis as a basis for pharmacotherapy. *Journal of Pharmacy and Pharmacology, 64*(5), 617-625. https://doi.org/10.1111/j.2042-7158.2012.01458.x.

Adetuyi, B. O., Odine, G. O., Olajide, P. A., Adetuyi, O. A., Atanda, O. O., & Oloke, J. K. (2022). Nutraceuticals: role in metabolic disease, prevention and treatment. *World News of Natural Sciences, 42,* 1–27.

Ahmed, S. (2010). Green tea polyphenol epigallocatechin 3-gallate in arthritis: Progress and promise. *Arthritis Research & Therapy, 12*(2), 1–9.

Ahn, H. Y., Cho, J.-H., Nam, D., Kim, E.-J., & Ha, I.-H. (2019). Efficacy and safety of Cortex Eucommia (*Eucommia ulmoides* Oliver) extract in subjects with mild osteoarthritis: Study protocol for a 12-week, multicenter, randomized, double-blind, placebo-controlled trial. *Medicine, 98*(50), 1–6.

Alluri, V. K., Kundimi, S., Sengupta, K., Golakoti, T., & Kilari, E. K. (2020). An anti-inflammatory composition of *Boswellia serrata* resin extracts alleviates pain and protects cartilage in monoiodoacetate-induced osteoarthritis in rats. *Evidence-Based Complementary and Alternative Medicine, 2020,* 7381625. https://doi.org/10.1155/2020/7381625.

Ansaripour, S., & Dehghan, M. (2020). Efficacy of some herbal medicines in osteoarthritis with a focus on topical agents: A systematic review. *Current Pharmaceutical Design, 26*(22), 2676–2681. https://doi.org/10.2174/1381612826666200429013728.

Aronson, J. K. (2017). Defining 'nutraceuticals': Neither nutritious nor pharmaceutical. *British Journal of Clinical Pharmacology, 83*(1), 8–19. https://doi.org/10.1111/bcp.12935.

Arora, R., Malhotra, P., Sharma, A., Haniadka, R., Yashawanth, H., & Baliga, M. (2013). Medicinal efficacy of Indian herbal remedies for the treatment of arthritis. In Bioactive food as dietary interventions for arthritis and related inflammatory diseases (pp. 601–617). Elsevier.

Asif, M., & Mohd, I. (2019). Prospects of medicinal plants derived nutraceuticals: a re-emerging new era of medicine and health aid. *Progress in Chemical and Biochemical Research, 2*(4), 150–169.

Bai, H., Yuan, R., Zhang, Z., Liu, L., Wang, X., Song, X., & Gao, L. (2021). Intra-articular injection of baicalein inhibits cartilage catabolism and NLRP3 inflammasome signaling in a posttraumatic OA model. *Oxidative Medicine and Cellular Longevity, 2021*, 1–11.

Bannuru, R. R., Osani, M. C., Al-Eid, F., & Wang, C. (2018). Efficacy of curcumin and Boswellia for knee osteoarthritis: Systematic review and meta-analysis. *Seminars in Arthritis and Rheumatism, 48*(3), 416–429. https://doi.org/10.1016/j.semarthrit.2018.03.001.

Barrera, P., van der Maas, A., van Ede, A. E., Kiemeney, B. A., Laan, R. F., van de Putte, L. B., & van Riel, P. L. (2002). Drug survival, efficacy and toxicity of monotherapy with a fully human anti-tumor necrosis factor-alpha antibody compared with methotrexate in long-standing rheumatoid arthritis. *Rheumatology (Oxford), 41*(4), 430–439. https://doi.org/10.1093/rheumatology/41.4.430.

Bartels, E. M., Folmer, V. N., Bliddal, H., Altman, R. D., Juhl, C., Tarp, S., & Christensen, R. (2015). Efficacy and safety of ginger in osteoarthritis patients: A meta-analysis of randomized placebo-controlled trials. *Osteoarthritis and Cartilage, 23*(1), 13–21. https://doi.org/10.1016/j.joca.2014.09.024.

Berköz, M., & Allahverdiyev, O. (2017). Punicalagin isolated from *Punica granatum* husk can decrease the inflammatory response in RAW 264.7 macrophages. *Eastern Journal of Medicine, 22*(2), 57.

Bischoff-Kont, I., & Furst, R. (2021). Benefits of ginger and its constituent 6-shogaol in inhibiting inflammatory processes. *Pharmaceuticals (Basel), 14*(6), 1–19. https://doi.org/10.3390/ph14060571.

Buhrmann, C., Brockmueller, A., Mueller, A. L., Shayan, P., & Shakibaei, M. (2021). Curcumin attenuates environment-derived osteoarthritis by Sox9/NF-kB signaling axis. *International Journal of Molecular Sciences, 22*(14), 7645. https://www.mdpi.com/1422-0067/22/14/7645 (accessed on 6 June 2024).

Calderón-Montaño, J. M., Burgos-Morón, E., Pérez-Guerrero, C., & López-Lázaro, M. (2011). A review on the dietary flavonoid kaempferol. *Mini Reviews in Medicinal Chemistry, 11*(4), 298–344. https://doi.org/10.2174/138955711795305335.

Chakrawarti, L., Agrawal, R., Dang, S., Gupta, S., & Gabrani, R. (2016). Therapeutic effects of EGCG: A patent review. *Expert Opinion on Therapeutic Patents, 26*(8), 907–916.

Chattopadhyay, I., Biswas, K., Bandyopadhyay, U., & Banerjee, R. K. (2004). Turmeric and curcumin: Biological actions and medicinal applications. *Current Science, 87*(1), 44–53. http://www.jstor.org/stable/24107978 (accessed on 6 June 2024).

Chen, A., Gupte, C., Akhtar, K., Smith, P., & Cobb, J. (2012). The global economic cost of osteoarthritis: How the UK compares. *Arthritis, 2012*, 1–6.

Chen, C., Zhang, C., Cai, L., Xie, H., Hu, W., Wang, T., & Chen, H. (2017). Baicalin suppresses IL-1β-induced expression of inflammatory cytokines via blocking NF-κB in human osteoarthritis chondrocytes and shows protective effect in mice osteoarthritis models. *International Immunopharmacology, 52*, 218–226. https://doi.org/10.1016/j.intimp.2017.09.017.

Chen, F. P., Chang, C. M., Hwang, S. J., Chen, Y. C., & Chen, F. J. (2014). Chinese herbal prescriptions for osteoarthritis in Taiwan: Analysis of National Health Insurance dataset. *BMC Complementary and Alternative Medicine, 14*, 91. https://doi.org/10.1186/1472-6882-14-91.

Chen, M. L., Yi, L., Jin, X., Xie, Q., Zhang, T., Zhou, X., & Mi, M. T. (2013). Absorption of resveratrol by vascular endothelial cells through passive diffusion and an SGLT1-mediated pathway. *Journal of Nutritional Biochemistry, 24*(11), 1823–1829. https://doi.org/10.1016/j.jnutbio.2013.04.003.

Chen, Z., Wu, G., & Zheng, R. (2020). A systematic pharmacology and in vitro study to identify the role of the active compounds of *Achyranthes bidentata* in the treatment of osteoarthritis. *Medical Science Monitor: International Medical Journal of Experimental and Clinical Research, 26*, e925545–925541.

Chin, K. Y. (2016). The spice for joint inflammation: Anti-inflammatory role of curcumin in treating osteoarthritis. *Drug Design, Development and Therapy, 10*, 3029–3042. https://doi.org/10.2147/DDDT.S117432.

Chopra, A., Lavin, P., Patwardhan, B., & Chitre, D. (2004). A 32-week randomized, placebo-controlled clinical evaluation of RA-11, an Ayurvedic drug, on osteoarthritis of the knees. *JCR: Journal of Clinical Rheumatology, 10*(5), 236–245.

Christensen, R., Bartels, E., Altman, R., Astrup, A., & Bliddal, H. (2008). Does the hip powder of *Rosa canina* (rosehip) reduce pain in osteoarthritis patients? – A meta-analysis of randomized controlled trials. *Osteoarthritis and Cartilage, 16*(9), 965–972.

Chun, J. M., Lee, A. Y., Nam, J. Y., Lim, K. S., Choe, M. S., Lee, M. Y., & Kim, J. S. (2021). Effects of *Dipsacus asperoides* extract on monosodium iodoacetate-induced osteoarthritis in rats based on gene expression profiling. *Frontiers in Pharmacology, 12*, 615157. https://doi.org/10.3389/fphar.2021.615157.

Cutler, R. (2003). Secondary metabolites: Medicinal and pharmaceutical uses, Elsevier, 716–726.

D'Adamo, S., Cetrullo, S., Panichi, V., Mariani, E., Flamigni, F., & Borzi, R. M. (2020). Nutraceutical activity in osteoarthritis biology: A focus on the nutrigenomic role. *Cells, 9*(5), 1–24. https://doi.org/10.3390/cells9051232.

Dar, N. J., Hamid, A., & Ahmad, M. (2015). Pharmacologic overview of *Withania somnifera*, the Indian ginseng. *Cellular and Molecular Life Sciences, 72*(23), 4445–4460.

Deng, Z., Li, Y., Liu, H., Xiao, S., Li, L., Tian, J., & Zhang, F. (2019). The role of sirtuin 1 and its activator, resveratrol in osteoarthritis. *Bioscience Reports, 39*(5), 1–11. https://doi.org/10.1042/BSR20190189.

Eghbali, S., Askari, S. F., Avan, R., & Sahebkar, A. (2021). Therapeutic effects of *Punica granatum* (pomegranate): An updated review of clinical trials. *Journal of Nutrition and Metabolism, 2021*, 1–22.

Elder, S. H., Mosher, M. L., Jarquin, P., Smith, P., & Chironis, A. (2021). Effects of short-duration treatment of cartilage with punicalagin and genipin and the implications for treatment of osteoarthritis. *Journal of Biomedical Materials Research Part B: Applied Biomaterials, 109*(6), 818–828.

Elmali, N., Esenkaya, I., Harma, A., Ertem, K., Turkoz, Y., & Mizrak, B. (2005). Effect of resveratrol in experimental osteoarthritis in rabbits. *Inflammation Research, 54*(4), 158–162. https://doi.org/10.1007/s00011-004-1341-6.

Feng, K., Ge, Y., Chen, Z., Li, X., Liu, Z., Li, X., & Wang, X. (2019). Curcumin inhibits the PERK-eIF2α-CHOP pathway through promoting SIRT1 expression in oxidative stress-induced rat chondrocytes and ameliorates osteoarthritis progression in a rat model. *Oxidative Medicine and Cellular Longevity, 2019*, 8574386. https://doi.org/10.1155/2019/8574386.

Ganesan, K., Sehgal, P. K., Mandal, A. B., & Sayeed, S. (2011). Protective effect of *Withania somnifera* and *Cardiospermum halicacabum* extracts against collagenolytic degradation of collagen. *Applied Biochemistry and Biotechnology, 165*(3), 1075–1091.

Gao, X., Xu, Y. X., Janakiraman, N., Chapman, R. A., & Gautam, S. C. (2001). Immunomodulatory activity of resveratrol: Suppression of lymphocyte proliferation, development of cell-mediated cytotoxicity, and cytokine production. *Biochemical Pharmacology, 62*(9), 1299–1308. https://doi.org/10.1016/s0006-2952(01)00775-4.

Gautam, R. K., Gupta, G., Sharma, S., Hatware, K., Patil, K., Sharma, K., & Dua, K. (2019). Rosmarinic acid attenuates inflammation in experimentally induced arthritis in Wistar rats, using Freund's complete adjuvant. *International Journal of Rheumatic Diseases, 22*(7), 1247–1254.

Ge, G., Bai, J., Wang, Q., Liang, X., Tao, H., Chen, H., & Xu, Y. (2022). Punicalagin ameliorates collagen-induced arthritis by downregulating M1 macrophage and pyroptosis via NF-κB signaling pathway. *Science China Life Sciences, 65*(3), 588–603.

Gong, L. L., Yang, S., Liu, H., Zhang, W., Ren, L. L., Han, F. F., & Liu, L. H. (2019). Antinociceptive and anti-inflammatory potentials of Akebia saponin D. *European Journal of Pharmacology, 845*, 85–90.

Goswami, S., Mitra, S., Paul, P., Dey, D., & Das, S. (2019). Biochemic system of medicine: Oldest form of nutraceutical therapy. In *Nutraceutical and Functional Foods in Disease Prevention* (pp. 403–431). IGI Global.

Gowd, V., Karim, N., Shishir, M. R. I., Xie, L., & Chen, W. (2019). Dietary polyphenols to combat the metabolic diseases via altering gut microbiota. *Trends in Food Science & Technology, 93*, 81–93.

Gruenwald, J., Uebelhack, R., & Moré, M. I. (2019). *Rosa canina*–Rose hip pharmacological ingredients and molecular mechanics counteracting osteoarthritis–A systematic review. *Phytomedicine, 60*, 152958.

Gupta, P., Samarakoon, S., Chandola, H., & Ravishankar, B. (2011). Clinical evaluation of *Boswellia serrata* (Shallaki) resin in the management of Sandhivata (osteoarthritis). *Ayu, 32*(4), 478.

Hadipour-Jahromy, M., Mozaffari-Kermani, R., & Nobakht, F. (2009). Influence of *Commiphora mukul* resin on the knee articular cartilage of rats in experimental osteoarthritis induced by iodoacetate. *Pakistan Journal of Medical Sciences April-June, 25*(2), 269–273.

Haghighian, M. K., Rafraf, M., Hemmati, S., Haghravan, S., & Asghari-Jafarabadi, M. (2021). Effects of pomegranate (*Punica granatum* L.) peel extract supplementation on serum lipid profile and oxidative stress in obese women with knee osteoarthritis: A double blind, randomized, placebo-controlled study. *Advances in Integrative Medicine, 8*(2), 107–113.

Hazra, A. K., Sur, T., Chakraborty, B., & Seal, T. (2018). HPLC analysis of phenolic acids and antioxidant activity of some classical ayurvedic Guggulu formulations. *International Journal of Research in Ayurveda and Pharmacy, 9*(1), 112–117.

He, Y., Li, Z., Alexander, P. G., Ocasio-Nieves, B. D., Yocum, L., Lin, H., & Tuan, R. S. (2020). Pathogenesis of osteoarthritis: Risk factors, regulatory pathways in chondrocytes, and experimental models. *Biology, 9*(8), 194.

Hewlings, S. J., & Kalman, D. S. (2017). Curcumin: A review of its effects on human health. *Foods, 6*(10), 1–11, https://doi.org/10.3390/foods6100092.

Huang, H. T., Cheng, T. L., Yang, C. D., Chang, C. F., Ho, C. J., Chuang, S. C., & Shen, H. Y. (2021). Intra-articular injection of (-)-Epigallocatechin 3-Gallate (EGCG) ameliorates cartilage degeneration in guinea pigs with spontaneous osteoarthritis. *Antioxidants, 10*(2), 178.

Huang, Z., Mao, X., Chen, J., He, J., Shi, S., Gui, M., & Hong, Z. (2022a). The efficacy and safety of Zhengqing Fengtongning for knee osteoarthritis: A systematic review and meta-analysis of randomized clinical trials. *Evidence-Based Complementary and Alternative Medicine, 2022*, 2768444. https://doi.org/10.1155/2022/2768444.

Huang, Z., Mao, X., Chen, J., He, J., Shi, S., Gui, M., & Hong, Z. (2022b). Sinomenine hydrochloride injection for knee osteoarthritis: A protocol for systematic review and meta-analysis. *Medicine, 101*(2), e28503. https://doi.org/10.1097/md.0000000000028503.

Hung, T. M., Jin, W., Thuong, P. T., Song, K. S., Seong, Y. H., & Bae, K. (2005). Cytotoxic saponins from the root of *Dipsacus asper* Wall. *Archives of Pharmacal Research, 28*(9), 1053–1056. https://doi.org/10.1007/BF02977401.

Hunter, D. J., McDougall, J. J., & Keefe, F. J. (2008). The symptoms of osteoarthritis and the genesis of pain. *Rheumatic Disease Clinics of North America, 34*(3), 623–643.

Hunter, D. J., Schofield, D., & Callander, E. (2014). The individual and socioeconomic impact of osteoarthritis. *Nature Reviews Rheumatology, 10*(7), 437–441.

Hussain, S. A., Marouf, B. H., Ali, Z. S., & Ahmmad, R. S. (2018). Efficacy and safety of co-administration of resveratrol with meloxicam in patients with knee osteoarthritis: A pilot interventional study. *Clinical Interventions in Aging, 13*, 1621–1630. https://doi.org/10.2147/CIA.S172758.

Hussain, T., Tan, B. E., Liu, G., Oladele, O. A., Rahu, N., Tossou, M. C., & Yin, Y. (2016). Health-promoting properties of *Eucommia ulmoides*: A review. *Evidence-Based Complementary and Alternative Medicine, 2016*, 5202908. https://doi.org/10.1155/2016/5202908.

Iancu, P., Soare, R., Dinu, M., Soare, M., Bonea, D., & Popescu, M. (2020). Analysis of the existing research regarding the use of the species *Rosa canina* L. *Scientific Papers. Series B. Horticulture, 64*(2), 325–331

Jiang, R., Hao, P., Yu, G., Liu, C., Yu, C., Huang, Y., & Wang, Y. (2019). Kaempferol protects chondrogenic ATDC5 cells against inflammatory injury triggered by lipopolysaccharide through down-regulating miR-146a. *International Immunopharmacology, 69*, 373–381. https://doi.org/10.1016/j.intimp.2019.02.014.

Jung, H. W., Jung, J. K., Son, K. H., Lee, D. H., Kang, T. M., Kim, Y. S., & Park, Y. K. (2012). Inhibitory effects of the root extract of *Dipsacus asperoides* CY Cheng et al TM Ai on collagen-induced arthritis in mice. *Journal of Ethnopharmacology, 139*(1), 98–103.

Kamble, S., Patil, A., Shinde, S., & Ankush, H. (2021). A review on current nutraceuticals in the management of osteoarthritis. *International Journal of Horticulture & Food Science, 3*(1), 22–28.

Keservani, R. K., & Sharma, A. K. (2014). Flavonoids: Emerging trends and potential health benefits. *Journal of Chinese Pharmaceutical Sciences, 23*(12), 815.

Keservani, R. K., Kesharwani, R. K., Vyas, N., Jain, S., Raghuvanshi, R., & Sharma, A. K. (2010a). Nutraceutical and functional food as future food: A review. *Der Pharmacia Lettre, 2*(1), 106–116.

Keservani, R. K., Sharma, A. K., & Kesharwani, R. K. (2016a). Nutraceutical and functional foods for cardiovascular health. In *Food Process Engineering* (pp. 291–312). Apple Academic Press, CRC Press.

Keservani, R. K., Sharma, A. K., & Kesharwani, R. K. (2016b). Medicinal effect of nutraceutical fruits for the cognition and brain health. *Scientifica*, Article ID 3109254, 10 pages. https://doi.org/10.1155/2016/3109254.

Keservani, R. K., Sharma, A. K., & Kesharwani, R. K. (2017). An overview and therapeutic applications of nutraceutical and functional foods. In *Recent Advances in Drug Delivery Technology* (pp. 160–201). ISBN: 9781522507543.

Keservani, R. K., Sharma, A. K., & Kesharwani, R. K. (Eds.). (2020). *Nutraceuticals and Dietary Supplements: Applications in Health Improvement and Disease Management*, 1–344. CRC Press. ISBN: 9781771888738.

Keservani, R.K., Kesharwani, R.K., Sharma, A.K., Vyas, N., & Chadoker, A. (2010b). Nutritional supplements: An overview. *International Journal of Current Pharmaceutical Review and Research, 1*(1), 59–75.

Kesharwani, R. K., & Misra, K. (2011). Prediction of binding site for curcuminoids at human topoisomerase II α protein; an in-silico approach. *Current Science, 10*(8), 1060–1065.

Kesharwani, R. K., Singh, D. B., Singh, D. V., & Misra, K. (2018). Computational study of curcumin analogues by targeting DNA topoisomerase II: A structure-based drug designing approach. *Network Modeling Analysis in Health Informatics and Bioinformatics, 7*(1), 1–7.

Kesharwani, R. K., Srivastava, V., Singh, P., Rizvi, S. I., Adeppa, K., & Misra, K. (2015). A novel approach for overcoming drug resistance in breast cancer chemotherapy by targeting new synthetic curcumin analogues against aldehyde dehydrogenase 1 (ALDH1A1) and glycogen synthase kinase-3 β (GSK-3β). *Applied Biochemistry and Biotechnology, 176*(7), 1996–2017.

Khan, N. M., Ahmad, I., Ansari, M. Y., & Haqqi, T. M. (2017). Wogonin, a natural flavonoid, intercalates with genomic DNA and exhibits protective effects in IL-1β stimulated osteoarthritis chondrocytes. *Chemico-Biological Interactions, 274*, 13–23.

Khan, N. M., Haseeb, A., Ansari, M. Y., & Haqqi, T. M. (2017). A wogonin-rich-fraction of *Scutellaria baicalensis* root extract exerts chondroprotective effects by suppressing IL-1β-induced activation of AP-1 in human OA chondrocytes. *Scientific Reports, 7*(1), 1–14.

Khan, N. M., Haseeb, A., Ansari, M. Y., Devarapalli, P., Haynie, S., & Haqqi, T. M. (2017). Wogonin, a plant-derived small molecule, exerts potent anti-inflammatory and chondroprotective effects through the activation of ROS/ERK/Nrf2 signaling pathways in human osteoarthritis chondrocytes. *Free Radical Biology and Medicine, 106*, 288–301.

Khan, S., & Shah, R. A. (2016). Assessment of genetic diversity among India Ginseng, *Withania somnifera* (L) Dunal using RAPD and ISSR markers. *Research in Biotechnology, 7*, 1–10.

Khan, S., Pandotra, P., Qazi, A. K., Lone, S. A., Muzafar, M., Gupta, A. P., & Gupta, S. (2016). Medicinal and nutritional qualities of *Zingiber officinale*. In *Studies in Natural Products Chemistry, 25*, 525–550. https://doi.org/10.1016/B978-0-12-802972-5.00025-1.

Kim, S. H., Park, J. G., Lee, J., Yang, W. S., Park, G. W., Kim, H. G., & Cho, J. Y. (2015). The dietary flavonoid kaempferol mediates anti-inflammatory responses via the Src, Syk, IRAK1, and IRAK4 molecular targets. *Mediators of Inflammation, 2015*, 904142. https://doi.org/10.1155/2015/904142.

Kimmatkar, N., Thawani, V., Hingorani, L., & Khiyani, R. (2003). Efficacy and tolerability of *Boswellia serrata* extract in treatment of osteoarthritis of knee–a randomized double-blind placebo-controlled trial. *Phytomedicine, 10*(1), 3–7.

Kok, T. W., Yue, P. Y., Mak, N. K., Fan, T. P., Liu, L., & Wong, R. N. (2005). The antiangiogenic effect of sinomenine. *Angiogenesis, 8*(1), 3–12. https://doi.org/10.1007/s10456-005-2892-z.

Kong, J., Wang, J., Gong, X., Zheng, X., & Chen, T. (2020). Punicalagin inhibits tert-butyl hydroperoxide-induced apoptosis and extracellular matrix degradation in chondrocytes by activating autophagy and ameliorates murine osteoarthritis. *Drug Design, Development and Therapy, 14*, 5521.

Kotha, R. R., & Luthria, D. L. (2019). Curcumin: Biological, Pharmaceutical, Nutraceutical, and Analytical Aspects. *Molecules, 24*(16), 2930. https://www.mdpi.com/1420-3049/24/16/2930 (accessed on 6 June 2024).

Kunnumakkara, A. B., Banik, K., Bordoloi, D., Harsha, C., Sailo, B. L., Padmavathi, G., & Aggarwal, B. B. (2018). Googling the Guggul (*Commiphora* and *Boswellia*) for prevention of chronic diseases. *Frontiers in Pharmacology, 9*, 686.

Kunnumakkara, A. B., Bordoloi, D., Padmavathi, G., Monisha, J., Roy, N. K., Prasad, S., & Aggarwal, B. B. (2017). Curcumin, the golden nutraceutical: Multitargeting for multiple chronic diseases. *British Journal of Pharmacology, 174*(11), 1325–1348. https://doi.org/10.1111/bph.13621.

Lee, C. J., Chen, L. G., Liang, W. L., Hsieh, M. S., & Wang, C. C. (2018). Inhibitory effects of punicalagin from *Punica granatum* against type II collagenase-induced osteoarthritis. *Journal of Functional Foods, 41*, 216–222.

Lee, D., Ju, M.-K., & Kim, H. (2020). Commiphora extract mixture ameliorates monosodium iodoacetate-induced osteoarthritis. *Nutrients, 12*(5), 1477.

Lee, M. K., Kim, M. J., Cho, S. Y., Park, S. A., Park, K. K., Jung, U. J., & Choi, M. S. (2005). Hypoglycemic effect of *Du-zhong* (*Eucommia ulmoides* Oliv.) leaves in streptozotocin-induced diabetic rats. *Diabetes Research and Clinical Practice, 67*(1), 22–28.

Li, F., Nishidono, Y., Tanaka, K., Watanabe, S., & Tezuka, Y. (2020). A New Monoterpenoid Glucoindole Alkaloid from *Dipsacus asper*. *Natural Product Communications, 15*(4), 1934578X20917292.

Li, L., Liu, H., Shi, W., Liu, H., Yang, J., Xu, D., & Wu, L. (2017). Insights into the action mechanisms of traditional Chinese medicine in osteoarthritis. *Evidence-Based Complementary and Alternative Medicine, 2017*, 1–13.

Li, W., Cai, L., Zhang, Y., Cui, L., & Shen, G. (2015). Intra-articular resveratrol injection prevents osteoarthritis progression in a mouse model by activating SIRT1 and thereby silencing HIF-2alpha. *Journal of Orthopaedic Research, 33*(7), 1061–1070. https://doi.org/10.1002/jor.22859.

Li, X. Z., & Zhang, S. N. (2020). Recent advance in treatment of osteoarthritis by bioactive components from herbal medicine. *Chinese Medicine, 15*, 80. https://doi.org/10.1186/s13020-020-00363-5.

Li, X., Wu, D., Hu, Z., Xuan, J., Ding, X., Zheng, G., & Wu, A. (2018). The protective effect of ligustilide in osteoarthritis: An in vitro and in vivo study. *Cellular Physiology and Biochemistry, 48*(6), 2583–2595.

Li, Y., Kamo, S., Metori, K., Koike, K., Che, Q. M., & Takahashi, S. (2000). The promoting effect of eucommiol from *Eucommia cortex* on collagen synthesis. *Biological and Pharmaceutical Bulletin, 23*(1), 54–59. https://doi.org/10.1248/bpb.23.54.

Liao, H., Ye, J., Gao, L., & Liu, Y. (2021). The main bioactive compounds of *Scutellaria baicalensis* Georgi. for alleviation of inflammatory cytokines: A comprehensive review. *Biomedicine & Pharmacotherapy, 133*, 110917.

Liu, F., Yang, H., Li, D., Wu, X., & Han, Q. (2021). Punicalagin attenuates osteoarthritis progression via regulating Foxo1/Prg4/HIF3α axis. *Bone, 152*, 116070.

Liu, W., Zhai, Y., Heng, X., Che, F. Y., Chen, W., Sun, D., & Zhai, G. (2016). Oral bioavailability of curcumin: Problems and advancements. *Journal of Drug Targeting, 24*(8), 694–702.

Loeser, R. F., Goldring, S. R., Scanzello, C. R., & Goldring, M. B. (2012). Osteoarthritis: A disease of the joint as an organ. *Arthritis and Rheumatism, 64*(6), 1697.

Logie, E., & Vanden Berghe, W. (2020). Tackling chronic inflammation with withanolide phytochemicals—A withaferin A perspective. *Antioxidants, 9*(11), 1107.

Mahdavi, A. M., & Javadivala, Z. (2021). Systematic review of the effects of pomegranate (*Punica granatum*) on osteoarthritis. *Health Promotion Perspectives, 11*(4), 411.

Majeed, M., Majeed, S., Narayanan, N. K., & Nagabhushanam, K. (2019). A pilot, randomized, double-blind, placebo-controlled trial to assess the safety and efficacy of a novel *Boswellia serrata* extract in the management of osteoarthritis of the knee. *Phytotherapy Research, 33*(5), 1457–1468.

Majumdar, A. S., & Somani, S. J. (2018). Chapter 12 – Natural Products in Lifestyle Diseases: In Vitro Screening. In S. C. Mandal, V. Mandal, & T. Konishi (Eds.), *Natural Products and Drug Discovery* (pp. 327–347). Elsevier. https://doi.org/10.1016/B978-0-08-102081-4.00012-5.

Meng, T., Xiao, D., Muhammed, A., Deng, J., Chen, L., & He, J. (2021). Anti-Inflammatory Action and Mechanisms of Resveratrol. *Molecules, 26*(1), 1–15. https://doi.org/10.3390/molecules26010229.

Mirjalili, M. H., Moyano, E., Bonfill, M., Cusido, R. M., & Palazón, J. (2009). Steroidal lactones from *Withania somnifera*, an ancient plant for novel medicine. *Molecules, 14*(7), 2373–2393.

Mishra, H., Kesharwani, R. K., Singh, D. B., Tripathi, S., Dubey, S. K., & Misra, K. (2019). Computational simulation of inhibitory effects of curcumin, retinoic acid and their conjugates on GSK-3 beta. *Network Modeling Analysis in Health Informatics and Bioinformatics, 8*(1), 3.

Mobasheri, A. (2012). Intersection of inflammation and herbal medicine in the treatment of osteoarthritis. *Curr Rheumatol Rep, 14*(6), 604–616. https://doi.org/10.1007/s11926-012-0288-9.

Moga, M. A., Dimienescu, O. G., Bălan, A., Dima, L., Toma, S. I., Bîgiu, N. F., & Blidaru, A. (2021). Pharmacological and therapeutic properties of *Punica granatum* phytochemicals: possible roles in breast cancer. *Molecules, 26*(4), 1054.

Mohd Sahardi, N. F. N., & Makpol, S. (2019). Ginger (*Zingiber officinale* Roscoe) in the prevention of ageing and degenerative diseases: Review of current evidence. *Evid Based Complement Alternat Med., 2019*, 5054395. https://doi.org/10.1155/2019/5054395.

Mozaffari-Khosravi, H., Naderi, Z., Dehghan, A., Nadjarzadeh, A., & Fallah Huseini, H. (2016). Effect of Ginger Supplementation on Proinflammatory Cytokines in Older Patients with Osteoarthritis: Outcomes of a Randomized Controlled Clinical Trial. *J. Nutr. Gerontol. Geriatr., 35*(3), 209–218. https://doi.org/10.1080/21551197.2016.1206762.

Nai, J., Zhang, C., Shao, H., Li, B., Li, H., Gao, L., & Sheng, H. (2021). Extraction, structure, pharmacological activities and drug carrier applications of *Angelica sinensis* polysaccharide. *International Journal of Biological Macromolecules, 183*, 2337–2353.

Neogi, T. (2013). The epidemiology and impact of pain in osteoarthritis. *Osteoarthritis Cartilage, 21*(9), 1145–1153.

Nybom, H., & Werlemark, G. (2017). Realizing the potential of health-promoting rosehips from dogroses (*Rosa sect. Caninae*). *Curr Bioact Compd, 13*(1), 3–17.

Oppedisano, F., Bulotta, R. M., Maiuolo, J., Gliozzi, M., Musolino, V., Carresi, C., & Mollace, V. (2021). The Role of Nutraceuticals in Osteoarthritis Prevention and Treatment: Focus on n-3 PUFAs. *Oxid Med Cell Longev, 2021*, 4878562. https://doi.org/10.1155/2021/4878562.

Park, J. S., Lee, H. J., Lee, D. Y., Jo, H. S., Jeong, J. H., Kim, D. H., & Hwang, S. C. (2015). Chondroprotective effects of wogonin in experimental models of osteoarthritis in vitro and in vivo. *Biomolecules & Therapeutics, 23*(5), 442.

Piao, T., Ma, Z., Li, X., & Liu, J. (2015). Taraxasterol inhibits IL-1β-induced inflammatory response in human osteoarthritic chondrocytes. *Eur. J. Pharmacol., 756*, 38–42. https://doi.org/10.1016/j.ejphar.2015.03.012.

Qin, N., Wei, L., Li, W., Yang, W., Cai, L., Qian, Z., & Wu, S. (2017). Local intra-articular injection of resveratrol delays cartilage degeneration in C57BL/6 mice by inducing autophagy via AMPK/mTOR pathway. *J. Pharmacol. Sci., 134*(3), 166–174. https://doi.org/10.1016/j.jphs.2017.06.002.

Ragavi, R., & Surendran, S. A. (2018). *Commiphora mukul*: An overview. *Research Journal of Pharmacy and Technology, 11*(7), 3205–3208.

Rahmani, A. H., Alsahli, M. A., Aly, S. M., Khan, M. A., & Aldebasi, Y. H. (2018). Role of Curcumin in disease prevention and treatment. *Adv. Biomed. Res., 7*, 38. https://doi.org/10.4103/abr.abr_147_16.

Rajendran, P., Rengarajan, T., Nandakumar, N., Palaniswami, R., Nishigaki, Y., & Nishigaki, I. (2014). Kaempferol, a potential cytostatic and cure for inflammatory disorders. *European Journal of Medicinal Chemistry, 86*, 103–112. https://doi.org/10.1016/j.ejmech.2014.08.011.

Ramesh, C. G. (2016). Chapter 13 – Nutraceuticals in Arthritis. In R. K. Kesharwani, R. K. Keservani, & A. K. Sharma (Eds.), *Nutraceuticals in Arthritis* (pp. 161–176), Apple Academic Press. https://doi.org/10.1016/B978-0-12-802147-7.00013-9.

Rane, B. R., Bharath, M. S., Patil, R. R., Keservani, R. K., & Jain, A. S. (2020a). Novel Approaches in Nutraceuticals. In R. K. Kesharwani, R. K. Keservani, & A. K. Sharma (Eds.), *Enhancing the Therapeutic Efficacy of Herbal Formulations through Novel Drug Delivery Systems* (pp. 241–266). IGI Global. ISBN13: 9781799844532.

Rane, B. R., Patil, A. S., Keservani, R. K., & Jain, A. S. (2020b). Novel Approaches in Herbal Formulation. In R. K. Kesharwani, R. K. Keservani, & A. K. Sharma (Eds.), *Enhancing the Therapeutic Efficacy of Herbal Formulations through Novel Drug Delivery Systems* (pp. 43–68). IGI Global. ISBN13: 9781799844532.

Rane, B. R., Tadavi, S. A., & Keservani, R. K. (2020). Naturopathy. In A. K. Sharma, R. K. Keservani, & S. P. Gautam (Eds.), *Herbal Product Development* (pp. 321–347). Apple Academic Press, CRC Press, Taylor & Francis Group. ISBN: 9781771888776.

Roach, H. I., & Tilley, S. (2007). The pathogenesis of osteoarthritis. In *Bone and Osteoarthritis* (pp. 1–18). London: Springer London.

Rondanelli, M., Fossari, F., Vecchio, V., Gasparri, C., Peroni, G., Spadaccini, D., & Perna, S. (2020). Clinical trials on pain lowering effect of ginger: A narrative review. *Phytother. Res., 34*(11), 2843–2856. https://doi.org/10.1002/ptr.6730.

Saad, J., & Mathew, D. (2023). Nonsteroidal Anti-Inflammatory Drugs Toxicity. In: StatPearls. StatPearls Publishing, Treasure Island (FL); PMID: 30252262.

Saldanha, E., Saxena, A., Kaur, K., Kalekhan, F., Venkatesh, P., Fayad, R., & Baliga, M. S. (2019). Polyphenols in the Prevention of Ulcerative Colitis: A Revisit. In R. R. Watson

& V. R. Preedy (Eds.), *Dietary Interventions in Gastrointestinal Diseases* (pp. 277–287). Academic Press. https://doi.org/10.1016/B978-0-12-814468-8.00023-5.

Schwager, J., Hoeller, U., Wolfram, S., & Richard, N. (2011). Rose hip and its constituent galactolipids confer cartilage protection by modulating cytokine, and chemokine expression. *BMC Complement Altern Med, 11*, 105. https://doi.org/10.1186/1472-6882-11-105.

Shaito, A., Posadino, A. M., Younes, N., Hasan, H., Halabi, S., Alhababi, D., & Pintus, G. (2020). Potential Adverse Effects of Resveratrol: A Literature Review. *Int J Mol Sci, 21*(6), 1–26. https://doi.org/10.3390/ijms21062084.

Shakibaei, M., Csaki, C., Nebrich, S., & Mobasheri, A. (2008). Resveratrol suppresses interleukin-1beta-induced inflammatory signaling and apoptosis in human articular chondrocytes: potential for use as a novel nutraceutical for the treatment of osteoarthritis. *Biochem. Pharmacol, 76*(11), 1426–1439. https://doi.org/10.1016/j.bcp.2008.05.029.

Sharma, A. K., Keservani, R. K., & Gautam, S. P. (Eds.). (2020). *Herbal Product Development*. Apple Academic Press, CRC Press, 1–376, Taylor & Francis Group. ISBN: 9781771888776.

Shields, M. (2017). Chemotherapeutics. In S. Badal & R. Delgoda (Eds.), *Pharmacognosy* (pp. 295–313). Academic Press. https://doi.org/10.1016/B978-0-12-802104-0.00014-7.

Shin, N. R., Lee, A. Y., Park, G., Ko, J. W., Kim, J. C., Shin, I. S., & Kim, J. S. (2019). Therapeutic Effect of *Dipsacus asperoides* C. Y. Cheng et T. M. Ai in Ovalbumin-Induced Murine Model of Asthma. *International Journal of Molecular Sciences, 20*(8), 1855. https://www.mdpi.com/1422-0067/20/8/1855 (accessed on 6 June 2024).

Shivnath, N., Rawat, V., Siddiqui, S., Verma, S., Gupta, P., Rais, J., & Arshad, M. (2021). Antiosteoarthritic effect of *Punica granatum L.* peel extract on collagenase induced osteoarthritis rat by modulation of COL-2, MMP-3, and COX-2 expression. *Environmental Toxicology, 36*(1), 5–15.

Siddiqui, M. Z. (2011). *Boswellia serrata*, a potential anti-inflammatory agent: An overview. *Indian Journal of Pharmaceutical Sciences, 73*(3), 255–261. https://doi.org/10.4103/0250-474X.93507.

Singh, B. B., Mishra, L. C., Vinjamury, S. P., Aquilina, N., & Shepard, N. (2003). The effectiveness of *Commiphora mukul* fir osteoarthritis of the knee: An Outcomes Study. *Alternative Therapies in Health & Medicine, 9*(3), 74–79.

Singh, D. B., Gupta, M. K., Kesharwani, R. K., & Misra, K. (2013). Comparative docking and ADMET study of some curcumin derivatives and herbal congeners targeting β-amyloid. *Network Modeling Analysis in Health Informatics and Bioinformatics, 2*(1), 13–27.

Singh, D. V., Agarwal, S., Kesharwani, R. K., & Misra, K. (2013). 3D QSAR and pharmacophore study of curcuminoids and curcumin analogs: Interaction with thioredoxin reductase. *Interdisciplinary Sciences: Computational Life Sciences, 5*(4), 286–295.

Singh, N., Bhalla, M., de Jager, P., & Gilca, M. (2011). An overview on *ashwagandha*: A Rasayana (rejuvenator) of Ayurveda. *African Journal of Traditional, Complementary and Alternative Medicines, 8*(5S), 208–213.

Singh, P., Kesharwani, R. K., Misra, K., & Rizvi, S. I. (2015). The modulation of erythrocyte Na+/K+-ATPase activity by curcumin. *Journal of Advanced Research, 6*(6), 1023–1030.

Singh, P., Kesharwani, R. K., Misra, K., & Rizvi. S. I. (2016). Modulation of erythrocyte plasma membrane redox system activity by curcumin. *Biochemistry Research International, 2016*(1), ArticleID 702039.

Sirong, S., Yang, C., Taoran, T., Songhang, L., Shiyu, L., Yuxin, Z., & Xiaoxiao, C. (2020). Effects of tetrahedral framework nucleic acid/wogonin complexes on osteoarthritis. *Bone Research, 8*(1), 1–13.

Smith, J. F., Starr, E. G., Goodman, M. A., Hanson, R. B., Palmer, T. A., Woolstenhulme, J. B., & Nelson, T. K. (2020). Topical application of wogonin provides a novel treatment of knee osteoarthritis. *Frontiers in Physiology, 11*, 80.

Sumantran, V. N., Kulkarni, A., Boddul, S., Chinchwade, T., Koppikar, S. J., Harsulkar, A., & Wagh, U. V. (2007). Chondroprotective potential of root extracts of *Withania somnifera* in osteoarthritis. *Journal of Biosciences, 32*(2), 299–307.

Sun, Y., Huang, K., Mo, L., Ahmad, A., Wang, D., Rong, Z., & Liu, G. (2021). *Eucommia ulmoides* polysaccharides attenuate rabbit osteoarthritis by regulating the function of macrophages [Original Research]. *Frontiers in Pharmacology, 12*, 1–9. https://doi.org/10.3389/fphar.2021.730557.

Tetali, S. D., Acharya, S., Ankari, A. B., Nanakram, V., & Raghavendra, A. S. (2021). Metabolomics of *Withania somnifera* (L.) Dunal: advances and applications. *Journal of Ethnopharmacology, 267*, 113469.

Upadhyaya, J., Kesharwani, R. K., & Misra, K. (2009). Metabolism, pharmacokinetics and bioavailability of ascorbic acid; synergistic effect with tocopherols and curcumin. *J. ComputIntellBioinform, 2*(1), 77–84.

Vyas, N., Keservani, R. K., Nayak, A., Jain, S., & Singhal, M. (2010). Effect of *Tamarindus indica* and *Curcuma longa* on stress-induced Alopecia. *Pharmacology online, 1*, 377–384.

Wang, D., Özen, C., Abu-Reidah, I. M., Chigurupati, S., Patra, J. K., Horbanczuk, J. O., & Atanasov, A. G. (2018). Vasculoprotective effects of pomegranate (*Punica granatum* L.). *Frontiers in Pharmacology, 9*, 544.

Wang, P., Zhu, P., Liu, R., Meng, Q., & Li, S. (2020). Baicalin promotes extracellular matrix synthesis in chondrocytes via the activation of hypoxia-inducible factor-1α. *Experimental and Therapeutic Medicine, 20*(6), 1-1.

Wang, Z. L., Wang, S., Kuang, Y., Hu, Z. M., Qiao, X., & Ye, M. (2018). A comprehensive review on phytochemistry, pharmacology, and flavonoid biosynthesis of *Scutellaria baicalensis*. *Pharmaceutical Biology, 56*(1), 465–484.

Weiskirchen, S., & Weiskirchen, R. (2016). Resveratrol: How much wine do you have to drink to stay healthy? *Advances in Nutrition, 7*(4), 706–718. https://doi.org/10.3945/an.115.011627.

Witkamp, R., & Norren, K. (2018). Let thy food be thy medicine…. when possible. *European Journal of Pharmacology, 836*, 102–114. https://doi.org/10.1016/j.ejphar.2018.06.026.

Wu, Y., Lin, Z., Yan, Z., Wang, Z., Fu, X., & Yu, K. (2019). Sinomenine contributes to the inhibition of the inflammatory response and the improvement of osteoarthritis in mouse-cartilage cells by acting on the Nrf_2/HO-1 and NF-κB signaling pathways. *International Immunopharmacology, 75*, 105715. https://doi.org/10.1016/j.intimp.2019.105715.

Xiang, Q., Wang, J., Wang, T., & Zuo, H. (2021). Combination of baicalein and miR-106a-5p mimics significantly alleviates IL-1β-induced inflammatory injury in CHON-001 cells. *Experimental and Therapeutic Medicine, 21*(4), 1–1.

Xiao, Y., Liu, L., Zheng, Y., Liu, W., & Xu, Y. (2021). Kaempferol attenuates the effects of XIST/miR-130a/STAT3 on inflammation and extracellular matrix degradation in osteoarthritis. *Future Medicinal Chemistry, 13*(17), 1451-1464.

Xie, G. P., Jiang, N., Wang, S. N., Qi, R. Z., Wang, L., Zhao, P. R., & Yu, B. (2015). *Eucommia ulmoides* Olive. bark aqueous extract inhibits osteoarthritis in a rat model of osteoarthritis. *Journal of Ethnopharmacology, 162*, 148–154. https://doi.org/10.1016/j.jep.2014.12.061.

Xu, C., Ni, S., Zhuang, C., Li, C., Zhao, G., Jiang, S., & Wang, Y. (2021). Polysaccharide from *Angelica sinensis* attenuates SNP-induced apoptosis in osteoarthritis chondrocytes by inducing autophagy via the ERK1/2 pathway. *Arthritis Research & Therapy, 23*(1), 1–13.

Xu, S., Chang, L., Zhao, X., Hu, Y., Lin, Y., Chen, Z., & Mei, X. (2022). Preparation of epigallocatechin gallate decorated Au-Ag nano-heterostructures as NIR-sensitive nano-enzymes for the treatment of osteoarthritis through mitochondrial repair and cartilage protection. *Acta Biomaterialia, 144,* 168–182.

Yamasaki, H. (1976). Pharmacology of sinomenine, an anti-rheumatic alkaloid from *Sinomenium acutum*. *Acta Medica Okayama, 30*(1), 1–20.

Yang, F., Lin, Z., Huang, T., Chen, T., Cui, J., Li, M., & Hua, Y. (2019). Ligustilide, a major bioactive component of *Angelica sinensis*, promotes bone formation via the GPR30/EGFR pathway. *Scientific Reports, 9*(1), 1–10.

Yang, X., Zhang, Q., Gao, Z., Yu, C., & Zhang, L. (2018). Baicalin alleviates IL-1β-induced inflammatory injury via down-regulating miR-126 in chondrocytes. *Biomedicine & Pharmacotherapy, 99,* 184–190.

Yang, Y., Gu, Y., Zhao, H., & Zhang, S. (2019). Loganin attenuates osteoarthritis in rats by inhibiting il-1beta-induced catabolism and apoptosis in chondrocytes via regulation of phosphatidylinositol 3-kinases (PI3K)/Akt. *Medical Science Monitor, 25,* 4159–4168. https://doi.org/10.12659/MSM.915064.

Yi, N., Mi, Y., Xu, X., Li, N., Zeng, F., Yan, K., & Lu, M. (2021). Baicalein Alleviates Osteoarthritis progression in mice by protecting subchondral bone and suppressing chondrocyte apoptosis based on network pharmacology. *Frontiers in Pharmacology, 12,* 1–11.

Yu, G., Xiang, W., Zhang, T., Zeng, L., Yang, K., & Li, J. (2020). Effectiveness of Boswellia and Boswellia extract for osteoarthritis patients: A systematic review and meta-analysis. *BMC Complementary Medicine and Therapies, 20*(1), 225. https://doi.org/10.1186/s12906-020-02985-6.

Zeng, L., Yu, G., Hao, W., Yang, K., & Chen, H. (2021). The efficacy and safety of *Curcuma longa* extract and curcumin supplements on osteoarthritis: A systematic review and meta-analysis. *Bioscience Reports, 41*(6), 1–20. https://doi.org/10.1042/BSR20210817.

Zhang, M., Zhao, R., Wang, D., Wang, L., Zhang, Q., Wei, S., & Wu, C. (2021). Ginger (*Zingiber officinale* Rosc.) and its bioactive components are potential resources for health beneficial agents. *Phytotherapy Research, 35*(2), 711–742.

Zhang, Y., & Zeng, Y. (2019). Curcumin reduces inflammation in knee osteoarthritis rats through blocking TLR4/MyD88/NF-κB signal pathway. *Drug Development Research, 80*(3), 353–359.

Zhao, T., Tang, H., Xie, L., Zheng, Y., Ma, Z., Sun, Q., & Li, X. (2019). *Scutellaria baicalensis* Georgi. (Lamiaceae): a review of its traditional uses, botany, phytochemistry, pharmacology and toxicology. *Journal of Pharmacy and Pharmacology, 71*(9), 1353–1369.

Zheng, Y., Xiao, L., Yu, C., Jin, P., Qin, D., Xu, Y., & Du, Q. (2019). Enhanced antiarthritic efficacy by nanoparticles of (−)-Epigallocatechin gallate–Glucosamine–Casein. *Journal of Agricultural and Food Chemistry, 67*(23), 6476–6486.

Zhou, M., Wang, D., & Tang, J. (2021). Identification of the resveratrol potential targets in the treatment of osteoarthritis. *Evidence-Based Complementary and Alternative Medicine, 2021,* 9911286.

Zhuang, C., Wang, Y., Zhang, Y., & Xu, N. (2018). Oxidative stress in osteoarthritis and antioxidant effect of polysaccharide from *Angelica sinensis*. *International Journal of Biological Macromolecules, 115*, 281–286.

Zhuang, Z., Ye, G., & Huang, B. (2017). Kaempferol alleviates the Interleukin-1β-Induced inflammation in rat osteoarthritis chondrocytes via suppression of NF-κB. *Medical Science Monitor, 23*, 3925–3931.

CHAPTER 7

MARINE BOTANICALS AS NUTRACEUTICALS FOR ARTHRITIS

PANKAJ KUMAR

Professor, Department of Pharmacology, Adesh Institute of Pharmacy and Biomedical Science, Adesh University, Bathinda, Punjab, India

ABSTRACT

The word "arthritis" is used to refer to any type of joint pain, regardless of its etiology or origin. There are around 100 different categories and forms of arthritis. Currently, 1 in 4 adults suffers from arthritis in the US. A few common examples of arthritis are Osteoarthritis, Rheumatoid arthritis, Gout, Lupus Arthritis, Ankylosing Spondylitis, Juvenile Arthritis, Psoriatic Arthritis, and Fibromyalgia. The major types of arthritis are RA, OA, and gout. For the treatment of different types of arthritis, non-steroidal anti-inflammatory drugs are mainly used. But because of their side effects, more natural remedies are preferred. Common people are moving towards natural foods which provide nutrients to fight against arthritis. Nutraceuticals are these kinds of foods. Given its enormous biodiversity and ability to manufacture a range of bioactive substances in order to adapt to the marine environment, the ocean is one of the main sources of nutraceuticals. Such species include *Lithothamnion corallioide, Perna canaliculus,* Marine sponge-derived fungi, Pestalotiopsis species, krill, various fishes, *Sargassum wightii, Mytilus edulis, Isostichopus badiontus,* shellfish, *Turbinaria ornate, Caulerpa Racemosa,* soft coral *Sinularia querciformis,* seaweed *Undaria pinnatifida, Halichondria sitiens*, and *Paphia malabarica*. This chapter will include certain nutraceuticals obtained from marine origins that will be useful in the treatment of arthritis.

Nutraceuticals in Arthritis and Psoriasis: Management and Prevention of Diseases.
Meenakshi Jaiswal, Raj K. Keservani, Rajesh K. Kesharwani, and Swati G. Talele (Eds.)
© 2025 Apple Academic Press, Inc. Co-published with CRC Press (Taylor & Francis)

7.1 INTRODUCTION

Arthritis originated in Latin and Greek languages. The word Arthron means joints and it means inflammation, so the literal meaning of the word arthritis is inflammation of joints. Arthritis is used collectively for joint pain of different origins and pathophysiology. Currently, 1 in 4 adults suffers from arthritis in the US. A huge financial burden is imposed globally on the general public through wage loss as well as the cost of medicines (Mitra, 2015). Osteoarthritis (OA), Rheumatoid arthritis (RA), Gout, Lupus arthritis (LA), Ankylosing Spondylitis (AS), Juvenile arthritis (JA), Psoriatic arthritis (PA), and Fibromyalgia are a few frequent types of arthritis. Gout, RA, and OA are the most common types of arthritis (Lawrence, 2008). Mainly joint pain is involved in arthritis.

7.1.1 OSTEOARTHRITIS

The most prevalent kind of arthritis is osteoarthritis as more than 30 million Americans suffer from it. Among all the forms of disability, OA ranks 5th (Sun, 2021). Athletes, military personnel, and individuals who do physically demanding jobs are more prone to OA. Any joint in the human body might develop OA, but mostly knee, hip, and neck joints are affected. Bones in normal joints are covered with cartilage tissue. In OA, cartilage loses its elasticity due to slow damage which causes stiffness and severe pain. Joints cannot absorb shock properly. This causes gradual erosion of joints due to the gradual friction of bones. As age increases, symptoms become worse, making it difficult to do everyday work. Slight movement in joints causes pain (Mitsuyama, 2007). As the disease progresses, joints lose flexibility causing an itching sensation while moving. In more severe cases, hard lumps or bone spurs develop in joints of the knee, elbow, or hips (Kean, 2004). Currently, there is no treatment for OA. More than half of patients suffering from OA may need knee replacement (Deshpande, 2016). There are several reasons behind the onset of OA like poor physical activity, advanced age, genetics, obesity, gender, bone density, and trauma. A woman who is more than 60 years of age has twice the risk of having OA than men (Maiese, 2016).

7.1.2 RHEUMATOID ARTHRITIS

RA is mainly known as an inflammatory disease of joints (Aletaha, 2010). When someone has RA, their immune system assaults their joints, creating inflammation and pain; hence it is also called an autoimmune disease (Guy,

2010). Repeated attacks of immunity can damage cartilage, soft tissue around joint bones, and bones as well. The spacing between the joints becomes smaller. This can cause joints to lose their mobility and become painful. RA mainly affects the joints of the arms, knees, wrists, fingers, and legs. RA can also affect different body systems, hence it is also called systemic arthritis. This disease involves extraarticular manifestations like rheumatoid nodules, vasculitis, and systemic comorbidities (Smolen, 2016). Women are more prone (two to three times) to get RA than men. One in 12 women can develop RA while 1 in 20 men can develop RA (Vollenhoven, 2018).

7.1.3 GOUT

Gout is also a form of arthritis affecting the joints present in the extremities of the body like toes and hands. Gout is not an autoimmune disease. It is a type of metabolic malfunction inflammatory disease. The main reason behind gout is the deposition of needle-like uric acid crystals in joints causing pain and inflammation. The key factors for gout are faulty purine metabolism as well as faulty excretion of uric acid through the kidney (Mitra, 2012). Also, persons who have a high level of uric acid in the blood are more prone to gout. The deposited crystals may cause extreme pain episodes which may last for hours to weeks, making day-to-day activities difficult. The disease is more prevalent in men than in females, but the ratio matches when a woman reaches menopause, showing the strong role of estrogen in the prevention of gout (Mitra, 2012). About 4% of US adults have gout (Zhu, 2011). Men are three times more likely to get gout than females. Black males are at a higher risk of gout (Wilson, 2016).

7.1.4 ANKYLOSING SPONDYLITIS (AS)

This disease mainly affects joints between the spine or joints between the spine and pelvis (Prakash, 1984). Inflamed joints experience excruciating pain that becomes worse with time. Ultimately, spine bones fuse and are unable to move with respect to each other. The exact cause is unknown but may be attributed to genetics. Males are more prone to develop AS compared with females, especially at an early age (Calin, 1999; Jaakkola, 2006). Pain is more intense at night and in the morning due to less physical activity, but it subsides as physical activity increases. Other symptoms associated with AS are swelling of the eyes, hip pain, loss of appetite, and low-grade fever (Calin, 1994). Men are twice as likely to be at risk of AS than females. About 80% of patients show symptoms of AS below the age of 30 (Louie, 2017).

7.1.5 LUPUS ARTHRITIS (LA)

The disease produces pain and swelling of the joints accompanied by morning stiffness due to the accumulation of fluid. It is an autoimmune disorder affecting about 1.5 million people in the US. Areas that are away from the body like fingers, wrists, feet, and toes are mostly affected. LA produces a symmetric effect, meaning the pain will be felt in the same area on both sides of the body. According to a study, anti-histone antibodies are possibly linked with LA (Hoffman, 2004).

Apart from the above-mentioned arthritis, several other types of arthritis exist, such as Infectious arthritis (infection inside the synovium caused by bacteria, fungi, or viruses), Juvenile arthritis (arthritis in children), Psoriatic arthritis (involving inflammation due to psoriasis), Fibromyalgia (a disorder of musculoskeletal pain along with fatigue).

Treatments available for arthritis include non-steroidal anti-inflammatory drugs like Ibuprofen, Naproxen, and COX-2 inhibitors, Disease-modifying drugs like methotrexate, hydroxychloroquine, minocycline, and immuno-suppressants like azathioprine, cyclosporine, and cyclophosphamide, TNF α inhibitors like Infliximab and Golimumab.

Each of these therapies has its adverse effects. Therefore, finding an alternative to these therapies is vital. Natural treatments include the use of food or parts of food that are termed nutraceuticals for the treatment of arthritis.

7.2 NUTRACEUTICAL

"Nutraceutical" term was coined by Dr. Stephen DeFelice in the year 1989 from "Nutrition" and "Pharmaceutical." DeFelice defines nutraceutical as, "a part of food or whole food that provides medical or health benefits like the prevention and treatment of a disease." But in general, terms used in the market, it has no definite definition (Kalra, 2003). Nutraceuticals and food that function as dietary supplements are similar in many ways (Keservani et al., 2010a, b, 2017, 2020). A number of proposed definitions of nutraceutical exist, which are summarized in Table 7.1.

TABLE 7.1 Nutraceutical Definitions

Author	Definition
DeFelice (1989); Kalra (2003)	"A nutraceutical is any substance that is a food or part of a food and provides medical or health benefits, including the prevention and treatment of disease."
U.S. Nutraceutical Research and Education	"A dietary supplement, food or medical food that has a benefit, which prevents or reduces the risk of a disease or health condition, including the management of a disease or health condition or the improvement of health; and is safe for human consumption in the quantity, and with the frequency required to realize such properties."
Corzo (2020)	"Nutraceuticals are biological substances extracted from natural sources by non-denaturing processes to preserve their original properties without any chemical manipulation."

These nutraceuticals can be obtained from various natural sources like terrestrial botanicals, marine botanicals, and marine animals.

This chapter will mainly focus on nutraceuticals of arthritis medication made from marine sources. The ocean has enormous biodiversity, which accounts for 80% of the world's animal and plant species. From these plants, a variety of biological/chemical components are derived (McCarthy, 2004; Safina, 2016). Various types of stresses are present in the marine environment, which cause marine organisms to produce various types of chemicals to fight against a variety of hazards. Hence, the metabolism of these organisms produces a unique type of bioactive compound (Ahmad, 2019; Kathiresan, 2008). These metabolites can be used as pharmacologically active compounds to treat a variety of diseases and disorders (Haefner, 2003). Marine sources for bioactive compounds were unexplored until recent years. Lately, a variety of new molecules of marine origin have been discovered, developed, and also patented. Almost 25,000 marine chemicals are reported (Newman, 2016). In the upcoming years, there are high chances of the discovery and development of a variety of bioactive compounds and supplements for the treatment of a variety of human diseases (Haefner, 2003). A variety of studies indicate the use of these marine bioactive compounds as anti-diabetic, for the treatment of chronic pain, and cardiovascular diseases, as antibacterial, antiprotozoal, antifungal, and antiviral activity (Mayer, 2020). Also, these marine-derived biologicals can be used for their immunomodulatory and anti-inflammatory properties for the treatment of a variety of arthritic conditions as a nutraceutical.

7.2.1 LITHOTHAMNION CORALLIOIDE

Lithothamnion corallioide is a marine red algae species that is rich in seawater-derived minerals such as calcium and magnesium (AquaminF®). These sea algae-derived minerals have been recently explored for potential impact on the usage of non-steroidal anti-inflammatory drugs. The patients suffering from OA who have undergone a randomized trial of AquaminF® with NSAIDs were found to have more physical performance as compared to NSAIDs (Frestedt, 2009). Also, the combination of this seaweed extract Mg $(OH)^2$ (268 mg) with Lithothamnion (2668 mg) and pine bark extract (120 mg) reduced the dose of analgesics by 72% (Heffernan, 2020). This red algae species can decrease the NFκB pathway, and reduce the activity of inflammatory cytokines like TNF-α, interleukin 1 beta (IL-1β), and COX2, along with reduced serum TNF-α (Murphy, 2014). The above results indicate the use of *Lithothamnion corallioide* for the reduction of doses of NSAIDs for the treatment of OA. This marine-derived nutraceutical on large-scale replication can be utilized for the early treatment of arthritis (Figure 7.1).

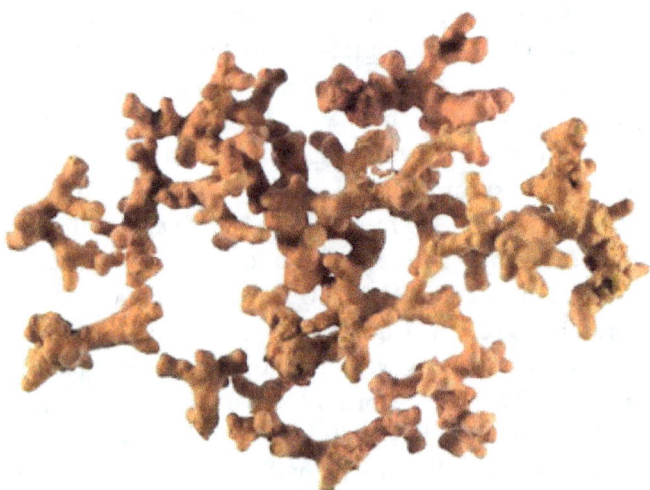

FIGURE 7.1   Marine red algae *"Lithothamnion corallioide."*

7.2.2 PERNA CANALICULUS

Lyprinol® is a lipid extract obtained from the New Zealand Green Lipped Mussel which is enriched in omega-3 fatty acids shown to have anti-inflammatory effects in animal studies as well as in *in-vitro* studies. Lau et al., compared the effects of Lyprinol® with placebo in the treatment of knee OA as well as on the signs and symptoms of OA. Around 80 patients who were suffering from knee OA were treated with Lyprinol® or a placebo in a randomized manner for six months. All 80 patients were allowed paracetamol rescue treatment during the trial and periodically reviewed at 0, 2, 4, 8, 12, 18, and 24 weeks for assessment and safety evaluation of arthritis. Patients were assessed for arthritis on various scales like patient's and physician's global assessment of arthritis, a 100 mm visual analog scale (VAS) for pain, the Oxford Knee Score (OKS) validated Chinese version, a validated Chinese version of the Arthritis Impact Measurement Scale 2-short form (CAIMS2-SF), erythrocyte sedimentation rate (ESR), and C-reactive protein (CRP). All of the arthritis assessment parameters were improved in almost both groups. However, patients treated with Lyprinol® showed greater improvement in the perception of pain on the VAS scale, and the patient's global assessment of arthritis as compared with controls after week 4. Patients treated with only Lyprinol® showed improved scores after week 4 in the CAIMS2-SF physical function and psychological status domains. After six months, Lyprinol® was found to be safe and well-tolerated without any serious side effects. From the study, it can be concluded that Lyprinol®, which is a lipid extract of the green-lipped mussel, may be used for the treatment of OA safely (Lau, 2004) (Figure 7.2).

According to a different study, a fatty preparation of *Perna canaliculus* contains furan fatty acids (F-acids) which are naturally occurring and show potent antioxidant activity. This study found that lipids had strong antioxidant action and the extract may contribute to the anti-inflammatory activity for the OA treatment. Authors found more anti-inflammatory activity in F-acids as compared to eicosatetraenoic acid (EPA) (Wakimoto, 2011) (Figure 7.3).

7.2.3 MARINE SPONGE-DERIVED FUNGI, PESTALOTIOPSIS SPECIES

Lee et al. studied immunosuppressive compounds obtained from *Pestalotiopsis* species of marine sponge-derived fungi secreted in the culture broth. The authors isolated 4-(hydroxymethyl) catechol (4-HMC) from *Pestalotiopsis* species, and by using a murine collagen-induced arthritis (CIA) model, they evaluated the anti-rheumatoid arthritis effects. Additionally, the authors studied the anti-rheumatoid arthritis effects on tumor necrosis factor-α-stimulated human RA synovial fibroblasts. The clinical score of arthritis pain was found to be decreased along with paw thickness, histologic and radiologic changes, and serum IgG1 and IgG2a levels. 4-HMC prohibited the propagation of helper T (Th) 1/Th17 CD4+ lymphocytes, hence reducing

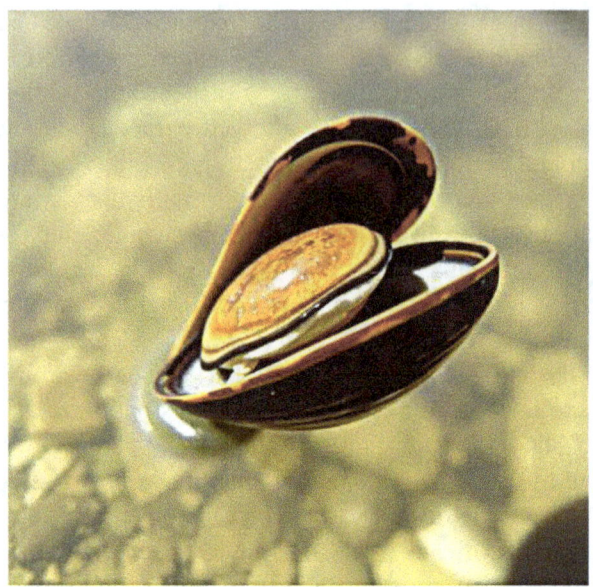

FIGURE 7.2 *Perna canaliculus*, green-lipped mussel.

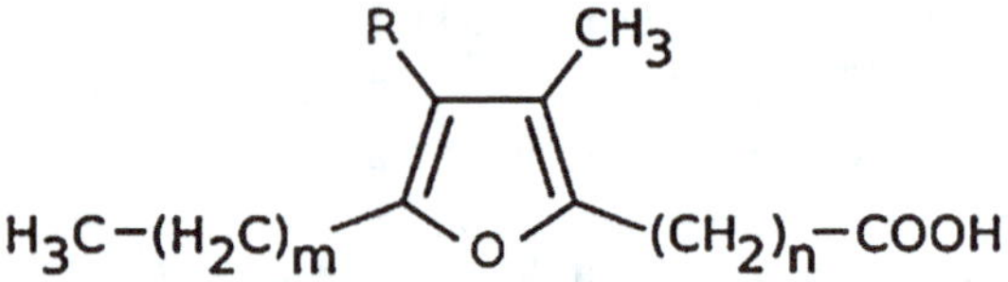

FIGURE 7.3 Furan fatty acid structure.

the production of inflammatory cytokines in CIA mice. 4-HMC showed an *in-vitro* and *in-vivo* decrease in the expression of inflammatory mediators like cytokines and matrix metalloproteinases (MMPs). The authors observed that 4-HMC, by modulating the PI3K/Akt/NF-κB pathway, reduces rheumatoid arthritis (Lee, 2018) (Figure 7.4).

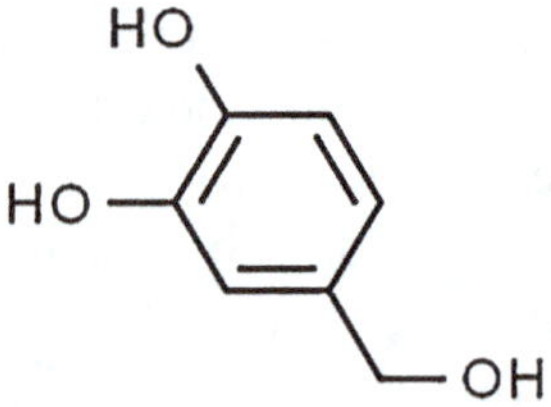

FIGURE 7.4 4-(hydroxymethyl) catechol structure.

7.2.4 KRILL OIL

Krill is a small red-colored crustacean from the Antarctic Ocean from which krill oil is extracted and is edible. Administration of this oil is reported to mitigate pain associated with RA or OA. In the present study, the authors assessed the effect of krill oil on knee pain.

Around 50 adults aged 38 to 85 with mild knee pain were investigated through randomized, double-blind, placebo-controlled trials. Participants were given 2 g per day of either krill oil or an identical placebo for 30 days in a randomized manner.

The reduction of knee discomfort was evaluated using the Japanese Knee Osteoarthritis Measure (JKOM) and Japanese Orthopedic Association score (JOA). Blood and urine biochemical parameters were also studied as secondary outcomes.

The study indicated that both the placebo and krill oil administration showed notable improvements in the JKOM and JOA scores. The krill oil group showed more improvements than the placebo group regarding pain and stiffness in the knees in the JKOM. From this study, it can be concluded that the administration of krill oil (2 g/day for 30 days) enhanced the specific symptoms of adult patients with minor knee discomfort (Suzuki, 2016) (Figure 7.5).

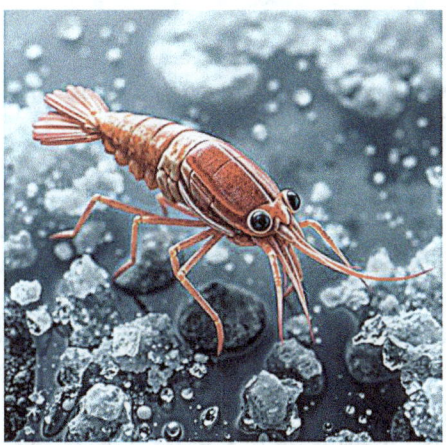

FIGURE 7.5 Antarctic krill.

7.2.5 MARINE N-3 PUFAS FROM FISH OIL

Marine n-3 polyunsaturated fatty acids, mainly eicosatetraenoic acid (EPA) and docosahexaenoic acid (DHA) which are found in oily fish and fish oils, were found to decrease the Arachidonic acid (ARA) content of cells involved in immune responses, also decreasing the generation of eicosanoids responsible for inflammation from ARA. EPA produces eicosanoid mediators that are less inflammatory than those generated from ARA. EPA and DHA produce resolvins that show anti-inflammatory and inflammation-resolving activity. Immunity and inflammation related to RA can also be decreased by Marine n-3 PUFAs, which also affect dendritic cell and T-cell function, causing a decrease in the production of inflammatory cytokines and reactive oxygen species. Fish oil has decreased the development of arthritis in animal models and reduced disease severity. Several studies have been performed on the effect of marine n-3 PUFAs in patients with RA. A methodical review included 23 studies. An indication is observed for the advantage of marine n-3 PUFAs on joint pain and swelling, and the use of non-steroidal anti-inflammatory drugs (Miles, 2012) (Figure 7.6).

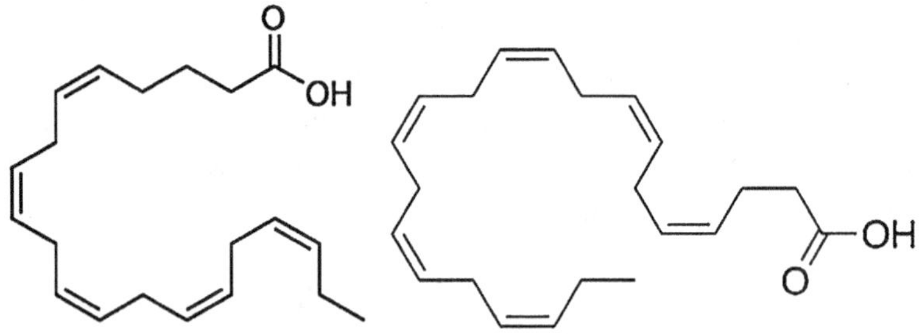

FIGURE 7.6 Structure of eicosatetraenoic acid and docosahexaenoic acid, respectively.

7.2.6 BROWN ALGAE, SARGASSUM WIGHTII

The authors assessed the possible anti-inflammatory and antioxidant use of arthritis-prone rats that were given alginic acid from the brown algae *Sargassum wightii*. Rats were evaluated in various parameters like paw edema volume, cyclooxygenase enzyme, lipoxygenase, and myeloperoxidase, as well as the levels of C-reactive protein and rheumatoid factor for the anti-rheumatic activity of *Sargassum wightii*. Alginic acid, derived from *Sargassum wightii*, treatment (100 mg/kg) in arthritic rats showed decreased paw edema volume and a decrease in levels of various enzymes responsible for inflammation like cyclooxygenase, lipoxygenase, and myeloperoxidase. It was observed that alginic acid also caused a reduction in the levels of CRP and rheumatoid factor. Lipid peroxidation was also reduced, and the activity of the antioxidant enzyme was increased. The histopathological analysis also indicated a reduction in paw edema due to treatment with alginic acid. Experimental findings suggest that

Sargassum wightii-derived alginic acid shows potent anti-inflammatory and antioxidant activity, and this marine alga can be developed as a nutraceutical for the treatment of arthritis (Figures 7.7 and 7.8).

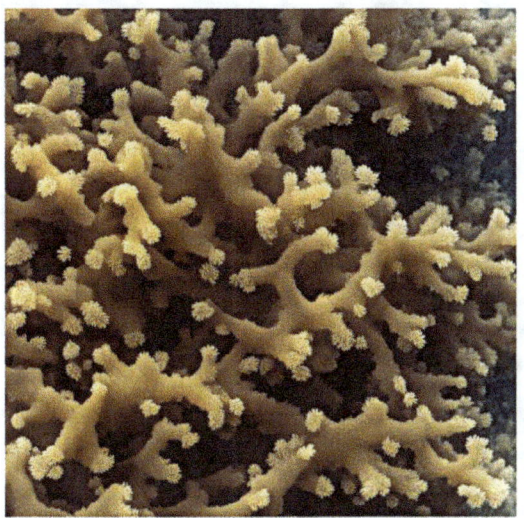

FIGURE 7.7 Brown algae, *Sargassum wightii*.

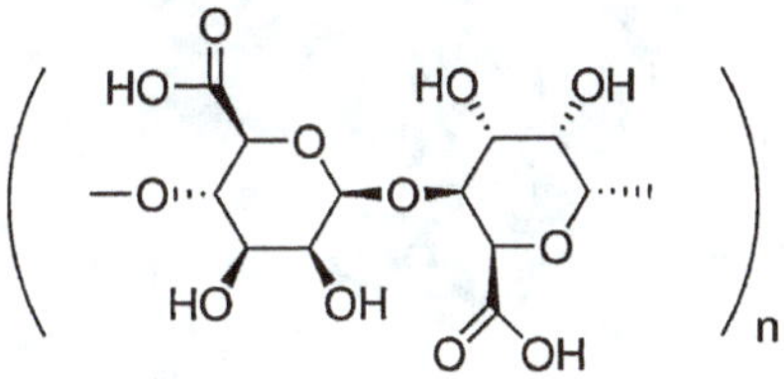

FIGURE 7.8 Structure of alginic acid.

7.2.7 *MYTILUS EDULIS*

Mytilus edulis, blue mussel, also called the common mussel, is a medium-sized eatable marine bivalve mollusk from the family Mytilidae, the mussels. This mussel contains bioactive compounds such as proteins, lipids, and carbohydrates. A higher content of glycogen and lipids is present. Also, it contains PUFAs like eicosapentaenoic acid, which shows anti-inflammatory activity and is useful in the treatment of arthritis. The peptide portion above 5000 Dalton prevents nitric oxide synthase, Prostaglandin E2, and cyclo-oxygenase-2, which are responsible for inflammation. This lipid extract of *Mytilus edulis* is high in non-polar lipids and has anti-inflammatory action. Pet food encompassing extracts of *Mytilus edulis* is used for the preservation of healthy joints and to assuage arthritic symptoms in animals (Bui, 2003) (Figure 7.9).

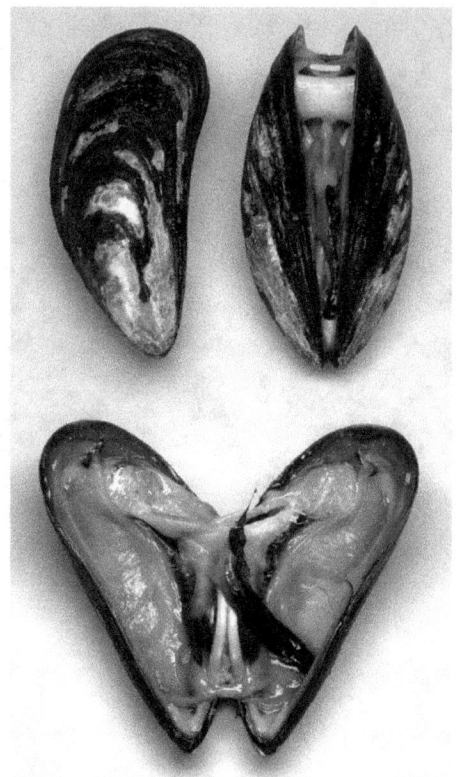

FIGURE 7.9 *Mytilus edulis.*
Image courtesy: Rainer Zenz. https://creativecommons.org/licenses/by-sa/3.0/

7.2.8 ISOSTICHOPUS BADIONTUS

It is also called chocolate chip cucumber and cookie dough sea cucumber of the same family as *Stichopus*. The expression of pro-inflammatory genes of TNFα, iNOS, COX2, NFκB, or IL-6 is suppressed along with the enhancement of the expression of anti-inflammatory genes. Several formulations having anti-inflammatory activity contain sea cucumber. A composition including separate parts of the sea cucumber-like body wall, flower, and epithelial layer shows an anti-inflammatory effect for which they are used as anti-inflammatory agents. The active ingredients present are sulfated polysaccharides, sterol glycosides, saponins, lactones, peptides, and glycogens. It helps in increasing elasticity and shows anti-inflammatory activity against arthritis (Leticia, 2018) (Figure 7.10).

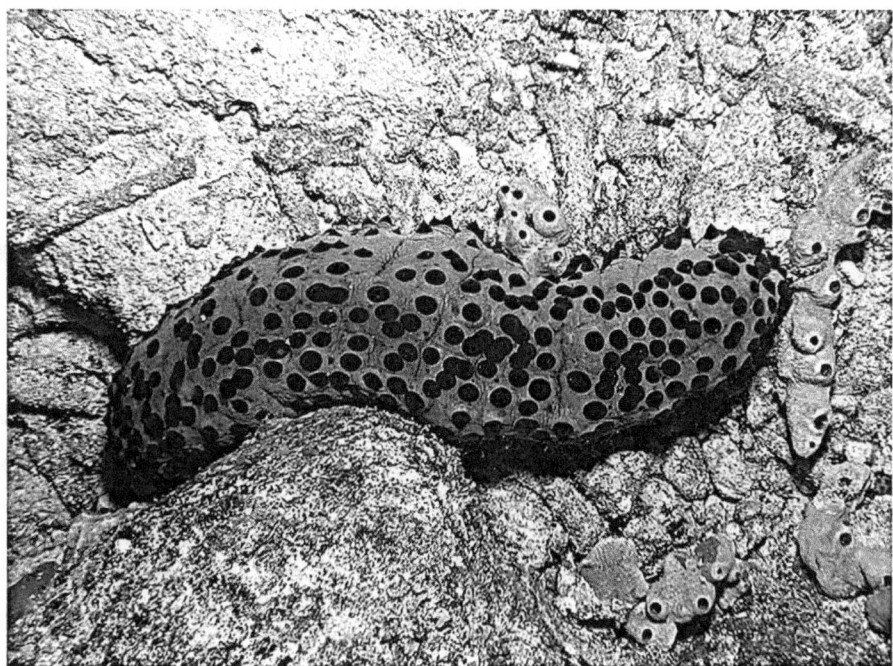

FIGURE 7.10 *Isostichopus badiontus*.

Image courtesy: Daniel Hershman from Federal Way, US. https://creativecommons.org/licenses/by/2.0/

7.2.9 SHELLFISH-DERIVED GLUCOSAMINE

Glucosamine is derived from chitin, which is obtained from the shells of shellfish and is very popular among consumers for the treatment of OA. Glucosamine is an essential non-cellular component of connective tissue, cartilage, ligaments, and other structures. Nutraceuticals rich in glucosamine generate a precursor, one of the major components of joint cartilage, called glycosaminoglycans. Supplements rich in glucosamine help to rebuild cartilage. Glucosamine is generally used in the form of glucosamine sulfate. A typical dosage of glucosamine is 1,500 mg per day. Glucosamine is also extensively used in veterinary medicine as an unregulated but widely accepted supplement. Glucosamine is found to play a role in a variety of diseases like osteoporosis, pain, psoriasis, depression, fibromyalgia, athletic injuries, back pain, kidney stones, and spondylosis deformation. Glucosamine also acts as an immunosuppressant for autoimmune diseases (Figure 7.11).

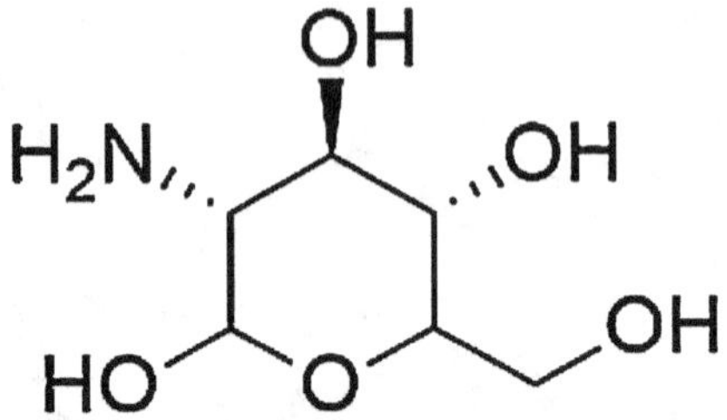

FIGURE 7.11 Structure of glucosamine.

A randomized, double-blind, placebo-controlled study using glucosamine was conducted by Reginster et al., which indicated that the use of glucosamine improved symptoms of OA by WOMAC scoring in a three-year study (Reginster, 2001).

Pavelká et al., performed randomized, double-blind placebo-controlled trials of glucosamine for arthritis with a 1,500 mg dose, which showed prevention of loss of articular space and amelioration of pain as assessed by WOMAC scoring in a three-year follow-up (Pavelká, 2002).

Herrero-Beaumont et al. investigated the effect of 1,500 mg daily through a randomized, double-blind, placebo-controlled study. They observed that glucosamine can be used for symptomatic treatment of knee OA (Herrero-Beaumont, 2007).

7.2.10 TURBINARIA ORNATE MICROALGAE

T. ornata macroalgae possesses various biological activities because of the various biomolecules present in it. Ananthi et al. performed a study to assess the anti-arthritic effect of the aqueous extract and the sulfated polysaccharide isolated from *T. ornata* by use of Complete Freund's Adjuvant (CFA)-induced arthritis in rats. The anti-arthritic effect of aqueous *T. ornata* & *T. ornata* sulfated polysaccharide was demonstrated by the noteworthy drop in paw volume and arthritic score. Levels of inflammatory and antioxidant markers were decreased in the drug-treated groups when compared with dexamethasone. The antiarthritic potential of aqueous *T. ornata* & *T. ornata* sulfated polysaccharide was found to be supported by histopathological and radiological examination. It is observed that sulfated polysaccharide in a very low dose stops inflammation and bone damage. Hence, TSP could be a potential candidate for chronic inflammatory diseases like rheumatoid arthritis management (Ananthi, 2017) (Figure 7.12).

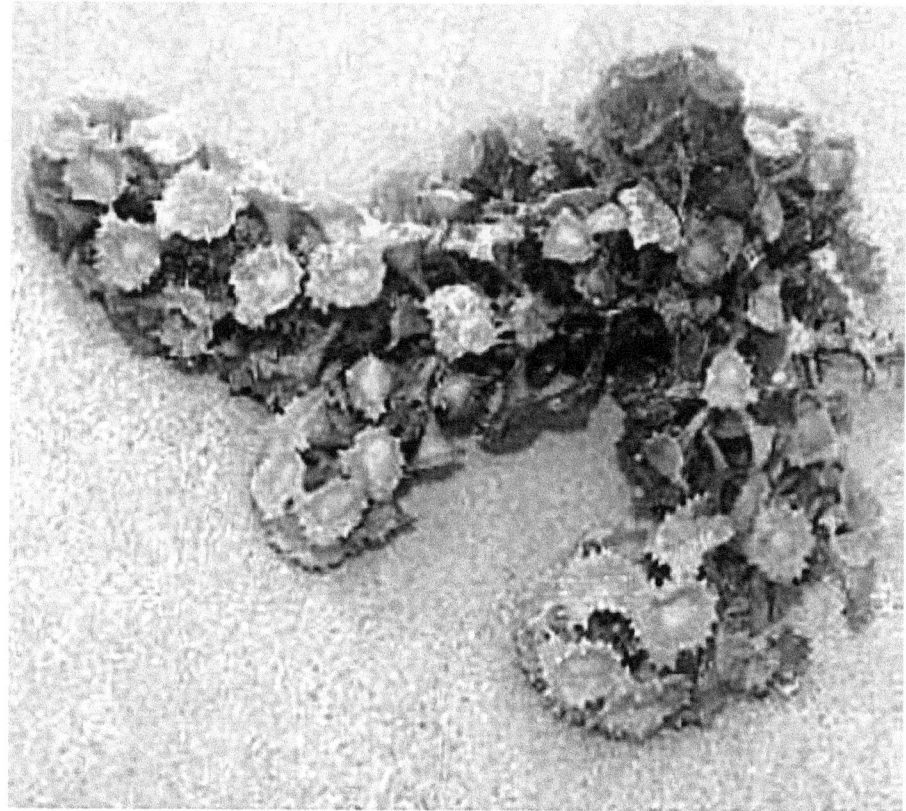

FIGURE 7.12 *Turbinaria ornate* microalgae.

Source: Reprinted from Deyab et al., 2012. http://creativecommons.org/licenses/by/4.0/.

7.2.11 MARINE GREEN ALGAE, CAULERPA RACEMOSA

Lavanya R. and her co-workers evaluated the antioxidant and anti-arthritic activity of *Caulerpa racemosa* methanolic extract. The protein denaturation method was used to study the *in-vitro* anti-arthritic activity. The methanolic extract showed 49.33±0.597% percentage inhibition at 1,000 μg/0.05 ml by the protein denaturation method. Results indicated that the methanolic extract of *Caulerpa racemosa* possesses significant antioxidant and antiarthritic activity (Lavanya, 2014) (Figure 7.13).

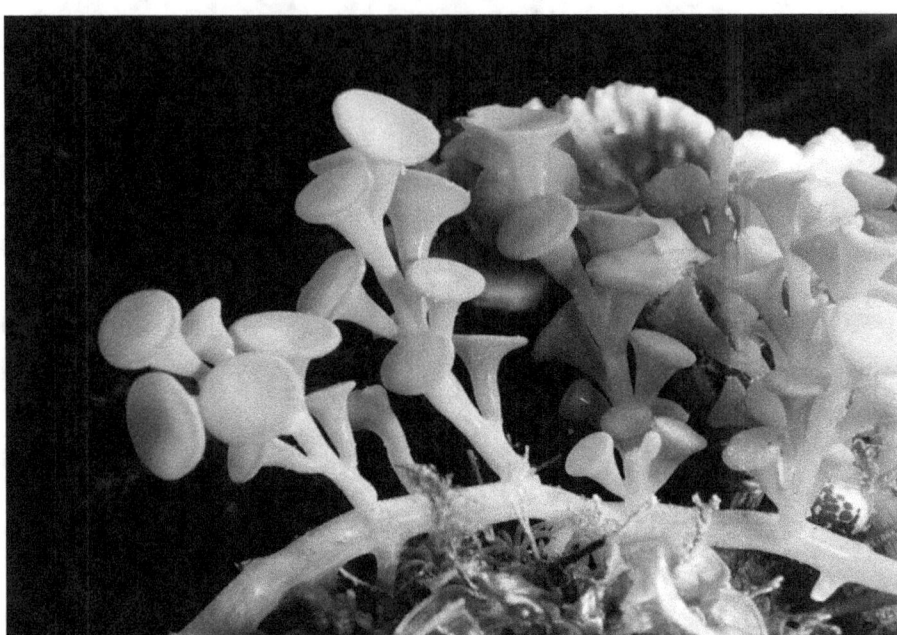

FIGURE 7.13 *Caulerpa racemose.*
Image courtesy: Nhobgood Nick Hobgood. https://creativecommons.org/licenses/by-sa/3.0/

7.2.12 FORMOSA SOFT CORAL SINULARIA QUERCIFORMIS

Lin and co-workers isolated 11-epi-sinulariolide acetate (Ya-s11, a cembrane-type compound) from the Formosa soft coral *Sinularia querciformis* having anti-inflammatory effects. An initial study showed inhibition of expression of the pro-inflammatory proteins induced nitric oxide synthase and cyclo-oxygenase-2 in lipopolysaccharide-stimulated murine macrophages because of Ya-s11. The authors also studied the therapeutic properties of Ya-s11 on adjuvant-induced arthritis in female Lewis rats. Animal experiments discovered that Ya-s11 in the dose of 9 mg/kg subcutaneously once every 2 days significantly inhibited adjuvant-induced arthritis characteristics. Furthermore, Ya-s11 also weakened the protein appearance of cathepsin K, matrix metalloproteinases-9 (MMP-9), tartrate-resistant acid phosphatase (TRAP), and tumor necrosis factor-α (TNF-α) in ankle tissues of adjuvant-induced arthritis rats. Based on its weakening of the expression of proinflammatory proteins and disease progression in adjuvant-induced arthritis rats, the marine-derived compound Ya-s11 may help as a therapeutic agent for the treatment of RA (Lin, 2013) (Figure 7.14).

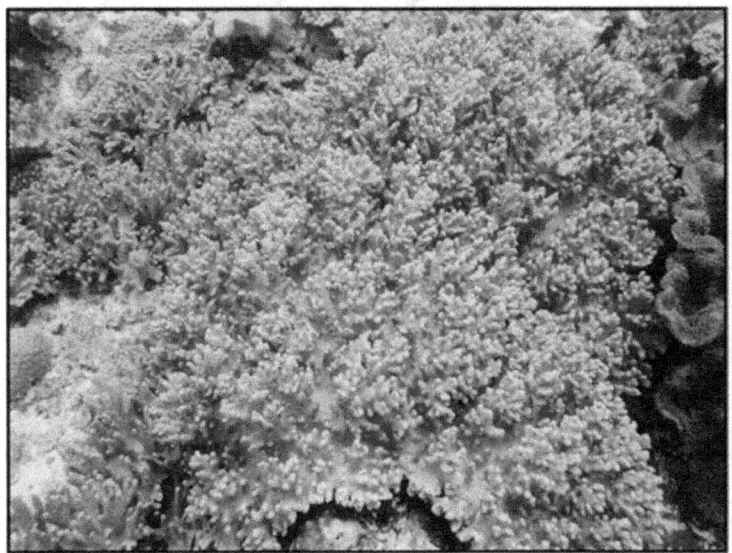

FIGURE 7.14 *Sinularia querciformis.*
Source: Reprinted from Cooper et al., 2024. https://creativecommons.org/licenses/by/3.0/

7.2.13 UNDARIA PINNATIFIDA

Undaria pinnatifida is a type of edible seaweed that belongs to the Alariaceae family. This alga contains polysaccharides, fucoxanthin, and a considerable number of proteins, as well as stearidonic acid, Eicosa Pentaenoic Acid (EPA), and arachidonic acid. Low concentrations of arachidonic acid and stearidonic acid have been proven to be effective against ear irritation. The anti-inflammatory mechanism of fucoxanthin is similar to that of fucoidans and analogous to that of steroidal anti-inflammatory medications (Figure 7.15).

Several anti-inflammatory compositions based on microalgae have received patent protection. A composition containing monogalactosyldiacylglycerol (GDG-EPA) and algae from the genera *Chlorella, Chaetoceros, Cyclotella, Ellipsoidon, Isochrysis, Nannochloris, Nannochloropsis* is reported to have an anti-inflammatory effect (Hui, 2014).

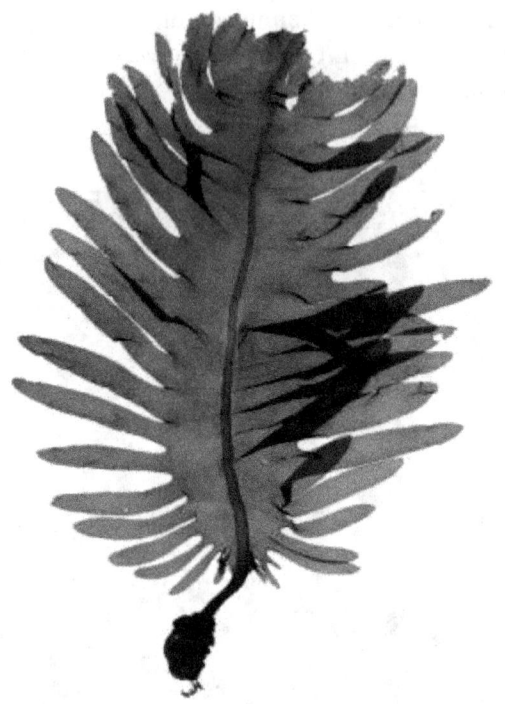

FIGURE 7.15 *Undaria pinnatifida.*

Image courtesy: Te Papa. https://marinebiosecurity.org.nz/undaria-pinnatifida-harvey-suringar/

Skin irritation can also be treated with a topical dermal anti-inflammatory microalgal lipid formulation. An anti-inflammatory skin spray formulation based on *Undaria pinnatifida* extract has been patented. Stearidonic acid (SDA) and -linolenic acid (GLA) dihydroxyoxylipins derived from microalgae operate as substrates for the generation of new oxylipins and also as anti-inflammatory compounds.

A composition containing an algae-based oil derived from the microalgae *N. oculata, Thalassiosira* sp., *Tetraselmis* sp., *Chaetoceros* sp., *Isochrysis* sp. containing a mixture of glycolipids, phospholipids, and Eicosapentaenoic (EPA) fatty acids in combination with astaxanthin in an oral dosage.

7.2.14 HALICHONDRIA SITIENS

From the *Halichondria sitiens* species, several bioactive compounds with anti-inflammatory potential have been identified from the lipophilic fractions. Dendritic cells secrete less IL-12 and IL-6, and their potential to generate a Th1 response in allogeneic CD4$^+$ T cells is reduced by lipophilic fractions (Die, 2017).

Several anti-inflammatory compositions have included marine sponges. Anti-inflammatory effects can be achieved with a therapeutically effective combination of manoalide, seco-manoalide, or dehydro-secomanoalide. One of the patents proposes a method for assessing the anti-inflammatory capabilities of a marine sponge compound based on cell aggregation inhibition.

Bis-heterocyclic alkaloid compounds identified from marine sponges, such as topsentins, bromotopsentins, homocarbonyltopsentins, nortopsentins, hamacanthins, bis-indoleethylamines, or dragmacidins, have anti-inflammatory effects.

Collagen nanoparticles produced from marine sponges are effective in reducing inflammation caused by cyclooxygenase. A skincare product containing peptides obtained from sponges functions as a UV ray protector and/or antiphlogistic agent.

The anticancer, antiviral, and anti-inflammatory properties of a formulation containing the novel bioactive chemical Sorbicillactone A from marine sponges have been studied (Bringmann, 2004) (Figure 7.16).

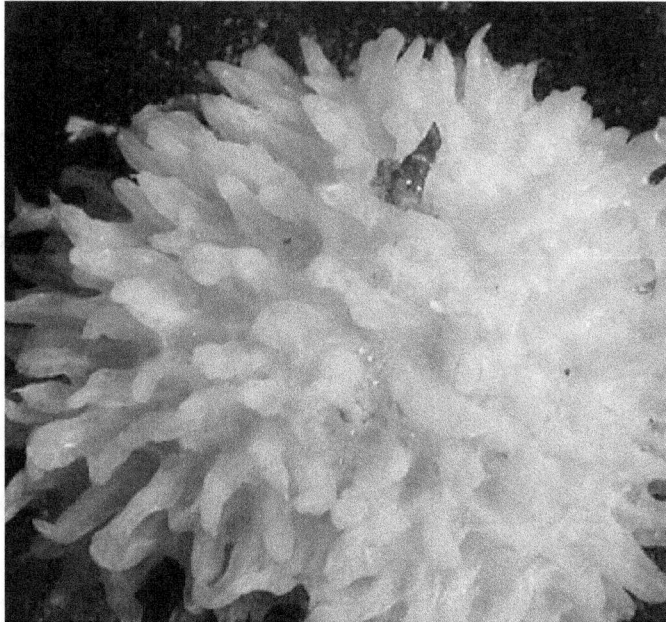

FIGURE 7.16 *Halichondria sitiens.*
Source: Reprinted from Gerasimova and Ereskovsky, 2007.

7.2.15 PAPHIA MALABARICA

Marine bivalves make up a large portion of the total edible mollusks found around the coasts of Southeast Asia, and they have been proven to have substantial nutritional and ecological potential. Various *in-vitro* evaluations for antioxidant and anti-inflammatory activity guided purification of the ethyl acetate-methanol (EtOAc-MeOH) extract from the bivalve clam *Paphia malabarica*, which resulted in the identification of two new sterol derivatives: 23-gem-dimethylcholesta-5-en-3-ol (1) and (22E)-24^1,24^2-methyldihomocholest-5,22-dien-3β-ol. Based on 1D, and 2D NMR spectroscopy, and mass spectrometry, their structures were unambiguously assigned.

The antioxidant and anti-inflammatory properties of the above 2 were substantially stronger (IC_{50} 1 mg/mL) than 1 (IC_{50} > 1 mg/mL) as evaluated by DPPH/ABTS+ radical scavenging and anti-cyclooxygenase-2/5-lipoxygenase assays. The bioactivities of these compounds were precisely related to the electronic and lipophilic characteristics, according to a structure-activity relationship analysis. This is the first time that 23-gem-dimethyl-3-hydroxy-5-cholestane nucleus and C-30 dihomosterol have been found and characterized in marine creatures (Sukumaran, 2019) (Figure 7.17).

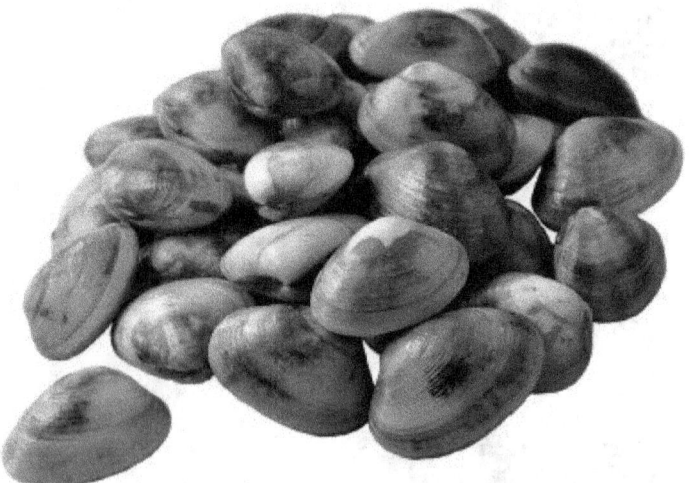

FIGURE 7.17 *Paphia malabarica.*

Source: Reprinted with permission from Sukumaran, 2019. Copyright © 2019 Elsevier B.V. All rights reserved.

7.3 CONCLUSION

About 70% of the Earth's area is covered by the ocean. The ocean is the home of numerous organisms including fish, algae, mollusks, seaweed, and other species. The marine source has a huge biodiversity. Adaptation of marine species to the marine environment is quite difficult, and hence to adapt to this environment, marine species produce a variety of bioactive chemicals effective against a variety of disorders. Hence, these species have been utilized for ages as food for their benefit. Such food articles having health benefits are called nutraceuticals. These nutraceuticals are also utilized for the treatment of arthritis. A variety of marine sources like sponges, corals, mollusks, seaweed, algae, and microalgae have the potential to be used in the treatment of arthritis as an anti-inflammatory agent and as a nutraceutical. These sources contain a number of bioactive substances which, through different mechanisms like inhibition of various enzymes like COX, by decreasing the NFκB pathway and reducing the activity of inflammatory cytokines like TNF-α, interleukin 1β (IL-1β), act as an anti-inflammatory agent and reduce the pain and swelling in various types of arthritis. Nowadays, a number of commercial products are present in the market as nutraceuticals for the treatment of arthritis. Also, in the future, marine nutraceuticals will prove their usefulness in the treatment of a variety of disorders along with arthritis.

KEYWORDS

- anti-inflammatory agent
- arthritis
- C-reactive protein
- erythrocyte sedimentation rate
- Oxford knee score
- rheumatoid arthritis
- visual analog scale

REFERENCES

Act USNRaE. H.R.3001–Nutraceutical Research and Education Act. (106th Congress of 1999–2000): U.S. Congress; 1999 [Available from: https://www.congress.gov/bill/106th-congress/house-bill/3001?q=%7B%22search%22%3A%5B%22Nutraceutical+Research+and+Education+Act%22% (accessed on 6 June 2024).

Ahmad, B., Shah, M., & Choi, S. (2019). Oceans as a source of immunotherapy. *Marine Drugs, 17*(5), 282. https://doi.org/10.3390/md17050282.

Aletaha, D., Neogi, T., Silman, A. J., et al. (2010). Rheumatic arthritis classification criteria: An American College of Rheumatology/European League Against Rheumatism—A collaborative initiative. *Annals of the Rheumatic Diseases, 69*(9), 1580–1588. https://doi.org/10.1136/ard.2010.138461.

Ananthi, S., Gayathri, V., Malarvizhi, R., et al. (2017). The anti-arthritic potential of marine macroalgae *Turbinaria ornata* in Complete Freund's Adjuvant induced rats. *Experimental and Toxicologic Pathology, 69*(8), 672–680. https://doi.org/10.1016/j.etp.2017.06.006.

Bringmann, G., Gerhard, L., Muchlbacher, J., et al. (2004). New compounds sorbicillactone A and derivatives, useful as antitumor, antiviral, and anti-inflammatory agents, obtained, e.g., by culturing *Penicillium* fungi. DE10238257.

Bui, L. M., Bierer, T. L., Hodge, J., Bektash, R., & Blackwood, G. (2003). Pet food for maintenance of joint health and alleviation of arthritic symptoms in companion animals. US6596303.

Calin, A., Brophy, S., & Blake, D. (1999). Impact of sex on the inheritance of ankylosing spondylitis: A cohort study. *Lancet, 354*(9191), 1687–1690. https://doi.org/10.1016/S0140-6736(99)03219-5.

Calin, A., Garrett, S., Whitelock, H., Kennedy, L. et al. (1994). A new approach to defining disease status in ankylosing spondylitis. *Current Opinion in Rheumatology, 20*(4), 384–391.

Centers for Disease Control and Prevention (CDC). (2017). Library of Congress Catalog Number 76 –641496 For sale by Superintendent of Documents U. S. Government Printing Office Washington, DC 20402. https://www.ncbi.nlm.nih.gov/books/NBK453378/pdf/Bookshelf_NBK453378.pdf (accessed on 6 June 2024).

Cooper, E., Hirabayashi, K., Strychar K., Sammarco, P., (2014). Corals and Their Potential Applications to Integrative Medicine. Evidence-based Complementary and Alternative Medicine. 2014. 10.1155/2014/184959.

Corzo, L., Fernández-Novoa, L., Carrera, I., Martínez, O., Rodríguez, S., Alejo, R., & Cacabelos, R. (2020). Nutrition, health, and disease: Role of selected marine and vegetal nutraceuticals. *Nutrients, 12*(3), 747–749. https://doi.org/10.3390/nu12030747.

Deshpande, B. R., Katz, J. N., Solomon, D. H., et al. (2016). Number of persons with symptomatic knee osteoarthritis in the US: Impact of race and ethnicity, age, sex, and obesity. *Arthritis Care and Research, 68*(12), 1743–1750. https://doi.org/10.1002/acr.22897.

Deyab, M., Habbak, L., Ward, F. & Deyab,. (2012). ANTITUMOR ACTIVITY OF WATER EXTRACT AND SOME FATTY ACIDS OF TURBINARIA ORNATA (TURNER) J. AGARDH. 199–204.

Di, X., Oskarsson, J. T., Omarsdottir, S., et al. (2017). Lipophilic fractions from the marine sponge *Halichondria sitiens* decrease the secretion of pro-inflammatory cytokines by dendritic cells and decrease their ability to induce a Th1-type response by allogeneic CD4 + T cells. *Pharmaceutical Biology, 55*(1), 2116–2122. https://doi.org/10.1080/13880209.2017.1373832.

Fessel, W. J. (1974). Systemic lupus erythematosus in the community. Incidence, prevalence, outcome, and first symptoms; the high prevalence in black women. *Archives of Internal Medicine, 134*(6), 1027–1035. https://doi.org/10.1001/archinte.134.6.1027.

Frestedt, J. L., Kuskowski, M. A., & Zenk, J. L. (2009). A natural seaweed derived mineral supplement (Aquamin F) for knee osteoarthritis: A randomized, placebo-controlled pilot study. *Nutrition Journal, 8*, 7. https://doi.org/10.1186/1475-2891-8-7.

Gerasimova, & Ereskovsky, Alexander. (2007). Reproduction of two species of Halichondria (Demospongiae: Halichondriidae) in the White Sea.

Guy, T., & Michaelstein, C. (2010) Ch.-R. In *The Encyclopedia of Arthritis* (2nd ed) (pp. 228–255). Infobase Publishing, Inc.

Haefner, B. (2003). Drugs from the deep: Marine natural products as drug candidates. *Drug Discovery Today, 8*(12), 536–544. https://doi.org/10.1016/s1359-6446(03)02713-2.

Heffernan, S. M., McCarthy, C., Eustace, S., et al. (2020). Mineral-rich algae with pine bark improved pain, physical function and analgesic use in mild-knee joint osteoarthritis, compared to glucosamine: A randomized controlled pilot trial. *Complementary Therapies in Medicine, 50*, 102349. https://doi.org/10.1016/j.ctim.2020.102349.

Herrero-Beaumont, G., Ivorra, J. A., Del Carmen Trabado, M., et al. (2007). Glucosamine sulfate in the treatment of knee osteoarthritis symptoms: A randomized, double-blind, placebo-controlled study using acetaminophen as a side comparator. *Arthritis and Rheumatism, 56*(2), 555–567. https://doi.org/10.1002/art.22371.

Hoffman, I. E., Peene, I., Meheus, L., et al. (2004). Specific anti-nuclear antibodies are associated with clinical features in systemic lupus erythematosus. *Annals of the Rheumatic Diseases, 63*(9), 1155–1158. https://doi.org/10.1136/ard.2003.013417.

Jaakkola, E., Herzberg, I., Laiho, K., et al. (2006). Finnish HLA studies confirm the increased risk conferred by HLA–B27 homozygosity in ankylosing spondylitis. *Annals of the Rheumatic Diseases, 65*(6), 775–780. https://doi.org/10.1136/ard.2005.041103.

Kalra, E. K. (2003). Nutraceutical definition and introduction. *AAPS PharmSci, 5*(3), E25. https://doi.org/10.1208/ps050325.

Kathiresan, K., Nabeel, M. A., & Manivannan, S. (2008). Bioprospecting of marine organisms for novel bioactive compounds. *Sci. Trans. Enviorn. Technovation, 1*, 107–120.

Kean, W. F., Kean, R., & Buchanan, W. W. (2004). Osteoarthritis: Symptoms, signs, and source of pain. *Inflammopharmacology, 12*(1), 3–31. https://doi.org/10.1163/156856004773121347.

Keservani, R. K., Kesharwani, R. K., Sharma, A. K., Vyas, N., & Chadoker, A. (2010b). Nutritional Supplements: An Overview. *International Journal of Current Pharmaceutical Review and Research, 1*(1), 59–75.

Keservani, R. K., Kesharwani, R. K., Vyas, N., Jain, S., Raghuvanshi, R., & Sharma, A. K. (2010a). Nutraceutical and functional food as future food: a review. *Der Pharmacia Lettre, 2*(1), 106–116.

Keservani, R. K., Sharma, A. K., & Kesharwani, R. K. (2017). An overview and therapeutic applications of nutraceutical and functional foods. *Recent Advances in Drug Delivery Technology, 1*, 160–201. ISBN:9781522507543.

Keservani, R. K., Sharma, A. K., & Kesharwani, R. K. (Eds.). (2020). *Nutraceuticals and Dietary Supplements: Applications in Health Improvement and Disease Management*, Apple Academic Press, CRC Press. pp. 1–344. ISBN: 9781771888738.

Lau, C. S., Chiu, P. K. Y., Chu, E. M. Y., et al. (2004). Treatment of knee osteoarthritis with Lyprinol®, lipid extract of the green-lipped mussel – A double-blind placebo-controlled study. *Progress in Nutrition, 6*(1), 17–31.

Lawrence, R. C., Felson, D. T., Helmick, et al. (2008). Estimates of the prevalence of arthritis and other rheumatic conditions in the United States. Part II. *Arthritis and Rheumatism, 58*(1), 26–35. https://doi.org/10.1002/art.23176.

Lee, J. Y., Kim, G. J., Choi, J. K., et al. (2018). 4-(Hydroxymethyl) catechol extracted from fungi in marine sponges attenuates rheumatoid arthritis by inhibiting PI3K/Akt/NF-κB signaling. *Frontiers in Pharmacology, 9*, 726. https://doi.org/10.3389/fphar.2018.00726.

Lin, Y. Y., Jean, Y. H., Lee, H. P., et al. (2013). A soft coral-derived compound, 11-epi-Sinulariolide acetate suppresses the inflammatory response and bone destruction in adjuvant-induced arthritis. *PLOS ONE, 8*(5), e62926. https://doi.org/10.1371/journal.pone.0062926.

Louie, G. (2024). Ankylosing spondylitis. Retrieved from: https://www.hopkinsarthritis.org/arthritis-info/ankylosing-spondylitis/ (accessed on 6 June 2024). Johns Hopkins University.

Maiese, K. (2016). Picking a bone with WISP1 (CCN4): New strategies against degenerative joint disease. *Journal of Translational Science, 1*(3), 83–85. https://doi.org/10.15761/JTS.1000120.

Mayer, A. M. S., Guerrero, A. J., Rodríguez, A. D., Taglialatela-Scafati, O., Nakamura, F., & Fusetani, N. (2019). Marine pharmacology in 2014–2015: Marine compounds with antibacterial, antidiabetic, antifungal, anti-inflammatory, antiprotozoal, antituberculosis, antiviral, and anthelmintic activities; Affecting the immune and nervous systems, and other miscellaneous mechanisms of action. *Marine Drugs, 18*(1), 5. https://doi.org/10.3390/md18010005.

McCarthy, P. J., & Pomponi, S. (2004). A search for new pharmaceutical drugs from marine organisms. *Biomedical Research, March, 22*, 1–2.

Miles, E. A., & Calder, P. C. (2012). Influence of marine n-3 polyunsaturated fatty acids on immune function and a systematic review of their effects on clinical outcomes in rheumatoid arthritis. *British Journal of Nutrition, 107*(Suppl. 2), S171–S184. https://doi.org/10.1017/S0007114512001560.

Mitra, S. P. (2012). The biochemical and physiological implication of Gout—A review. *American Journal of Bio pharmacology, Biochemistry, and Life Sciences, 1*, 1–35.

Mitsuyama, H., Healey, R. M., Terkeltaub, R. A., et al. (2007). Calcification of human articular knee cartilage is primarily an effect of aging rather than osteoarthritis. *Osteoarthritis and Cartilage, 15*(5), 559–565. https://doi.org/10.1016/j.joca.2006.10.017.

Murphy, C. T., Martin, C., Doolan, A. M., et al. (2014). The marine-derived, multi-mineral formula, AquaPT reduces TNF-α levels in osteoarthritis patients. *Journal of Nutrition Health Food Science, 2*, 1–3.

Newman, D. J., & Cragg, G. M. (2016). Drugs and drug candidates from marine sources: An assessment of the current "state of play." *Planta Medica, 82*(9–10), 775–789. https://doi.org/10.1055/s-0042-101353.

Olivera-Castillo, L., Grant, G., Kantún-Moreno, N., et al. (2018). Sea cucumber (*Isostichopus badionotus*) body-wall preparations exert anti-inflammatory activity in vivo. *PharmaNutrition, 6*(2), 74–80. https://doi.org/10.1016/j.phanu.2018.03.002.

Pavelká, K., Gatterová, J., Olejarová, M., et al. (2002). Glucosamine sulfate use and delay of progression of knee osteoarthritis: A 3-year, randomized, placebo-controlled, double-blind study. *Archives of Internal Medicine, 162*(18), 2113–2123. https://doi.org/10.1001/archinte.162.18.2113.

Prakash, S., Mehra, N. K., Bhargava, S., Vaidya, M. C., & Malaviya, A. N. (1984). Ankylosing spondylitis in North India: A clinical and immunogenetic study. *Ann. Rheumat, 43*(3), 381–385. https://doi.org/10.1136/ard.43.3.381.

Reginster, J. Y., Deroisy, R., Rovati, L. C., et al. (2001). Long-term effects of glucosamine sulfate on osteoarthritis progression: A randomized, placebo-controlled clinical trial. *Lancet, 357*(9252), 251–256. https://doi.org/10.1016/S0140-6736(00)03610-2.

Safina, C., & Paladines, P. (2016). Oceans: Abode of nutraceuticals, pharmaceuticals, and biotoxins. In *Routledge Handbook of Religion and Ecology* (pp. 153–174). Elsevier.

Sankar, M. (2013). Arthritis: Classification, nature & cause – A review. *American Journal of Bio-Pharmacology Biochemistry and Life Sciences, 2*(3), 01–19.

Sarithakumari, C. H., Renju, G. L., & Kurup, G. M. (2013). Anti-inflammatory and antioxidant potential of alginic acid isolated from the marine algae, Sargassum wightii on adjuvant-induced arthritic rats. *Inflammopharmacology, 21*(3), 261–268. https://doi.org/10.1007/s10787-012-0159-z.

Smolen, J. S., Aletaha, D., & McInnes, I. B. (2016). Rheumatoid arthritis. *The Lancet, 388*(10055), 2023–2038. https://doi.org/10.1016/S0140-6736(16)30173-8.

Sukumaran, S., Mohamed, K. S., Asokan, P. K., et al. (2019). Morphological and molecular investigations reveal that *Paphia malabarica* from Indian waters is not synonymous with Paphia (Protapes) gallus. *Regional Studies in Marine Science, 27*, 2019. https://doi.org/10.1016/j.rsma.2019.100549.

Sumanya, H., Lavanya, R., & Umamaheswara Reddy, C. (2015). Evaluation of in vitro antioxidant and anti-arthritic activity of methanolic extract of marine green algae *Caulerpa racemosa*. *International Journal of Pharmacy and Pharmaceutical Sciences, 7*(7), 340–343.

Sun, Q., Zhen, G., Li, T. P., Guo, Q., et al. (2021). Parathyroid hormone attenuates osteoarthritis pain by remodeling subchondral bone in mice. *eLife, 10*, e66532. https://doi.org/10.7554/eLife.66532.

Suzuki, Y., Fukushima, M., Sakuraba, K., et al. (2016). Krill oil improves mild knee joint pain: A randomized control trial. *PLOS ONE, 11*(10), e0162769. https://doi.org/10.1371/journal.pone.0162769.

Van Vollenhoven, R., Dore, R. K., Chen, K., et al. (2018). Impact of 12 weeks of Upadacitinib treatment on individual and composite disease measures in patients with rheumatoid arthritis and inadequate response to conventional synthetic or biologic DMARDs. *Arthritis and Rheumatology, 70*(Suppl. 10), 1–4.

Wakimoto, T., Kondo, H., Nii, H., et al. (2011). Furan fatty acid as an anti-inflammatory component from the green-lipped mussel *Perna canaliculus*. *Proceedings of the National Academy of Sciences of the United States of America, 108*(42), 17533–17537. https://doi.org/10.1073/pnas.1110577108.

Wilson, L., & Saseen, J. J. (2016). Gouty arthritis: A review of acute management and prevention. *Pharmacotherapy, 36*(8), 906–922. https://doi.org/10.1002/phar.1788.

Zhang, H., Pang, Z., & Han, C. (2014). *Undaria pinnatifida* (wakame): A seaweed with pharmacological properties. *Science International, 2*(2), 32–36. https://doi.org/10.17311/sciintl.2014.32.36.

Zhu, Y., Pandya, B. J., & Choi, H. K. (2011). Prevalence of gout and hyperuricemia in the U.S. general population: The National Health and Nutrition Examination Survey 2007-2008. *Arthritis Rheumatology, 63*(10), 3136–3141. https://doi.org/10.1002/art.30520.

PART II
NUTRACEUTICALS IN PSORIASIS MANAGEMENT AND PREVENTIONS

CHAPTER 8

A COMPREHENSIVE REVIEW ON DIET AND PSORIASIS

PANKAJ G. JAIN,[1] AFSAR S. PATHAN,[1] EKNATH D. AHIRE,[2] KHEMCHAND R. SURANA,[3] RAJ K. KESERVANI,[4] and SWATI G. TALELE[5]

[1]Department of Pharmacology, R.C. Patel Institute of Pharmaceutical Education and Research, Shirpur, Maharashtra, India

[2]Department of Pharmaceutics, MET's Institute of Pharmacy, Bhujbal Knowledge City, Adgaon, Nashik, Maharashtra, India

[3]Department of Pharmaceutical Chemistry, Divine College of Pharmacy, Satana, Maharashtra, India

[4]Associate Professor, Faculty of B. Pharmacy, CSM Group of Institutions, Prayagraj, Uttar Pradesh, India

[5]Department of Pharmaceutics, Sandip Institute of Pharmaceutical Sciences, Mahiravani, Nashik, Maharashtra, India

ABSTRACT

Psoriasis is defined as a persistent, non-communicable skin condition that has no known origin or cure. With a major impact on people's lives, psoriasis affects all ages. The reported prevalence of psoriasis in countries ranges from 0.09% to 11.43%, making it one of the most common skin diseases that affects both males and females. There are uncertain symptoms with a variety of causes, such as environmental causes and comorbidity with other diseases. It is necessary to address this situation, but most treatments have no results or time-dependent results. Some of the pathophysiology behind psoriasis is oxidation and reactive oxygen species. We all know that a healthy diet containing nutrition with biologically active ingredients and having antioxidant, anti-inflammatory, and anti-aging properties is useful for improving skin tone and condition. In this chapter, we will focus on insights from psoriasis and what constitutes a good diet for psoriasis.

8.1 INTRODUCTION

Psoriasis is regarded as an autoimmune disease; the disease's name comes from the Greek word "psora," which means "itch." Psoriasis is a non-contagious, dehydrated, inflammatory, and unsightly skin disorder that can affect a person's entire system. It is characterized by highly marginated scaly, erythematous patches that grow in a somewhat symmetrical pattern and are mostly hereditary (Unissa et al., 2019). The most commonly affected places include the scalp, fingertips and toes, palms, soles, genital area, gluteus, underneath the breasts and genitals, wrists, knees, shins, and sacrum. This is a chronic disease with a propensity for relapse. It is irritating and might cause pain throughout the affected region in rare cases ('What is psoriasis?' 1999). Psoriasis has a long history, dating back to when psoriasis, leprosy, and other inflammatory skin conditions were all supposed to be the same thing. Psoriasis was not recognized as a separate entity until the 19th century after clinical descriptions differentiated it from other cutaneous disorders (Cowden & Van Voorhees, 2008). Psoriasis may occur at any age, with cases reported as early as infancy and as late as senior age. Precisely determining the age of onset of psoriasis is difficult because most research relies on a patient's memory of when lesions first appeared or on the physician's diagnosis as documented on the initial visit (Langley, Krueger, & Griffiths, 2005). Alcoholism, obesity, mental stress, repeated infections, and genetic predisposition are all risk factors for psoriasis. Regular cigarette use raises not only the likelihood of acquiring psoriasis but also the severity of the disease. The impact of psoriasis on a patient is generally determined by the affected areas of the body and the existence of systemic co-morbidities (Narkhede & Mahajan, 2019). There are numerous therapy methods available. Some are costly, while others are only available through specialized care; all require constant monitoring. The active topical treatments are the first step in this guideline's treatment route. The Guideline Development Group (GDG) recognized that emollients were already widely used in psoriasis, thus the evidence review was limited to active topical psoriasis therapy ('Psoriasis: assessment and management,' 2021) (Figure 8.1).

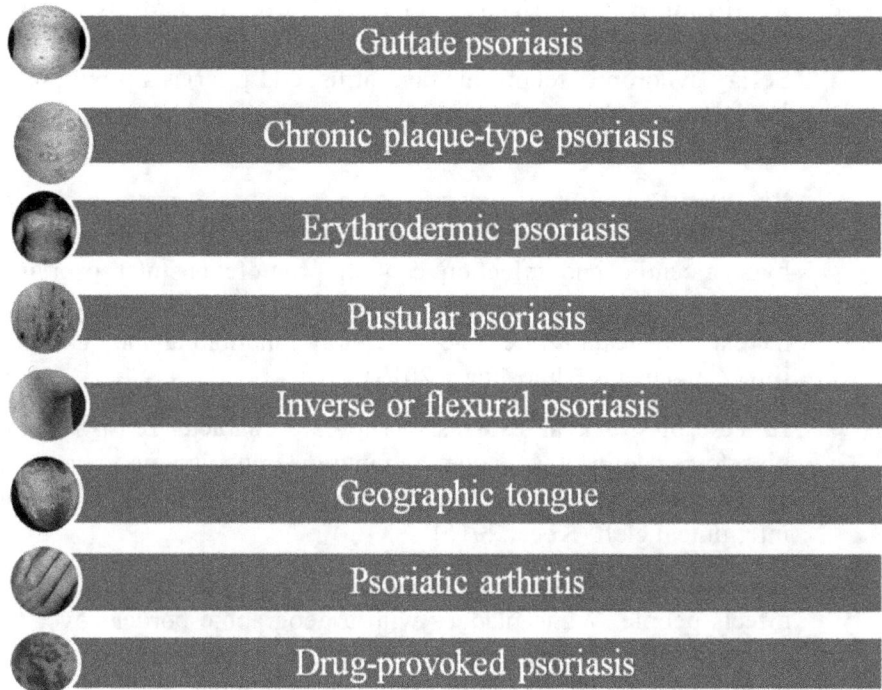

FIGURE 8.1 Different types of psoriasis.

8.2 TYPES OF PSORIASIS

Psoriasis typically appears as stubborn plaques containing silvery scale on extensor areas like the elbows and knees. The disease's severity is proportional to the amount of body surface area affected. Although plaque-type psoriasis seems to be the most common (Clebak et al., 2020), there are different types of psoriasis as follows.

1. **Chronic Plaque-Type Psoriasis:** The most prevalent variety is characterized by symmetrically distributed finely delineated pink papules and plaques with a silvery scale on extensor surfaces, scalp, trunk, and lumbosacral areas (Guidelines, 2005).

2. **Guttate Psoriasis:** Small pink scaly papules (typically less than 1 cm) arise unexpectedly. It is more frequent in children and is often preceded by an upper respiratory tract infection, most commonly caused by Streptococcus (Fry & Baker, 2007).

3. **Erythrodermic Psoriasis:** At most 75% of the body is covered in erythema and scaling. Atopic dermatitis, a medication reaction, Sezary syndrome, seborrheic dermatitis, and pityriasis rubra pilaris are just a few of the disorders that can cause erythroderma (World Health Organization psoriasis, 2016).

4. **Pustular Psoriasis:** Bright erythema and sterile pustules characterize this condition. Pregnancy, abrupt tapering of corticosteroids, hypocalcemia, and infection can all promote pustular psoriasis. Palm and sole involvement combined with severe desquamation can have a significant influence on everyday functioning and quality of life (Zangeneh & Shooshtary, 2013).

5. **Inverse or Flexural Psoriasis:** They are characterized by bright, pink-to-red delineated plaques and involve intertriginous areas, such as the groin, inguinal crease, axilla, inframammary regions, and intergluteal cleft (Koca, 2016).

6. **Geographic Tongue:** Tongue psoriasis is a type of psoriasis that affects people. White plaques with a geographic border cover the mucosa of the tongue. Moisture on the tongue promotes hyperkeratosis, which appears white instead of scale (Clebak et al., 2020).

7. **Psoriatic Arthritis:** It can be debilitating and cause considerable joint damage. The majority of people who have psoriatic arthritis have a history of skin illness. Psoriasis does not have a specific lab test; however, radiologic examinations can reveal bulky syndesmophytes, central and marginal erosions, and periostitis (Zangeneh & Shooshtary, 2013). Joint involvement manifests itself in a variety of ways. Psoriatic arthritis is much more likely than rheumatoid arthritis to impact the distal interphalangeal joints, and it is more likely than osteoarthritis to harm the metacarpophalangeal joints. Psoriatic arthritis is generally regarded as providing discomfort instead of acute pain because it progresses slowly (Garg & Gladman, 2010).

8. **Drug-Provoked Psoriasis:** Is split into two categories: drug-induced and drug-exacerbated. Drug-induced psoriasis improves if the causative drug is stopped, and it is more common in people who have no personal or family history of psoriasis. Drug-aggravated psoriasis progresses even when the offending drug is stopped, and it is more common in people who have had psoriasis before (Dogra & Kamat, 2019).

8.3 EPIDEMIOLOGY

Although psoriasis is found all around the world, its prevalence varies greatly. In the United States, about 2% of the population is affected (Papp et al., 2021). People in the Faroe Islands have been reported to have high rates of psoriasis, with one study finding that 2.8% of the population is affected. Psoriasis is uncommon in some ethnic groups, such as the Japanese, and may be absent in Aboriginal Australians and South American Indians (Langley, Krueger, & Griffiths, 2005). Although the disease is believed to be more prevalent in the world's Polar Regions, its impact in a tropical/subtropical country like India should not be overlooked (Dogra & Mahajan, 2016). Epidemiological studies in India are listed in Table 8.1.

TABLE 8.1 Epidemiological Studies on Psoriasis in India (Dogra & Mahajan, 2016)

SL. No.	Name of Scientist	No. of Patients	Prevalence (Percentage of Total Dermatologic Outpatients)	Ratio (M:F)	Mean Age of Males and Female
1.	Okhandiar et al. (1963)	3,573	1.02	2.46:1	Comparable
2.	Bedi et al. (1977)	162	0.8	2.5:1	Lower in females
3.	Kaur et al. (1986)	782	1.4	2.3:1	Lower in females
4.	Bedi et al. (1995)	530	2.8	2.4:1	–
5.	Kaur et al. (1997)	1,220	2.3	2.03:1	Lower in females

Psoriasis is more common among people in their 40s and 50s. Females are more likely to suffer from it than males. Children are almost never impacted. White people suffer more than black people. Nearly a third of psoriasis patients suffer from arthritis. The condition usually begins when a person is around the age of 20. Psoriatic arthritis affects 10% to 15% of the population (Unissa et al., 2019).

8.3.1 RISK FACTORS

The hypothesis proposed for psoriasis causation is multifactorial heredity, which involves interactions between genetic and environmental factors. According to heritability studies, genetic factors are responsible for 50 to 90% of the psoriatic phenotype. Environmental factors account for the remainder of the variation (Naldi, 2013). Psoriasis is linked to a higher metabolic risk, which varies depending on the severity of the condition.

According to current research, psoriatic patients have a higher frequency of obesity and metabolic syndrome, which puts them at risk of developing heart disease (Ganzetti, 2016). Psoriasis risk factors can be split into two categories: extrinsic and intrinsic risk factors (Figure 8.2).

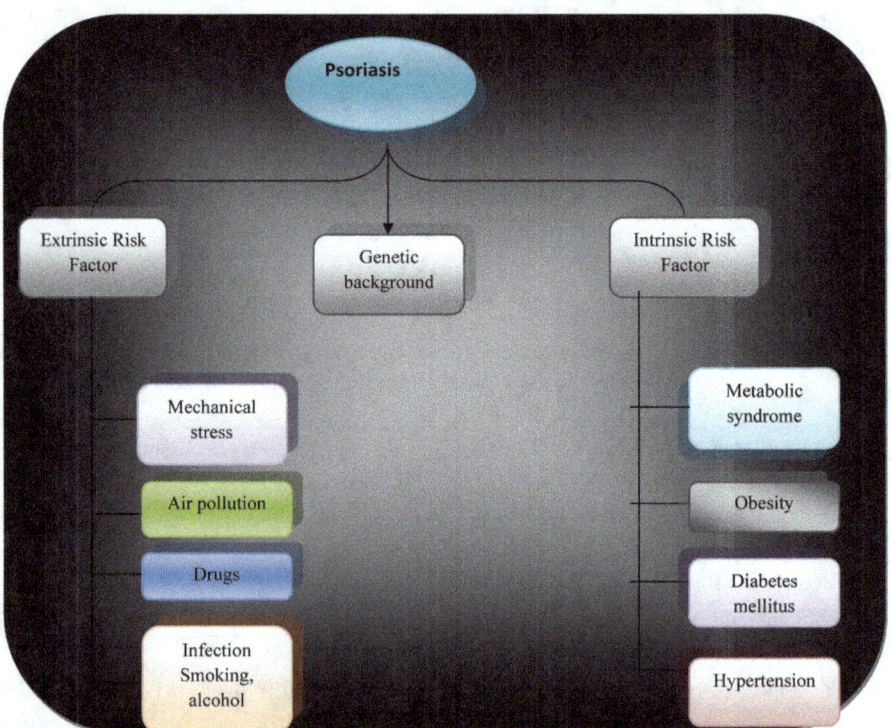

FIGURE 8.2 Risk factor for psoriasis.

8.3.1.1 GENETIC FACTORS

Psoriasis is a complex genetic disease, with hereditary variables accounting for approximately 70% of disease susceptibility. According to studies worldwide, psoriasis is more common in families (Naldi, 2013). According to twin studies, monozygotic twins have a tendency for psoriasis that is 2–3 times greater than dizygotic twins (Lønnberg et al., 2013). Psoriasis was linked to nine loci (PSORS1 through PSORS9) based on linkage studies. PSORS1 is known to be the most important indicator of psoriasis susceptibility; it is found in the MHC region, accounting for 35–50% of psoriasis heredity, and it is linked to early-onset psoriasis (Griffiths & Barker, 2007).

The susceptibility allele of PSORS1 has been found as HLA-Cw6, and the significance of detecting human leukocyte antigen (HLA) alleles related to psoriasis has been recognized (Ogawa & Okada, 2020).

8.3.1.2 MECHANICAL STRESS

The Koebner phenomenon occurs when psoriasis patients develop skin lesions in non-involved areas after various injuries (Arias-Santiago, Espiñeira-Carmona, & Aneiros-Fernández, 2013). New psoriasis lesions have been reported to be triggered by radiotherapy, ultraviolet (UV) B, and even minor skin irritation (Charalambous & Bloomfield, 2000). After injuries, however, psoriatic lesions are not usually visible in the unaffected skin. The pathophysiology of the Koebner phenomenon may be influenced by the type, location, depth, and degree of trauma.

8.3.1.3 LIFESTYLE

According to a systematic review and meta-analysis, psoriasis has been linked to both smoking and alcohol consumption. People with this condition are much more likely to be current or past smokers; the chance of having psoriasis is enhanced when you smoke (Naldi et al., 2005). Psoriasis pustular lesions are significantly linked with smoking and alcohol consumption. With more pack-years or smoking time, the risk of psoriasis rises. According to another research, the degree and/or duration of smoking had a positive relationship with the development of psoriasis. According to a comprehensive review, psoriasis appears to be linked to excessive alcohol drinking; nonetheless, there isn't enough evidence to say if alcohol causes psoriasis (Brenaut et al., 2013).

8.4 PATHOGENESIS

Psoriasis is now regarded as the most widespread autoimmune disease resulting from improper cellular immune system activation. The thing that happens in the evolution of Psoriasis has two primary hypotheses. The first views psoriasis as predominantly a skin condition, a condition characterized by increased skin cell proliferation and reproduction. Hyperproliferation with insufficient development of epidermal keratinocytes and reduced keratinocyte death describe the problem, which is simply considered as a flaw of the epidermis and its keratinocytes (Orton, 1996). The second hypothesis considers psoriasis to be an immune-mediated condition (immunosuppressant drugs can eliminate psoriasis plaques), in which excessive skin cell proliferation is caused by immune system components (Boehncke, 2015). T cells get activated, move to the dermis, and release cytokines, which promote inflammation and fast skin cell formation. It is unknown what causes T cells to become activated. The pathogenic input of T cells has now been investigated in clinical investigations using immune modulator biological agents in psoriasis patients, which first pointed to a key role of T lymphocytes as stimulants of the disease phenotype (Ogawa et al., 2018) (Figure 8.3).

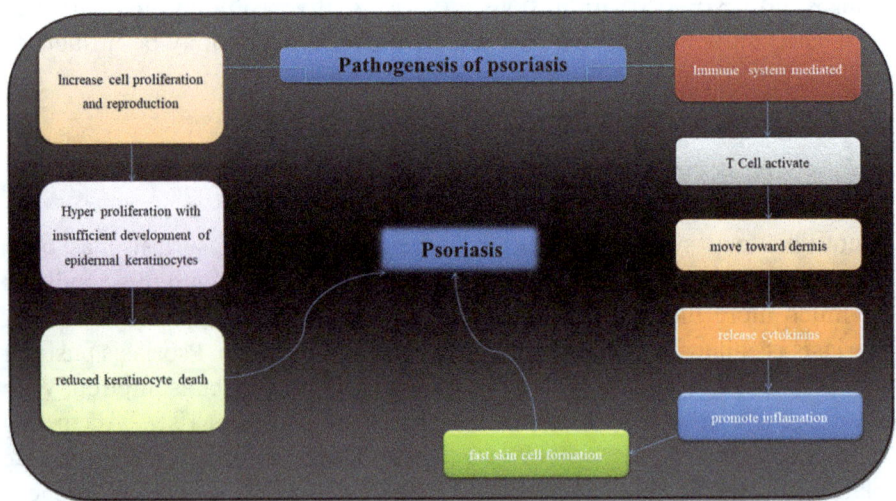

FIGURE 8.3 Pathogenesis of psoriasis.

8.5 CURRENT TREATMENT AND PROBLEMS

There are a number of treatments for psoriasis, and some of the most often used treatments for psoriasis include topical corticosteroids, tars, anthralin, vitamin D analogs, tazarotene, and salicylic acids. Herbal medications (Sharma et al., 2020; Rane et al., 2020a, b, c) are another traditional strategy; however, there is limited *in vivo* and safety data available, thus additional research into *in vivo* efficacy is required. According to a survey conducted by the National Psoriasis Foundation, only 26% of patients were pleased with traditional treatment (Rahman et al., 2012) (Figure 8.4).

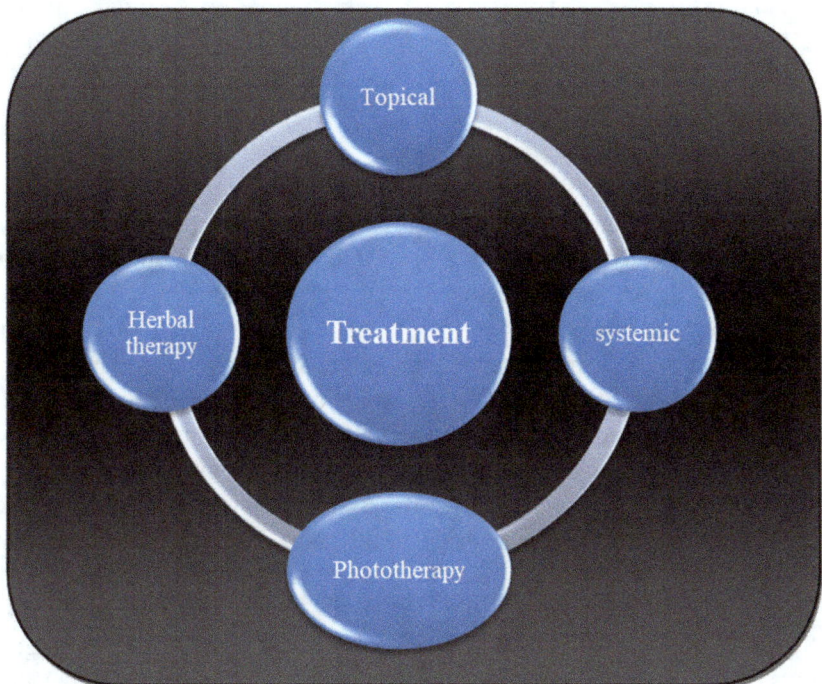

FIGURE 8.4 Various treatments for psoriasis.

8.5.1 TOPICAL TREATMENT

For most psoriasis patients, especially those with mild illness, topical therapy remains the backbone of treatment. Although it is effective for individual plaques, it is lengthy, and compliance is a major concern. As a result, it's critical to personalize and simplify topical therapy, as well as comprehend the many bases: creams, lotions, foams, sprays, ointments, and gels (Nakamizo, 1977). Some of the mainly used agents in topical therapy are Vitamin D analogs (Soleymani, Hung, & Soung, 2015), corticosteroids, dithranol, tars, retinoids, Tacrolimus, Babchi oil, and 8-methoxypsoralen. The use of topical medication minimizes the risk of side effects that come with systemic medicines (Menter & Griffiths, 2007). All of these treatments are effective, but they have some major side effects of topical treatment as follows (Nakamizo, 1977; Soleymani, Hung, & Soung, 2015; Menter & Griffiths, 2007):

- Irritant, hypercalcemia (vitamin D analogs);
- Short duration of remission myelosuppression, alopecia, teratogenic (corticosteroids);

- Dithranol stains skin, clothing, and skin Irritation (dithranol);
- Irritation, unpleasant odor, folliculitis, a possible carcinogen (tar).

8.5.2 SYSTEMIC TREATMENT

Traditional systemic medicines were available for the treatment of psoriasis, especially for moderate to severe cases that were refractory to topical medications or phototherapy. Since the US Food and Drug Administration approved methotrexate for the first time in 1971 (Boffa & Chalmers, 1996), retinoid has also been widely used. Retinoid, a form of vitamin A, is available in both natural and synthetic forms. Hyperkeratosis of the skin is caused by a nutrient shortage in the body. The impact of retinoids on nuclear receptors modulates gene transcription and decreases epidermal hyperplasia in psoriasis (Lee & Koo, 2005). Retinoid is classified into two generations, both of which are effective against psoriasis. Cyclosporine is also an effective short-term treatment for moderate-to-severe psoriasis, although it is ineffective for severe psoriatic arthritis. Its efficacy in arthritis was discovered by chance in 1979 during a study (Biren & Barr, 1986).

Some of the systemic drugs used in psoriasis have disadvantages as follows (Boffa & Chalmers, 1996; Lee & Koo, 2005; Biren & Barr, 1986):

- **Acitretin:** Teratogenicity, and raised plasma lipids.
- **Methotrexate:** Nausea, bone marrow suppression, hepatic fibrosis.
- **Cyclosporine:** Nephrotoxicity, immunosuppressant Hypertension.
- **Hydroxycarbamide (Hydroxyurea):** Bone marrow suppression.
- **Fumaric Acid Esters:** GIT complications (flushing episodes, diarrhea) and lymphopenia (usually mild).

8.5.3 BIOLOGICAL AGENTS

Biological agents comprise recombinant molecules that are created using genetic sequences from many organisms and are frequently comparable to or similar to proteins generated by humans. Fusion proteins, recombinant proteins (such as cytokines and selective receptors), and monoclonal antibodies are among them (Brownstone et al., 2021). Alefacept was the earliest biological agent to be developed particularly for the treatment of psoriasis and to be authorized by the FDA (in 2003, in the USA). It's a recombinant human leukocyte function-associated antigen-3/IgG1 fusion protein that binds to CD2 on memory effector T cells, specifically inhibiting antigen-presenting cell activity and, as a result, T-cell activation. Another significant mechanism of action is the apoptosis of memory-effector CD45RO-positive T cells in the skin (Chamian et al., 2005). Efalizumab is a humanized monoclonal antibody that binds to the CD11a component of LFA-1, preventing circulating T cells from entering the skin by reducing T cell activation and adherence to endothelial cells (Culp & Menter, 2008).

Example of biological side effect:

- A flu-like symptom that appears within the first two weeks of treatment is thrombocytopenia and hemolytic anemia.

8.6 IMPACT OF DIET ON PSORIASIS

There have been several dietary approaches for psoriasis over the years, but none has acquired widespread acceptance in the treatment of this disease. The therapies available for psoriasis have major side effects, which is a worldwide problem related to the treatment of psoriasis. This is the reason why people are now moving towards lifestyle changes, modifying habits, and also adjusting their diets because the diet is accessible and has no side effects. In terms of diet, a low-energy, low-calorie diet, and a gluten-free diet are most useful for improving symptoms of psoriasis. In a 2017 survey of 1206 psoriasis patients, 86% reported that they changed their diets. The most popular diets were Gluten-free (35.6%) (Wolters, 2005), low carbohydrate/high protein (16.6%), and Paleolithic diets (11.6%). In addition to these diets, a Mediterranean diet as well as a vegetarian diet have also been shown to help with psoriasis symptoms. Significant reductions in alcohol, gluten, nightshades, and fast-food consumption were linked to skin benefits in half of the patients.

8.6.1 MEDITERRANEAN DIET

The Mediterranean diet emphasizes fruits, vegetables, nuts and legumes, grains, and olive oil while limiting red meat, dairy products, and alcohol (except red wine) intake during meals. Anti-inflammatory qualities of dietary fiber, antioxidants, and polyphenols (Keservani & Sharma, 2014; Keservani et al., 2016a, b), all of which are abundant in the Mediterranean diet, could be one explanation for the Mediterranean diet's potential to lower chronic, systemic inflammation (Tsigalou et al., 2020). MUFAs, fish, vitamins A, C, D, and E, and omega-3 fatty acids are among the foods and nutrients indicated in the studies as possessing anti-inflammatory qualities. It's difficult to definitively classify the Mediterranean diet because of the huge array of influencing variables in dietary studies that rely on questionnaires as a psoriasis treatment (Phan et al., 2018).

Vitamin D and analog (Millsop et al., 2014; Wolters, 2006): Although the effectiveness of topical vitamin D in the management of psoriasis is well established, the significance of oral vitamin D supplements in the management of psoriasis is unknown. It has been claimed that low serum vitamin D levels are linked to increased psoriasis severity. In observational studies, oral vitamin D supplementation has been demonstrated to be safe and effective for the treatment of psoriatic lesions and psoriatic arthritis. However, in a recent randomized, placebo-controlled trial, patients treated with oral vitamin D showed no significant improvement in skin lesions when compared to controls.

8.6.2 GLUTEN-FREE DIET

Although the occurrence of gluten sensitivity in psoriasis patients is debated, data suggests that a gluten-free diet can relieve psoriasis lesions in certain patients before conclusive treatment recommendations can be made. Larger and more controlled investigations on the effectiveness of a gluten-free diet on this subgroup of psoriasis patients are needed (Rush & Bagel, 2011). The National Psoriasis Foundation (NPF) believes the verdict is still out on whether or not a gluten-free diet is a feasible psoriasis treatment. Gluten intolerance is prevalent in the psoriatic population, according to reports that range from 6.67% to 25.3% (Pona et al., 2019). According to Michaelsson and colleagues, a group of 33 antigliadin antibodies (AGA)-positive psoriasis patients was put on a gluten-free diet for three months. The Psoriasis Area Severity Index (PASI) scores of 73% of these individuals improved significantly (from an average of 9.0 to 5.5 in patients with an initial PASI greater than 5). Furthermore, when these individuals returned to their regular diets, their PASI scores returned to pre-diet levels (Michaëlsson et al., 2000).

8.6.3 VEGETARIAN DIET

The vegetarian diet is also studied to evaluate its effectiveness against inflammatory disorders. It was found that some psoriasis patients experienced a reduction in their symptoms when they followed a vegetarian or vegan diet ('magnesite dressing,' 2015). In comparison to omnivorous diets, vegetarian diets have been linked to higher ratios of anti-inflammatory to proinflammatory adipokines, as well as lower expression of proinflammatory genes inside the gut microbiota and lower expression levels of IgE (Ambroszkiewicz et al., 2018). Psoriasis symptoms may have been influenced by the diet's anti-inflammatory effects. The substantial rate of potassium ingested in a vegetarian diet has also been linked to the body's ability to manufacture cortisol, a traditional treatment for psoriasis. Supplementing with potassium has been proven to increase serum cortisol levels in patients. However, further research is needed to clarify the role of potassium in a vegetarian diet; all hypotheses are plausible explanations for the outcomes of these studies (Rastmanesh, 2009).

8.6.4 VERY-LOW-CALORIE KETOGENIC DIET

Since obesity and fat mass are linked to psoriasis, some patients resort to calorie-restricted diets to alleviate their symptoms. The Ketogenic diet is a very low, high-fat diet that resembles the Atkins and low-carb diets in many ways. In recent days, a Ketogenic diet (KD) has now been proposed as an alternative weight-loss technique (Katsimbri et al., 2021). Different types of KD include the standard ketogenic diet, very-low-carbohydrate ketogenic diet, Atkins diet, high-fat ketogenic diet, and very low-calorie ketogenic diet (VLCKD). Low carbohydrate intake (less than 30–50 g/day) and a rise in protein and fat are the major characteristics of KD. As a result, the metabolism shifts to relying on fat as a primary source of energy (Castellana et al., 2019). Due to the ketogenic diet, fatty acids, ketone bodies, and pyruvic acid levels rise. The ketogenic diet reduces oxidative stress by activating nuclear factor erythroid-derived 2 (NF-E2)-related factor 2 (Nrf2); it also reduces inflammation by activating peroxisome proliferator-activated receptor-gamma (PPAR-γ) and hydroxy-carboxylic acid receptor 2 (HCAR-2) (HCA2) (Verdile et al., 2015). Evaluation of whether the Ketogenic diet is useful or not requires performing a study on that.

8.7 CONCLUSION

Psoriasis is a common skin disease that has a huge impact on people's lives. The treatment of psoriasis has some dangerous side effects, so it's necessary to move toward an easy and harmless diet. Dietary changes have a complex multifactorial effect on psoriasis, which is often reliant on the patient's lifestyle, such as the degree of exercise, hobbies including drinking and smoking, and genetic susceptibilities to conditions like obesity. As a result, it's difficult to find a single diet that has a substantial impact on psoriasis symptoms for the vast majority of people. However, it appears that some foods or nutritional supplements can be removed from diets to improve overall health.

KEYWORDS

- guideline development group
- human leukocyte antigen
- proliferator-activated receptor-gamma
- psoriasis area severity index
- ultraviolet
- very-low-calorie ketogenic diet

REFERENCES

Ambroszkiewicz, J., et al. (2018). Anti-inflammatory and pro-inflammatory adipokine profiles in children on vegetarian and omnivorous diets. *Nutrients, 10*(9), 1241. https://doi.org/10.3390/nu10091241.

Arias-Santiago, S., Espiñeira-Carmona, M. J., & Aneiros-Fernández, J. (2013). The Koebner phenomenon: Psoriasis in tattoos. *Cmaj., 185*(7), 585. https://doi.org/10.1503/cmaj.111299.

Biren, T. A., & Barr, R. J. (1986). Dermatologic applications of cyclosporine. *Archives of Dermatology, 122*(9), 1028–1032. https://doi.org/10.1001/archderm.1986.01660210078022.

Boehncke, W. H. (2015). Etiology and pathogenesis of psoriasis. *Rheumatic Disease Clinics of North America, 41*(4), 665–675. https://doi.org/10.1016/j.rdc.2015.07.013.

Boffa, M. J., & Chalmers, R. J. G. (1996). Methotrexate for psoriasis. *Clinical and Experimental Dermatology, 21*(6), 399–408. https://doi.org/10.1111/j.1365-2230.1996.tb00142.x.

Brenaut, E., et al. (2013). Alcohol consumption and psoriasis: A systematic literature review. *Journal of the European Academy of Dermatology and Venereology, 27*(Suppl. 3), 30–35. https://doi.org/10.1111/jdv.12164.

Brownstone, N. D., et al. (2021). Biologic treatments of psoriasis: An update for the clinician. *Biologics: Targets and Therapy, 15*, 39–51. https://doi.org/10.2147/BTT.S252578.

Castellana, M., Conte, E., Cignarelli, A., Perrini, S., Giustina, A., Giovanella, L., & Trimboli, P. (2020). Efficacy and safety of very low calorie ketogenic diet (VLCKD) in patients with overweight and obesity: A systematic review and meta-analysis. *Reviews in Endocrine and Metabolic Disorders, 21*(1), 5–16.

Chamian, F., et al. (2005). Alefacept reduces infiltrating T cells, activated dendritic cells, and inflammatory genes in psoriasis vulgaris. *Proceedings of the National Academy of*

Sciences of the United States of America, *102*(6), 2075–2080. https://doi.org/10.1073/pnas.0409569102.

Charalambous, H., & Bloomfield, D. (2000). Psoriasis and radiotherapy: Exacerbation of psoriasis following radiotherapy for carcinoma of the breast (the Koebner phenomenon). *Clinical Oncology, 12*(3), 192–193. https://doi.org/10.1053/clon.2000.9149.

Clebak, K. T., et al. (2020). The many variants of psoriasis. *The Journal of Family Practice, 69*(4), 192–200.

Cowden, A., & Van Voorhees, A. S. (2008). Introduction: History of psoriasis and psoriasis therapy. *Treatment of Psoriasis, 1,* 1–9. https://doi.org/10.1007/978-3-7643-7724-3_1.

Culp, B., & Menter, M. A. (2008). Efalizumab in the treatment of psoriasis. *Moderate-to-Severe Psoriasis, Third Edition, 1*(3), 307–326. https://doi.org/10.2217/14750708.1.2.197.

Dogra, S., & Kamat, D. (2019). Drug-induced psoriasis. *Indian Journal of Rheumatology, 14*(5), S37–S43. https://doi.org/10.4103/0973-3698.272159.

Dogra, S., & Mahajan, R. (2016). Psoriasis: Epidemiology, clinical features, co-morbidities, and clinical scoring. *Indian Dermatology Online Journal, 7*(6), 471. https://doi.org/10.4103/2229-5178.193906.

Fry, L., & Baker, B. S. (2007). Triggering psoriasis: The role of infections and medications. *Clinics in Dermatology, 25*(6), 606–615. https://doi.org/10.1016/j.clindermatol.2007.08.015.

Ganzetti, G. (2016). Psoriasis, non-alcoholic fatty liver disease, and cardiovascular disease: Three different diseases on a unique background. *World Journal of Cardiology, 8*(2), 120. https://doi.org/10.4330/wjc.v8.i2.120.

Garg, A., & Gladman, D. (2010). Recognizing psoriatic arthritis in the dermatology clinic. *Journal of the American Academy of Dermatology, 63*(5), 733–748. https://doi.org/10.1016/j.jaad.2010.02.061.

Griffiths, C. E., & Barker, J. N. (2007). Pathogenesis and clinical features of psoriasis. *Lancet, 370*(9583), 263–271. https://doi.org/10.1016/S0140-6736(07)61128-3.

Guidelines, E. E. (2005). Entitlement eligibility guidelines for peptic ulcer disease.

Indian Minerals Yearbook 2015 (Part III : Mineral Reviews) 54th Edition Magnesite (Advance Release), *Magnesite Dressing,* 5–8. https://ibm.gov.in/writereaddata/files/01192017154907IMYB2015_Magnesite_19012017_Adv.pdf.

Katsimbri, P., et al. (2021). The effect of antioxidant and anti-inflammatory capacity of diet on psoriasis and psoriatic arthritis phenotype: Nutrition as a therapeutic tool? *Antioxidants, 10*(2), 1–28. https://doi.org/10.3390/antiox10020157.

Keservani, R. K., & Sharma, A. K. (2014). Flavonoids: Emerging trends and potential health benefits. *Journal of Chinese Pharmaceutical Sciences, 23*(12), 815.

Keservani, R. K., Sharma, A. K., & Kesharwani, R. K. (2016a). Nutraceutical and functional foods for cardiovascular health. In *Food Process Engineering* (pp. 291–312). Apple Academic Press, CRC Press, (pp. 257–278). ISBN: 9781771884020.

Keservani, R. K., Sharma, A. K., & Kesharwani, R. K. (2016b). Medicinal effect of nutraceutical fruits for cognition and brain health. *Scientifica,* 2016. Article ID 3109254, 10 pages. https://doi.org/10.1155/2016/3109254.

Koca, T. T. (2016). A summary of clinical types of psoriasis. *Northern Clinics of Istanbul, 3*(1), 79–82. https://doi.org/10.14744/nci.2016.16023.

Langley, R. G. B., Krueger, G. G., & Griffiths, C. E. M. (2005). Psoriasis: Epidemiology, clinical features, and quality of life. *Annals of the Rheumatic Diseases, 64*(Suppl. 2), 18–23. https://doi.org/10.1136/ard.2004.033217.

Lee, C. S., & Koo, J. (2005). A review of acitretin, a systemic retinoid for the treatment of psoriasis. *Expert Opinion on Pharmacotherapy, 6*(10), 1725–1734. https://doi.org/10.1517/14656566.6.10.1725.

Lønnberg, A. S., et al. (2013). Heritability of psoriasis in a large twin sample. *British Journal of Dermatology, 169*(2), 412–416. https://doi.org/10.1111/bjd.12375.

Menter, A., & Griffiths, C. E. (2007). Current and future management of psoriasis. *Lancet, 370*(9583), 272–284. https://doi.org/10.1016/S0140-6736(07)61129-5.

Michaëlsson, G., et al. (2000). Psoriasis patients with antibodies to gliadin can be improved by a gluten-free diet. *British Journal of Dermatology, 142*(1), 44–51. https://doi.org/10.1046/j.1365-2133.2000.03240.x.

Millsop, J. W., et al. (2014). Diet and psoriasis, part III: Role of nutritional supplements. *Journal of the American Academy of Dermatology, 71*(3), 561–569. https://doi.org/10.1016/j.jaad.2014.03.016.

Nakamizo, Y. (1977). Topical treatment of psoriasis. *Nishinihon Journal of Dermatology, 39*(6), 855–859. https://doi.org/10.2336/nishinihonhifu.39.855.

Naldi, L. (2013). Risk factors for psoriasis. *Current Dermatology Reports, 2*(1), 58–65. https://doi.org/10.1007/s13671-012-0034-6.

Naldi, L., Liliane Chatenoud, Dennis Linder, Anna Belloni Fortina, Andrea Peserico, Anna Rosa Virgili, Pier Luigi Bruni et al., (2005). Cigarette Smoking, Body Mass Index, and Stressful Life Events as Risk Factors for Psoriasis: Results from an Italian Case–Control Study, *Journal of Investigative Dermatology, 125*(1), 61–67.

Narkhede, G. D., & Mahajan, S. S. (2019). Study of clinical and epidemiological features of psoriasis at a tertiary care center. *MedPulse International Journal of Medicine, 11*(3), 206–209. https://doi.org/10.26611/102111313.

Ogawa, E., et al. (2018). Pathogenesis of psoriasis and development of treatment. *Journal of Dermatology, 45*(3), 264–272. https://doi.org/10.1111/1346-8138.14139.

Ogawa, K., & Okada, Y. (2020). The current landscape of psoriasis genetics in 2020. *Journal of Dermatological Science, 99*(1), 2–8. https://doi.org/10.1016/j.jdermsci.2020.05.008.

Ortonne, J. P. (1996). Aetiology and pathogenesis of psoriasis. *British Journal of Dermatology, Supplement, 135*(49), 1–5. https://doi.org/10.1111/j.1365-2133.1996.tb15660.x.

Papp, K. A., et al. (2021). Psoriasis prevalence and severity by expert elicitation. *Dermatology and Therapy, 11*(3), 1053–1064. https://doi.org/10.1007/s13555-021-00518-8.

Phan, C., et al. (2018). Association between Mediterranean anti-inflammatory dietary profile and severity of psoriasis: Results from the NutriNet-Santé cohort. *JAMA Dermatology, 154*(9), 1017–1024. https://doi.org/10.1001/jamadermatol.2018.2127.

Pona, A., et al. (2019). Diet and psoriasis. *Dermatology Online Journal, 25*(2), 1, https://doi.org/10.5070/d3252042883.

Psoriasis: Assessment and Management (2021), (October 2012), 1–57. https://www.ncbi.nlm.nih.gov/books/NBK553610.

Rahman, M., et al. (2012). Classical to current approach for treatment of psoriasis: A review. *Endocrine, Metabolic & Immune Disorders – Drug Targets, 12*(3), 287–302. https://doi.org/10.2174/187153012802002901.

Rane, B. R., Bharath, M. S., Patil, R. R., Keservani, R. K., & Jain, A. S. (2020b). Novel approaches in nutraceuticals. In R. K. Kesharwani, R. K. Keservani, & A. K. Sharma (Eds.), *Enhancing the Therapeutic Efficacy of Herbal Formulations through Novel Drug Delivery Systems* (Chapter 11, pp. 241–266). IGI Global International Publisher, Pennsylvania, USA. ISBN: 9781799844532.

Rane, B. R., Patil, A. S., Keservani, R. K., & Jain, A. S. (2020a). Novel approaches in herbal formulation. In R. K. Kesharwani, R. K. Keservani, & A. K. Sharma (Eds.), *Enhancing the Therapeutic Efficacy of Herbal Formulations through Novel Drug Delivery Systems* (Chapter 2, pp. 43–68). IGI Global International Publisher, Pennsylvania, USA. ISBN: 9781799844532.

Rane, B. R., Tadavi, S. A., & Keservani, R. K. (2020c). Naturopathy. In A. K. Sharma, R. K. Keservani, & S. P. Gautam (Eds.), *Herbal Product Development* (Chapter 12, pp. 321–347). Apple Academic Press, CRC Press, Taylor & Francis Group. ISBN: 9781771888776.

Rastmanesh, R. (2009). Psoriasis and vegetarian diets: A role for cortisol and potassium? *Medical Hypotheses, 72*(3), 368. https://doi.org/10.1016/j.mehy.2008.09.031.

Rush, M., & Bagel, J. (2011). The role of a gluten-free diet in psoriasis. *Psoriasis Forum, 17a* (4), 254–258. https://doi.org/10.1177/247553031117a00402.

Sharma, A. K., Keservani, R. K., & Gautam, S. P. (2020). *Herbal Product Development*. Apple Academic Press, CRC Press, Taylor & Francis Group. 1st Edition, pp. 376. ISBN: 9781003003182.

Soleymani, T., Hung, T., & Soung, J. (2015). The role of vitamin D in psoriasis: A review. *International Journal of Dermatology, 54*(4), 383–392. https://doi.org/10.1111/ijd.12790.

Tsigalou, C., et al. (2020). Mediterranean diet as a tool to combat inflammation and chronic diseases: An overview. *Biomedicines, 8*(8), 1–13.

Unissa, R., et al. (2019). Psoriasis: A comprehensive review. *Asian Journal of Research in Pharmaceutical Science, 9*(1), 29. https://doi.org/10.5958/2231-5659.2019.00005.5.

Verdile, G., et al. (2015). Inflammation and oxidative stress: The molecular connectivity between insulin resistance, obesity, and Alzheimer's disease. *Mediators of Inflammation, 2015*. https://doi.org/10.1155/2015/105828.

What is psoriasis? (1999). *Nursing Times, 95*(24), 17. https://www.nursingtimes.net/clinical-archive/dermatology/psoriasis-01–11–2002/.

Wolters, M. (2005). Diet and psoriasis: Experimental data and clinical evidence. *British Journal of Dermatology, 153*(4), 706–714.

Wolters, M. (2006). Die Bedeutung der Ernährung und begleitender Faktoren für die Psoriasis. *Hautarzt, 57*(11), 999–1004. https://doi.org/10.1007/s00105-006-1164-1.

World Health Organization psoriasis. (2016). Global report on. *Global Report on Psoriasis, 978*, 1–26.

Zangeneh, F. Z., & Shooshtary, F. S. (2013). Psoriasis—Types, causes, and medication. *Psoriasis – Types, Causes and Medication* (Table 1), Vol. 1, 3–38. https://doi.org/10.5772/54728.

CHAPTER 9

MARINE BOTANICALS AS NUTRACEUTICALS FOR PSORIASIS

KAJAL M. GAWADE,[1] BHARATI S. GARALE,[1] SWATI G. TALELE,[1] RAMDAS DOLAS,[1] and LAXMIKANT B. BORSE[2]

[1]Department of Pharmaceutics, Sandip Institute of Pharmaceutical Sciences, Nashik, Maharashtra, India

[2]Department of Pharmacology, Sandip Institute of Pharmaceutical Sciences, Nashik, Maharashtra, India

ABSTRACT

Psoriasis is a polygenic, chronic relapsing autoimmune skin disease that affects 1–3% of the world's population and is considered to be initiated by an immune system disorder that accelerates the life cycle of skin cells, mainly on the surface of the skin. A leading dermatologist has developed and validated a sophisticated animal model for psoriasis, enabling us to study the early stages of the disease and test new treatment methods. While there are various treatment approaches that provide symptom relief, it has been noted that there is no definitive cure for psoriasis. Additionally, due to poor treatment outcomes and high medication toxicity profiles, these drugs are less convenient to use in the management of psoriasis. Marine botanicals have been identified as a nutraceutical in the quest for alternative and complementary treatments for this condition, although only a few have been documented since ancient times. These include seaweeds such as Rhodophyta, Phaeophyta, Chlorophyta, Cyanobacteria, and Sea Moss, as well as Vitamin D. Incorporating appropriate marine botanicals into a patient's diet may improve their quality of life and have a positive impact on their overall health condition. This chapter focuses on the nutritional benefits of marine botanicals in the treatment of psoriasis.

9.1 INTRODUCTION

Stephen DeFelice coined the phrase "nutraceutical" in 1989 by merging the words "nutrition" and "pharmaceutical." Raw foods, fortified foods, and dietary supplements that contain purely energetic particles, also known as bioactive molecules (Palthur, Sajala Palthur, Chitta et al., 2010), which provide health benefits beyond basic nutrition, are referred bioactive molecules (Liu et al., 2003). Certain polysaccharides, peptides, phytochemicals (Keservani & Sharma, 2014; Keservani et al., 2016a, b), vitamins, and fatty acids are examples of bioactive substances that occur naturally in foods, can be added to foods to create fortified or functional foods, or can be produced as dietary supplements. These bioactive combinations can be extracted from natural sources or synthesized using chemical and biotechnological methods (Keith et al., 2009). Compared to terrestrial ecosystems, marine ecosystems offer a greater diversity of living species, providing more nutrients for human nourishment and health (Hill, Fenical et al., 2010). Maritime invertebrates are a diverse group that can be found in various ocean environments, from the intertidal zone to the deep sea (Thorpe, Sole-Cava, Watts et al., 2000).

9.2 PSORIASIS

Psoriasis is a vexing autoimmune illness that generates an increase in the growth of T-cells. Psoriatic scales are often whitish-silver in color and form a thick, crimson smear. Normal skin cells have a one-month life cycle; however, in psoriasis, the inflammation of skin cells can proliferate up to 10 times quicker than normal skin cells. Scales are found in any place on your body such as hands, feet, neck, scalp, and face, and are most typically found on joints like elbows and knees. Patches on the nails, lips, and region surrounding the genitals are less prevalent. Psoriasis affects approximately 1.5 to 2.0% of the world's population (Parisi, Symmons, Griffiths, Ashcroft et al., 2013), with more than 7.2 million persons in the US. Psoriasis vulgaris, often known as plaque psoriasis, is the most widespread type of illness, affecting 85–90% of individuals. Psoriasis is often classified as mild, moderate, or severe, depending on the degree and extent of skin involvement. Due to the quick destruction process, the silvery-white patches are caused by the accumulation and accelerated restoration of skin in predilection locations.

It is estimated that over 30% of psoriasis patients have a 1st- or 2nd-degree domestic past of the illness (Jain et al., 2012). The chances of having a child are 41% if both parents have psoriasis.

9.3 HISTORY

The origin of the disease name is from the Grecian word 'Psora.' 'Psora' means 'Itch.' Intellectuals are of the opinion that psoriasis is thought to have been comprised amid the various skin conditions called 'tzaraath' in the Hebrew Bible, a circumstance inflicted as retribution for defamation (Gruber, Kastelan, Brajac et al., 2004). The Grecians used the term 'lepra' for squamate skin circumstances. They passed down the turn of phrase 'psora' to describe the itchy skin circumstances. It became known as Willian's lepra in the late 18th century when English dermatologists Robert Willian and Thomas Bateman differentiated it from other skin diseases. Willian identified two categories: Leprosa graecorum and Psora leprosa (Meenan et al., 1955). Psoriasis is thought to have first been described in Ancient Rome by Cornelius Celsus (Benedek et al., 2013). In the 18th and 19th eras, Fowler's solution, which contains a toxic and cancer-causing arsenic compound, became utilized by dermatologists as a remedy for psoriasis (Gruber, Kastelan, Brajac et al., 2004). Mercury became moreover cast off for psoriasis at some stage during this period (Gruber, Kastelan, Brajac et al., 2004). Sulfur, iodine, and phenol were additionally typically used remedies for psoriasis at some point during this period when it became imperfectly understood that psoriasis became an infectious sickness (Gruber, Kastelan, Brajac et al., 2004). Coal tars had been extensively used with UV radioactivity as a relevant management technique in the early 1900s (Benedek et al., 2013).

9.4 TYPES OF PSORIASIS

There are five types of psoriasis.

9.4.1 PSORIASIS PLAQUE

Among the several types of psoriasis, plaque psoriasis is the most frequent. Psoriasis vulgaris (also known as chronic stationary psoriasis or plaque-like psoriasis) is the most common type of psoriasis, affecting 85–90% of people (Palfreeman, McNamee, McCann et al., 2013). Plaque psoriasis is defined by raised, inflammatory skin patches that are covered with silvery-white, rough scales. Plaques can be found on the elbows, knees, scalp, as well as back, and are the most common areas for plaques (Colledge, Walker, Ralston et al., 2010).

9.4.2 GUTTATE PSORIASIS

It is quite common among children. Numerous small, scaly, red or pink, droplet-like lesions characterize guttate psoriasis (papules). These psoriasis patches can be found all over the body, especially on the chest, but also on the limbs and scalp. A streptococcal infection, most commonly streptococcal pharyngitis, is a common cause of guttate psoriasis (Weigle, McBane et al., 2013).

9.4.3 PUSTULAR PSORIASIS

Adults are more likely to develop pustular psoriasis. Pustular psoriasis is characterized by raised bumps that contain noninfectious pus (pustules) (Robinson, Van Voorhees, Hsu, Korman, Lebwohl, Bebo, Kalb et al., 2012). The skin around the pustules is red and inflamed (Raychaudhuri, Maverakis, Raychaudhuri et al., 2014). Pustular psoriasis can be localized or spread out across the entire body. Both localized pustular psoriasis and acrodermatitis varieties of Hallopeau affect the hands and feet (Rendon, Schäkel et al., 2019).

9.4.4 ERYTHRODERMIC PSORIASIS

It is a simple and exceedingly unusual form of psoriasis, according to the National Psoriasis Foundation. Psoriasis that affects the skin is known as erythrodermic psoriasis. The skin is inflamed and exfoliated throughout the majority of the body's surface, frequently involving more than 90% of the body's surface area (Rendon, Schäkel et al., 2019). Severe dryness, itching, swelling, and discomfort may accompany it. Any sort of psoriasis can lead to it (Rendon, Schäkel et al., 2019). It's usually caused by an aggravation of unstable plaque psoriasis, especially when systemic glucocorticoids are abruptly stopped (Zattra, Belloni Fortina, Peserico, Alaibac et al., 2012). Because the high inflammation and exfoliation undermine the body's capacity to normalize heat and perform barrier functions, this kind of psoriasis can be lethal (Stanway et al., 2014). This form of infection can be fatal.

9.4.5 PSORIASIS INVERSE

Inverse Psoriasis is a type of psoriasis in which the Inverse psoriasis (sometimes called flexural psoriasis) is characterized by smooth, inflamed areas of skin. Skin folds surrounding the genitals (between the thigh and the groin), the armpits, the skin folds of an overweight belly (known as panniculus), the intergluteal cleft, and the inframammary fold beneath the breasts are all affected by the patches. Heat, stress, and infection are thought to play a role in the development of this unusual type of psoriasis (Weigle, McBane et al., 2013).

9.5 PSORIASIS ETIOLOGY

The particular etiology of psoriasis is unknown; however, researchers have a basic notion owing to decades of research: Genetics, Microbes, Medications, Lifestyle, and Marine botanicals.

9.5.1 GENETICS

About a third of patients with psoriasis have an intimate past of the disease, and researchers have discovered genetic loci linked to the disease. According to identical twin research, if one twin has psoriasis, the other twin has a 70% probability of having it as well. For nonidentical twins, the risk is roughly 20%. These data imply that psoriasis is caused by both a genetic vulnerability and an environmental reaction (Krueger, Ellis et al., 2005). Psoriasis has a high genetic element, and various genes are linked to it, but it's unknown how those genes interact. The majority of the genes discovered are associated with the immune system, specifically the MHC and T cells. Inborn investigations are significant because they can discover molecular appliances and passageways that can be studied further. Psoriasis is linked to nine loci on various chromosomes, according to traditional genome-wide linkage research.

They're known as psoriasis susceptibility 1 to 9 (PSORS1 through PSORS9). Genes involved in inflammatory pathways are found within those loci. Psoriasis is recurrently linked with certain variants (mutations) of particular genes (Nestle, Kaplan, Barker et al., 2009). Other genes that are mutated to distinctive variations in psoriasis have been discovered using genome-wide association scans. Some of these genes produce inflammatory signal proteins, which have an impact on immune cells involved in psoriasis. Other autoimmune illnesses are linked to some of these genes (Nestle, Kaplan, Barker et al., 2009). PSORS1 is the most important factor, accounting for 35–50% of psoriasis heredity (Smith, Barker et al., 2006). It regulates genes that impact the immune system or code for excessive skin proteins. PSORS1 affects essential immunological activities and is found on chromosome 6 of the MHC. Psoriasis is strongly linked to 3 genes in the PSORS1 locus.

9.5.2 MICROBES

Psoriasis is thought to mature after strep throat and can be exacerbated by skin or gut colonization with Staphylococcus aureus, Malassezia spp., or Candida albicans. Guttate psoriasis is a type of psoriasis that commonly affects children and teenagers and is caused by a recent group A streptococcal infection (tonsillitis or pharyngitis) (Rendon, Schakel et al., 2019).

9.5.3 MEDICATIONS

Beta-blockers, lithium, antimalarial medications, nonsteroidal anti-inflammatory drugs, terbinafine, calcium channel blockers, captopril, glyburide, granulocyte colony-stimulating factor, interleukins, interferons, (Jain et al., 2012) lipid-lowering medications, and paradoxically TNF inhibitors such as infliximab or adalimumab have all been linked to drug-induced psoriasis (Guerra, Gisbert et al., 2013). The rebound effect of stopping corticosteroids (topical steroid cream) can worsen psoriasis (Raychaudhuri, Maverakis, Raychaudhuri et al., 2014).

9.5.4 LIFESTYLE

Chronic conditions, stress, and seasonal variations have all been reported to aggravate the illness (Prieto-Pérez, Cabaleiro, Daudén, Ochoa, Roman, Abad-Santos et al., 2013). Hot water, scratching psoriasis skin lesions, skin dryness, extreme alcohol use, cigarette smoking, and obesity are all potential aggravators (Clarke et al., 2011; Richard, Barnetche, Horreau, Brenaut, Pouplard, Aractingi et al., 2013). As of 2019, no studies on the impacts of quitting smoking or alcohol abuse have been conducted (Ko, Chi, Yeh, Wang, Tsai, Hsu et al., 2019).

9.6 PATHOPHYSIOLOGY

The collection of pathological events in psoriasis is thought to begin with an initiation phase in which an event (skin trauma, infection, or drugs) leads to activation of the immune system and then the maintenance phase including chronic progression of the disease (Nestle, Kaplan, Barker et al., 2009). Skin cells are replaced every 3–5 days in psoriasis instead of the usual 28–30 days (Parrish et al., 2012). These changes are believed to result from the abnormal growth of keratinocytes triggered by an inflammatory cascade in the dermis involving dendritic cells, macrophages, and T cells (Cedeno-Laurent, Gómez-Flores, Mendez, Ancer-Rodríguez, Bryant, Gaspari, Trujillo et al., 2011). These immune cells migrate from the dermis to the epidermis and release inflammatory signaling molecules (cytokines) such as interleukin-36, tumor necrosis factor-alpha, interleukin-1ß, interleukin-6, and interleukin-22 (Baliwag, Barnes, Johnston et al., 2015). These secreted inflammatory molecules are believed to stimulate keratinocytes to proliferate (Nestle, Kaplan, Barker et al., 2009). One supposition is that psoriasis comprises an illness in governing T cells and within the regulatory cytokine interleukin-10 (Nestle, Kaplan, Barker et al., 2009). The inflammatory cytokines observed in psoriatic nails and joints (in psoriatic arthritis) are related to the ones of psoriatic pores and skin lesions, suggesting a common inflammatory mechanism. Gene mutations of proteins concerned with the skin's capability to function as a barrier have been identified as markers of susceptibility to the development of psoriasis (Roberson, Bowcock et al., 2010; Ramos-e-Silva, Jacques et al., 2012). DNA released from dying cells acts as an inflammatory stimulus in psoriasis (Dombrowski, Schauber et al., 2012) and stimulates the receptors on certain dendritic cells, which in turn produce the cytokine interferon-alpha. In response to these chemical signals from dendritic cells and T cells, keratinocytes also secrete cytokines such as interleukin-1, interleukin-6, and tumor necrosis factor-alpha, which signal downstream inflammatory cells to arrive and further stimulate inflammation (Nestle, Kaplan, Barker et al., 2009). Dendritic cells bridge the innate immune system and adaptive immune system. They interact with T cells (Ouyang et al., 2010) and type 1 helper T cells proliferate in psoriatic lesions, promoting their proliferation (Th1). Targeted immunotherapy, as well as psoralen and ultraviolet A (PUVA) therapy, can reduce the number of different types of dendritic cells, favoring a Th2 cell cytokine profile over a Th1/Th17 cellular cytokine profile (Wong, Hsu, Liao et al., 2013). Psoriatic T cells produce interferon and interleukin-22 as they migrate from the dermis to the epidermis. Interleukin-22 collaborates with interleukin-17 to induce keratinocytes to release neutrophil-attracting cytokines (Mudigonda, Mudigonda, Feneran, Alamdari, Sandoval, Feldman et al., 2012).

9.7 EPIDEMIOLOGY

Psoriasis is estimated to affect 2–4% of the residents of the western world (Parisi, Symmons, Griffiths, Ashcroft et al., 2013). Psoriasis rates vary by age, area, and ethnicity; these differences are assumed to be triggered by a mix of environmental and inherited factors. It can affect a person at any age, but it most frequently strikes people between the ages of 15 and 25. Psoriasis is diagnosed in about a third of adults before they reach the age of 20 (Benoit, Hamm et al., 2007). Psoriasis affects both men and women (Kupetsky, Keller et al., 2013). About 6.7 million Americans suffer from psoriasis, which is more common among adults. Persons of European heritage are around five times more likely than individuals of Asian origin to have psoriasis. Psoriasis is more likely to improve in those who have inflammatory bowel diseases, such as Crohn's disease or ulcerative colitis (Guerra, Gisbert et al., 2013). Psoriasis is more widespread in regions that are farther from the equator. Psoriasis is more common among people of white European descent, while it is very rare in African Americans and extremely rare in Native Americans (Weller, John AA Hunter, John Savin, Mark Dahl et al., 2013).

9.8 TREATMENT

Psoriasis is estimated to affect 2–4% of the residents of the western world (Parisi, Symmons, Griffiths, Ashcroft et al., 2013). Psoriasis rates vary by age, area, and ethnicity; these differences are assumed to be triggered by a mix of environmental and inherited factors. It can affect a person at any age, but it most frequently strikes people between the ages of 15 and 25. Psoriasis is diagnosed in about a third of adults before they reach the age of 20 (Benoit, Hamm et al., 2007). Psoriasis affects both men and women (Kupetsky, Keller et al., 2013). About 6.7 million Americans suffer from psoriasis, which is more common among adults. Persons of European heritage are around five times more likely than individuals of Asian origin to have psoriasis. Psoriasis is more likely to improve in those who have inflammatory bowel diseases, such as Crohn's disease or ulcerative colitis (Guerra, Gisbert et al., 2013).

Psoriasis is more widespread in regions that are farther from the equator. Psoriasis is more common among people of white European descent, while it is very rare in African Americans and extremely rare in Native Americans (Weller, John AA Hunter, John Savin, Mark Dahl et al., 2013). Tonsillectomy: Limited evidence shows that tonsillectomy may help individuals with persistent plaque and guttate psoriasis. Aquatic botanicals differ from marine botanicals. The name implies that they are constantly associated with the sea or the ocean. The active chemicals may be identified and harvested biologically from an assorted range of marine organisms, which serve as great repositories for these compounds. These compounds could be used as nutritional supplements, medicines, cosmeceuticals, cosmetics, fine chemicals, or enzymes (Pomponi et al., 1999). Marine botanicals are plants or plant parts native to the sea or ocean that are prized for their medical or therapeutic capabilities, flavor, and aroma, all of which are used to maintain or improve health.

Thalassotherapy is a term that first appeared in the early 1800s, resulting from the Greek words "thalasso" (sea) and "therapia" (treatment) (cure). The French were the first to utilize it in the middle of the past century, and it quickly spread over the world thanks to the results gained and published on the welfare and excellence of life of individuals who used it. Some of their properties were already known to the Chinese, Egyptians, and Romans, who had manufactured various panaceas from algae. Many therapies are given the thalassotherapy title, but not all of them are deserving of it. Due to its recent popularity, the phrase has been used to refer to so-called "spa" treatments. It may be required to limit its use to seawater, sand, and other similar treatments, macroalgae, and other marine goods. The reality is that the sea's elements (whether mineral or biological) have always been a part of our lives. Water, particularly seawater, is considered important for the survival of life on our planet since it contains all the compounds or elements required for the growth of living beings (minerals, catalysts, vitamins, amino acids, etc.). Seawater has been shown to be effective in dealing with disorders affecting skin tissues, including cutaneous (skin) and mucous membranes. Thalassotherapy, which originated in Ireland, was a seaweed bath made with warm freshwater, seawater, and fresh seaweed, primarily Fucus serratus (*Phaeophyceae*). Fucales comprise a diverse range of species, including F. serratus and F. vesiculosus, with beneficial components such as fatty acids, antioxidants, and iodine, among others. Seawater was one of the first therapies employed by man for both appealing and well-being objectives due to its alignment (salt and iodine). Algae have a lot of pharmacological and aesthetic potential because they are high in proteins, vitamins, and minerals that our skin needs. In addition to the skin advantages, algae can help decrease cholesterol and prevent hypertension when consumed. In addition to calcium (Ca), iron (Fe), magnesium (Mg), sodium (Na), zinc (Zn), and copper (Cu), seawater is also rejuvenating, anti-infective, anti-stress, analgesic, and beneficial for depression and other mood disorders. The salt also acts as a natural exfoliator and promotes cellular renewal. Iodine, an inorganic compound found in seawater, activates the thyroid gland, which normalizes metabolism. The need to adapt to infection changes serves to raise the rate of metabolism and has a very progressive effect on blood passage (Charlier, Chaineux et al., 2009).

Other advantages of thalassotherapy include:

- Increased skin permeability;
- While interacting with the skin, their ionic properties enhance the uptake of cosmetic components during or after these procedures;
- As an enzymatic cofactor, controls organic activities via the neuro-endocrine system;
- Relieves tense muscles, giving the skin a refreshed appearance;
- Tends to bring seborrheic secretion back to normal;
- Decreases hyperhidrosis (excessive sweating, especially on the feet);
- Encourages organic remineralization in cutaneous tissue; and
- Promotes indirect oxygenation and sustenance of these tissues by activating cutaneous metabolism and stimulating local blood circulation.

Water, particularly the ocean, is regarded as critical to the lifecycle of our planet. It contains all of the ingredients required for the growth of living beings (minerals, catalysts, vitamins, amino acids, etc.). Oceans span about 70% of the Earth's surface and are home to 90% of the planet's creatures. The water has many different ecosystems and characteristics to discover. Numerous marine creatures have the capacity to create bioactive chemicals that can be employed as nutraceuticals, medicines, or cosmetics. As a result, more research is required to discover, explore, comprehend, and ultimately employ live species from the oceans. In the 19th century, the French biologist René Quinton could prove experimentally the remarkable similarity between seawater and human plasma—"Our organism is a kind of aquarium whose internal environment is constituted by seawater" (Gomez, Lambrecht, Lozano, Rinaudo, Villar et al., 2009).

9.9 CLASSIFICATION OF MARINE PLANTS

9.9.1 MONERA

In the marine environment, fewer than 2,000 genera of germs exist out of 100,000 species. Despite their modest size, this group of organisms plays a vital role in energy transmission, nutrient cycles, and organic turnover. Members of the Monera have archaeal cytology, which means they lack membrane-bound organelles including green plastids, mitochondria or sarcosomes, nuclei, and complex flagella, distinguishing them from the other four kingdoms (Dawes, Clinton et al., 1998). Eubacteria and Archaebacteria are the two primary bacterial subkingdoms.

9.9.2 PROTISTA

Algae in this kingdom can be classified as Phaeophyta, *Rhodophyta*, or *Chlorophyta*, which are three macroalgae/seaweed families. Due to their simple structure and unicellular nature, the Protista kingdom comprises species that have been categorized. Protozoa, algae, and slime molds are all examples of these organisms. Macroalgae and microalgae make up the majority of photosynthetic organisms found in marine habitats. Based on these characteristics, algae can be further classified according to Storage products, Photosynthetic pigments, Chloroplast structure, Inclusions in the cell, Cell wall structure, Flagella structure, and Cell division (Dawes, Clinton et al., 1998).

9.9.3 PLANTAE

Angiosperms, or herbs that produce kernels or flowers as part of their genital system, make up the Plantae Kingdom. In marine-like habitats, about 0.85% of the 300,000 Angiosperms estimated to prevail can be discovered. Mosses, ferns, seagrasses, mangroves, and salt marsh plants are examples of this kingdom. Seagrasses are considered to be among the most essential marine ecosystems. It's the only genuine submerged angiosperm, and it can help scientists figure out how healthy an ecosystem is (Editors et al., 2016).

9.10 MARINE ECOLOGY AND MARINE BOTANY

The zones of marine ecology and marine botany are as follows (Dawes, Clinton et al., 1998):

- Benthic zone;
- Coral reef;
- Kelp forests;
- Mangroves;
- Phytoplankton;
- Salt marsh;
- Sea grass;
- Seaweed.

However, only sea grass and seaweed sections are included in all of these zones' marine botanicals.

9.10.1 SEAWEED

Taxonomy and Bioactivities of Algae–Algae, like the majority of plants, have pigmented cells that enable them to perform photosynthesis. This group of organisms has a wide geographic distribution, colonizing many different locations, but they are all linked to the presence of water. They can be found floating in the water, attached to rocks and walls, or in combination with other organisms, such as lichens and fungi. The algae are particularly numerous in the euphotic or photic zones of seas, rivers, and lagoons, where they live until light penetration allows photosynthesis, which can be up to 200 meters deep depending on the environment. Benthic algae are planktonic algae. The first, which live attached to a substrate, are macroscopic and can grow to be 50 meters long; the second, which dwell suspended in the water column, are very small (Pereira, L. Algae. Litoral of Viana do Castelo, Câmara Municipal de Viana do Castelo: Viana do Castelo, Portugal et al., 2010; Pereira, Correia, Algas Marinhas da Costa Portuguesa et al., 2015). Macroalgae are photosynthetic aquatic creatures that belong to the Eukaryota domain as well as the Plantae and Chromista kingdoms. Despite the fact that categorization systems have developed over time, it is generally agreed that red algae belong to the phylum Rhodophyta, and its photosynthetic pigments are chlorophyll a, phycobilins, and carotenoids. Brown algae belong to the *Ochrophyta phylum* and the *Phaeophyceae* family, with pigments such as chlorophylls a, c, and carotenoids. Green algae belong to the phylum Chlorophyta, and their coloring is similar to that of land plants (chlorophyll a, b, and carotenoids). Due to their diversity of constituents, algae have been widely used in many parts of the world as a source of essential compounds for human nutrition, and for the cosmetic and pharmaceutical industries. They are the basis of proteins of brilliant quality, for the reason that they contain all the needed amino acids, polyunsaturated fatty acids, especially the omega-3 fatty acid family and other essential fatty acids; carbohydrates, vitamins, minerals, dietary fibers, and bioactive secondary metabolites, among others. Seaweed as a simple diet item has been used in China, Korea, and Japan since prehistoric times. "Some seaweed is a delicacy suited for the most valued guests, and even for the king himself," wrote Sze Teu in China in 600 BC. In modern Japan, some 21 kinds of algae are used in common cooking, six of which have been utilized since the 8th century (Pereira et al., 2018; Holdt, Kraan et al., 2011). Under normal growth conditions, such as reproduction, macroalgae produce both primary and secondary metabolites, which are directly involved in physiological functions. Secondary metabolites are produced under different stress conditions, such as UV radiation, temperature, salinity, or environmental pollutants. Primary algal metabolites include proteins, amino acids, polysaccharides, and fatty acids. The secondary metabolites produced in algae tissues are phenolic compounds, pigments, sterols, vitamins, and other bioactive compounds (Vo, Ngo, Kim et al., 2012; Thomas, Kim et al., 2013). They are impervious to the harshest living situations due to their incredible adaptability. Because of their skin-care properties as true multi-talents, their use in cosmetics was identified. Algae moisturize the skin, raise skin resistance, promote blood circulation, activate cell renewal and metabolism, regulate sebaceous gland function, drain the tissues, have an anti-inflammatory action, and regulate sebaceous gland function. Seaweeds or Macroalgae are categories of millions of species of multicellular, macroscopic, marine plants. Many individuals with psoriasis have a deficiency of Omega-3 fatty acids, which is commonly linked to inflammation within the body – and thus psoriasis outbreaks. But, luckily for consumers, marine algae having high Omega-3 content could help to reduce painful psoriasis symptoms when topically applied to the skin. Reduced inflammation is one of the assistances of omega-3 for treating psoriasis. They lubricate body cells when they get involved in the bloodstream. During this process, the cells are lubricated and are able to heal. Inflammation can also be decreased by this lubrication (Schrammek et al., 2018; Joshi, Kumari, Upasani et al., 2018). The non-disputed treasures of the maritime are the algae (macro and microalgae) (Figure 9.1).

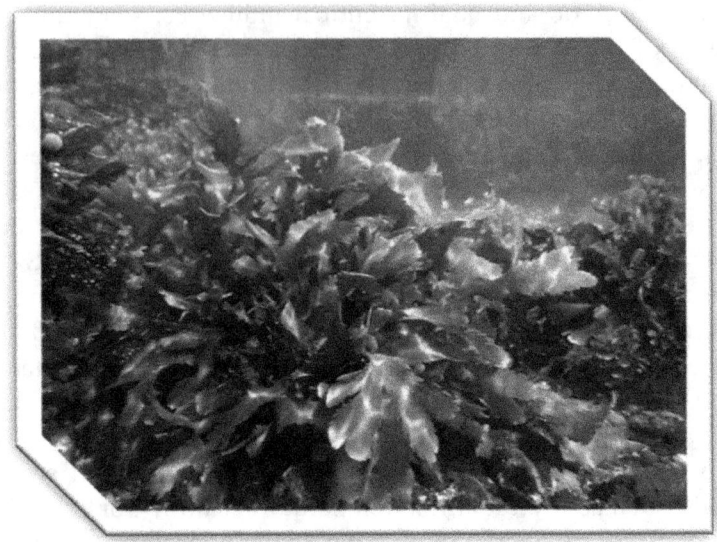

FIGURE 9.1 Seaweed.
Image courtesy: Grubio--1. https://creativecommons.org/licenses/by-sa/4.0/

9.10.2 RHODOPHYTA

Rhodophyta, also known as red algae, *Gracilaria* is a subfamily of scarlet macroalgae. Red algae have a high content of vitamin D and fatty acids, which are used in the therapy of psoriasis in patients with a deficiency of omega-3 fatty acids. It thins the plaque when applied directly to the skin due to vitamin D's ability to reduce the advancement of new cells. By reducing inflammation, alpha-linolenic acid helps manage psoriasis symptoms. Upon entering the bloodstream, fatty acids lubricate the dermis and reduce irritation. China, Japan, Germany, and the indigenous peoples of Latin America have been using red algae as food for centuries. They have also used red algae for its potent healing properties in the therapy of various diseases. Vitamin D is obtained from Rhodophyta, which is used in the therapy of psoriasis. People with compromised gut health, who find it hard to absorb vitamin D from the food they eat, benefit from vitamin D as it is a fat-soluble vitamin that can help treat psoriasis. *Gracilaria* algae is a red macroalgae that has shown considerable anti-inflammatory effects. The efficacy of a 3% *Gracilaria* algae topical cream and a 0.05% clobetasol cream were also used in the management of plaque psoriasis. (Mohammad Ali. Shatalebi, Safoura Bokaie Jazi, Afsaneh Yegdaneh, Fariba Iraji, Amir Hossein Saidat, Pegah Noorshargh et al., 2012) (Figures 9.2 and 9.3).

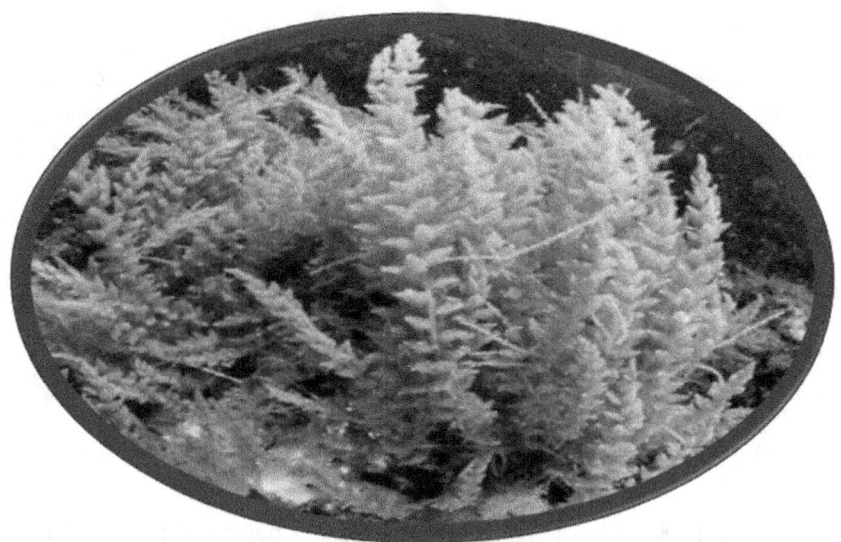

FIGURE 9.2   Rhodophyta.

Source: Indiamart.   https://www.indiamart.com/proddetail/red-algae-extract-n4338-2851934682833.html

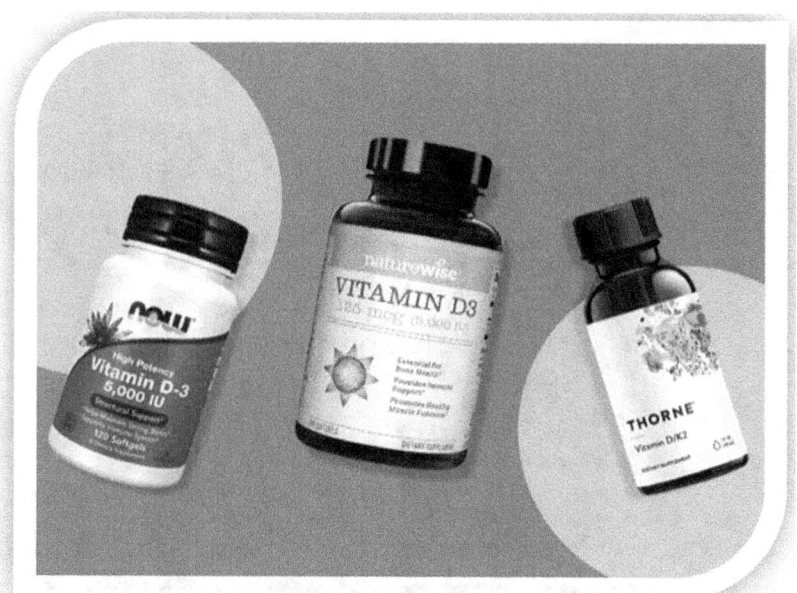

FIGURE 9.3   Marketed formulation of vitamin D.

Source: Greatist. https://greatist.com/health/best-vitamin-d-supplement#how-to-use

9.10.3 SEA MOSS

It is also identified as Irish moss (*Chondrus crispus*). It originates from red algae and benefits the skin in a variety of ways, essentially making it an all-purpose skincare product. It can soothe inflammatory conditions of the skin such as psoriasis because it contains minerals and vitamins. Sea moss contains high sulfur content, giving it antibacterial, antiviral, and antimicrobial properties that may help maintain the balance of skin microbiomes. Various nutrients and antioxidants in sea moss can enhance immunity and fight infections.

Marketed preparations of sea moss include (Figure 9.4):

i. **Serum:** Iceland moss drop, also known as Iceland moss. This sea moss serum is used to moisturize dry, irritated skin by replenishing moisture and soothing irritation.

ii. **Purple Sea Moss Gel:** Purple Sea moss carries a powerful antioxidant called anthocyanin. It supports the immune system and fights against infections.

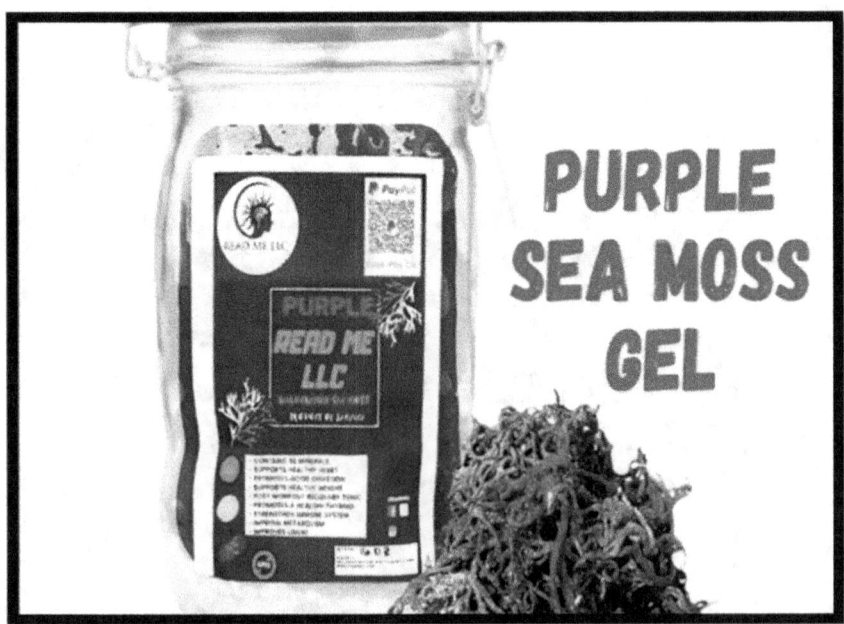

FIGURE 9.4 Marketed formulation of sea moss gel.
Source: Read Me LLC. https://readmesllc.com/wild-crafted-purple-sea-moss-from-jamaica.html

9.10.4 PHAEOPHYTA

Phaeophyta, also called Brown Algae, supports cellular energy production and thus promotes skin cell renewal. Furthermore, brown algae also contain helpful minerals and micro-nutrients and offer powerful anti-inflammatory, soothing, and hydrating properties. Brown macroalgae have sulfated, fucose-rich polymers called fucoidans (Kiple, Ornelas et al., 2000; Berteau, Mulloy et al., 2003). They were revealed in the early 20th century. Fucoidan was discovered to play a part in the biology of seaweed and was studied for its action in a variety of biological systems during the next few decades. Fucoidans have a high amount of fucose in the sugar backbone of the polymer in general. Sulfated, acetylated, and containing uronic acids are all possibilities. The yield of a crude first fraction of fucoidan is typically 2–10% by weight; however, *Cladosiphon* species can produce up to 20% by dry weight. Seaweed-derived fucoidans are all heavily branching. Echinoderms, in particular, provide a second source of linear rather than branching fucoidans, sea cucumbers, which are basically outside the scope of this analysis (Fitton, Irhimeh, Teas et al., 2008; Pomin, Mourao et al., 2008; Li, Lu, Wei, Zhao et al., 2008). Fucus vesiculosus, a frequent harvest crop of northern hemisphere kelp, is the most common source of experimental fucoidan used in the literature (Nishino, Nishioka, Ura, Nagumo et al., 1994). Fucus vesiculosus fucoidan is a sulfated fucoidan with a high fucose content. Other edible species that contain fucoidans include *Cladosiphon okamuranus*, *Laminaria japonica*, and *Undaria pinnatifida*. These seaweeds are gathered in large quantities throughout Asia and have a low toxicity level. Fucoidan is a chemical compound found in a variety of brown seaweed genera. Fucoidan is a type of sulfated polysaccharide that has a large amount of L-fucose. When it was first isolated from seaweeds by Kylin in 1913, fucoidan was known as 'fucoidan.' According to IUPAC standards, it was later dubbed fucoidan. Fucoidan comes in capsules, extracts, and powder form. Fucoidan is used to improve the immune system. Fucoidan can be simply 'cooked' from edible seaweed by boiling for 20 to 40 minutes in water. In addition to lessening inflammation, it promotes faster recovery of tissues when consumed. Current research has shown that the consumption of the sulfated polysaccharide fucoidan ameliorates the signs of Psoriasis (Figure 9.5).

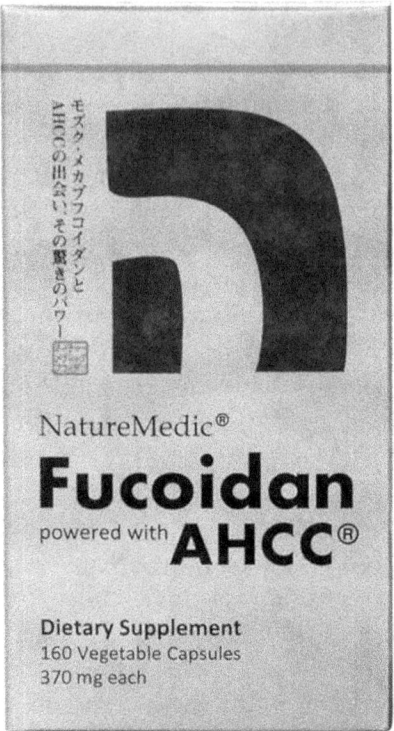 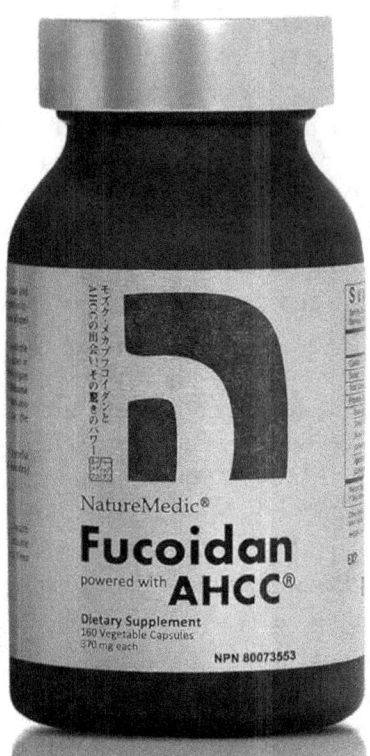

FIGURE 9.5 Marketed formulation of fucoidan.

Source: Amazon. https://www.amazon.com/NatureMedic-Fucoidan-Immunity-Supplement-Vegetable/dp/B016EFMPK2

9.11 CONCLUSION

There are numerous medications that are used to treat psoriasis currently have a number of side effects, which has shifted the researchers' attention to safer natural marine botanicals as a nutraceutical. We have to keep in mind that there are severe interactions that occur with the synthetic drugs available for the treatment of psoriasis; hence, there is a need to develop natural marine botanicals that seem to be a viable approach to explore for newer, safer, and more effective anti-psoriatic drugs. Marine botanicals such as Rhodophyta, Phaeophyta, Chlorophyta, Cyanobacteria, and Sea moss as seaweed have been used in traditional systems to offer relief in psoriasis, which has been scientifically proven for the traditional claims.

KEYWORDS

- algae
- cyanobacteria
- fucoidan
- inflammation
- marine botanical
- pathophysiology
- psoralen and ultraviolet A
- psoriasis
- Rhodophyta
- seaweed
- skin disease
- thalassotherapy

REFERENCES

Baliwag, J., Barnes, D. H., & Johnston, A. (2015). Cytokines in psoriasis. *Cytokine, 73*(2), 342–350.

Benedek, T. G. (2013). Psoriasis and psoriatic arthropathy, historical aspects: Part I. *Journal of Clinical Rheumatology, 19*(3), 135–140.

Benedek, T. G. (2013). Psoriasis and psoriatic arthropathy: historical aspects: Part II. *Journal of Clinical Rheumatology, 19*(4), 205–211.

Benoit, S., & Hamm, H. (2007). Childhood psoriasis. *Clinics in Dermatology, 25*(6), 555–562. https://doi.org/10.1016/j.clindermatol.2007.08.009.

Berteau, O., & Mulloy, B. (2003). Sulfated fucans, fresh perspectives: Structures, functions, and biological properties of sulfated fucans and an overview of enzymes active toward this class of polysaccharide. *Glycobiology, 13*, 29–40.

Cedeno-Laurent, F., Gómez-Flores, M., Mendez, N., Ancer-Rodríguez, J., Bryant, J. L., Gaspari, A. A., & Trujillo, J. R. (2011). New insights into HIV-1-primary skin disorders. *Journal of the International AIDS Society*, v.14; 2011.

Charlier, R. H., & Chaineux, M. C. P. (2009). The healing sea: A sustainable coastal ocean resource: Thalassotherapy. *Journal of Coastal Research, 25*, 838–856.

Clarke, P. (2011). Psoriasis. *Australian Family Physician, 40*(7), 468–473. https://www.racgp.org.au/getattachment/d011d1f0-ee93-47a4-8417-d731cc7d320e/Psoriasis.aspx

Colledge, N. R., Walker, B. R., & Ralston, S. H. (Eds.). (2010). *Davidson's Principles and Practice of Medicine* (21st ed.). Edinburgh: Churchill Livingstone/Elsevier. pp. 1360. ISBN: 9780702030857.

Dawes, C. J. (1998). *Marine Botany*. John Wiley & Sons. pp. 596. ISBN: 978-0-471-19208-4.

Dombrowski, Y., & Schauber, J. (2012). Cathelicidin LL-37: a defense molecule with a potential role in psoriasis pathogenesis. *Experimental Dermatology, 21*(5), 327–330.

Editors, B. D. (2016). "Eubacteria." *Biology Dictionary*. Retrieved 2020–11–23.

Fitton, J. H., Irhimeh, M. R., & Teas, J. (2008). Marine algae and polysaccharides with therapeutic applications. In C. Barrow & F. Shahidi (Eds.), *Marine Nutraceuticals and Functional Foods* (pp. 345–366). CRC Press, Taylor & Francis Group.

Gomez, C. G., Lambrecht, M. V. P., Lozano, J. E., Rinaudo, M., & Villar, M. A. (2009). Influence of the extraction-purification conditions on final properties of alginates obtained from brown algae (*Macrocystis pyrifera*). *International Journal of Biological Macromolecules, 44*, 365–371.

Gruber, F., Kastelan, M., & Brajac, I. (2004). Psoriasis treatment–yesterday, today, and tomorrow. *Acta Dermatovenerologica Croatica, 12*(1), 30–34.

Guerra, I., & Gisbert, J. P. (2013). Onset of psoriasis in patients with inflammatory bowel disease treated with anti-TNF agents. *Expert Review of Gastroenterology & Hepatology*.

Hill, R. T., & Fenical, W. (2010). Pharmaceuticals from marine natural products: Surge or ebb? *Current Opinion in Biotechnology, 21*, 777–779.

Holdt, S. L., & Kraan, S. (2011). Bioactive compounds in seaweed: Functional food applications and legislation. *Journal of Applied Phycology, 23*, 543–597.

Jain, S. (2012). *Dermatology: Illustrated Study Guide and Comprehensive Board Review*. Springer. pp. 83–87. Archived from the original on 8 September 2017, *7*(1), 41–48.

Joshi, S., Kumari, R., & Upasani, V. N. (2018). Applications of algae in cosmetics: An overview. *International Journal of Innovative Research in Science, Engineering and Technology, 7*, 1269–1278.

Keith, W. G. (2009). Marine products for healthcare: Functional and bioactive nutraceutical compounds from the ocean. In V. Venugopal (Ed.), *Functional Foods and Nutraceuticals Series*, 528. ACRC Press, Taylor and Francis Group.

Keservani, R. K., & Sharma, A. K. (2014). Flavonoids: emerging trends and potential health benefits. *Journal of Chinese Pharmaceutical Sciences, 23*(12), 815.

Keservani, R. K., Sharma, A. K., & Kesharwani, R. K. (2016a). Nutraceutical and Functional Foods for Cardiovascular Health. In *Food Process Engineering* (pp. 291–312). Apple Academic Press, CRC Press. ISBN: 9781771884020.

Keservani, R. K., Sharma, A. K., & Kesharwani, R. K. (2016b). Medicinal effect of nutraceutical fruits for cognition and brain health. *Scientifica*. Article ID 3109254. https://doi.org/10.1155/2016/3109254.

Kiple, K. F., & Ornelas, K. C. (2000). Important vegetable supplements. In S. V. Beck (Ed.), *The Cambridge World History of Food* (Vol. 1, pp. 231–249). Cambridge University Press.

Ko, S. H., Chi, C. C., Yeh, M. L., Wang, S. H., Tsai, Y. S., & Hsu, M. Y. (2019). Lifestyle changes for treating psoriasis. *The Cochrane Database of Systematic Reviews, 2019*(7), CD011972.

Krueger, G., & Ellis, C. N. (2005). Psoriasis–recent advances in understanding its pathogenesis and treatment. *Journal of the American Academy of Dermatology, 53*(1 Suppl 1): S94–100.

Kupetsky, E. A., & Keller, M. (2013). Psoriasis vulgaris: an evidence-based guide for primary care. *Journal of the American Board of Family Medicine, 26*(5), 698–710.

Kylin, H. (1913). Zur Biochemie der Meeresalgen. *Hoppe-Seyler's Zeitschrift für Physiologische Chemie, 83*, 171–197.

Li, B., Lu, F., Wei, X., & Zhao, R. (2008). Fucoidan: Structure and bioactivity. *Molecules, 13*, 1671–1695.
Liu, R. H. (2003). The health benefits of fruit and vegetables are from additive and synergistic combinations of phytochemicals. *American Journal of Clinical Nutrition, 78*, 517S–520S.
Meenan, F. O. (1955). A note on the history of psoriasis. *Irish Journal of Medical Science, 30*(3), 141–142.
Mohammad Ali, Shatalebi, S. B., Jazi, A. B., Yegdaneh, F., Iraji, F., Saidat, A. H., & Noorshargh, P. (2012). Comparative evaluation of Gracilaria algae 3% cream versus Clobetasol 0.0.5% cream in the treatment of plaque-type psoriasis. *33*(6), e14317.
Mudigonda, P., Mudigonda, T., Feneran, A. N., Alamdari, H. S., Sandoval, L., & Feldman, S. R. (2012). Interleukin-23 and interleukin-17: Importance in pathogenesis and therapy of psoriasis. *Dermatology Online Journal, 18*(10), 1.
Nestle, F. O., Kaplan, D. H., & Barker, J. (2009). Psoriasis. *The New England Journal of Medicine, 361*(5), 496–509.
Nishino, T., Nishioka, C., Ura, H., & Nagumo, T. (1994). Isolation and partial characterization of a novel amino sugar-containing fucan sulfate from commercial Fucus vesiculosus fucoidan. *Carbohydrate Research, 255*, 213–224.
Ouyang, W. (2010). Distinct roles of IL-22 in human psoriasis and inflammatory bowel disease. *Cytokine & Growth Factor Reviews, 21*(6), 435–441.
Palfreeman, A. C., McNamee, K. E., & McCann, F. E. (2013). New developments in the management of psoriasis and psoriatic arthritis: a focus on apremilast. *Drug Design, Development, and Therapy, 7*, 201–210.
Palthur, M. P., Sajala Palthur, S. S., & Chitta, S. K. (2010). Nutraceuticals: Concept and regulatory scenario. *International Journal of Pharmacy and Pharmaceutical Sciences, 2*, 14–20.
Parisi, R., Symmons, D. P., Griffiths, C. E., & Ashcroft, D. M. (2013). Global epidemiology of psoriasis: A systematic review of incidence and prevalence. *The Journal of Investigative Dermatology, 133*(2), 377–385.
Parrish, L. (2012). Psoriasis: Symptoms, treatments and its impact on quality of life. *British Journal of Community Nursing, 17*(11), 524, 526, 528.
Pereira, L. (2018). Seaweeds as Source of Bioactive Substances and Skin Care Therapy—Cosmeceuticals, Algotheraphy, and Thalassotherapy. *Cosmetics, 5*, 68.
Pereira, L. (2018). *Therapeutic and Nutritional Uses of Algae* (1st ed.). CRC Press, Boca Raton, FL, USA, pp. 2–64. ISBN: 9781315152844.
Pereira, L., & Correia, F. (2015). *Algae Marinhas da Costa Portuguesa: Ecologia, Biodiversidade e Utilizações*. Nota de Rodapé Editores: Paris, France, pp. 326–340. ISBN 978-989-20-5754-5.
Pomin, V. H., & Mourao, P. A. (2008). Structure, biology, evolution, and medical importance of sulfated fucans and galactans. *Glycobiology, 18*, 1016–1027.
Pomponi, S. A. (1999). The bioprocess-technological potential of the sea. *Journal of Biotechnology, 70*, 5–13.
Prieto-Pérez, R., Cabaleiro, T., Daudén, E., Ochoa, D., Roman, M., & Abad-Santos, F. (2013). Genetics of psoriasis and pharmacogenetics of biological drugs. *Autoimmune Diseases*.
Ramos-e-Silva, M., & Jacques, C. (2012). Epidermal barrier function and systemic diseases. *Clinics in Dermatology, 30*(3), 277–279.
Raychaudhuri, S. K., Maverakis, E., & Raychaudhuri, S. P. (2014). Diagnosis and classification of psoriasis. *Autoimmunity Reviews, 13*(4–5), 490–495.

Rendon, A., & Schäkel, K. (2019). Psoriasis pathogenesis and treatment. *International Journal of Molecular Sciences, 20*(6), 1475.

Richard, M. A., Barnetche, T., Horreau, C., Brenaut, E., Pouplard, C., Aractingi, S., et al. (2013). Psoriasis, cardiovascular events, cancer risk, and alcohol use: evidence-based recommendations based on systematic review and expert opinion. *Journal of the European Academy of Dermatology and Venereology, 27*(Suppl 3), 2–11.

Roberson, E. D., & Bowcock, A. M. (2010). Psoriasis genetics: Breaking the barrier. *Trends in Genetics, 26*(9), 415–423.

Robinson, A., Van Voorhees, A. S., Hsu, S., Korman, N. J., Lebwohl, M. G., Bebo, B. F., & Kalb, R. E. (2012). Treatment of pustular psoriasis: From the Medical Board of the National Psoriasis Foundation. *Journal of the American Academy of Dermatology, 67*(2), 279–288.

Schrammek Beauty News. (2018). Algae in Cosmetics—The All-Round Talents. https://www.schrammek.com/beautynews/algae-in-cosmetics/.

Smith, C. H., & Barker, J. N. (2006). Psoriasis and its management. *BMJ, 333*(7564), 380–384.

Stanway, A. (2014). Erythrodermic psoriasis. *DermNet NZ*. Retrieved from DermNet NZ (archived on 2 February 2014, retrieved 16 March 2014).

Thomas, N. V., & Kim, S. K. (2013). Beneficial effects of marine algal compounds in cosmeceuticals. *Marine Drugs, 11*, 146–164.

Thorpe, J. P., Sole-Cava, A. M., & Watts, P. C. (2000). Exploited marine invertebrates: Genetics and fisheries. *Hydrobiologia, 420*, 165–184.

Vo, T. S., Ngo, D. H., & Kim, S. K. (2012). Marine algae is a potential pharmaceutical source for anti-allergic therapeutics. *Process Biochemistry, 47*, 386–394.

Weigle, N., & McBane, S. (2013). Psoriasis. *American Family Physician*, 87(9), 626–633.

Weller, R., Hunter, J. A. A., Savin, J., & Dahl, M. (2008). *Clinical Dermatology* (4th ed.). Malden, MA: Blackwell. https://www.yumpu.com/en/document/view/21980162/clinical-dermatology-4th-ed-famona-site#google_vignette.

Wong, T., Hsu, L., & Liao, W. (2013). Phototherapy in psoriasis: A review of mechanisms of action. *Journal of Cutaneous Medicine and Surgery, 17*(1), 6–12.

Zattra, E., Belloni Fortina, A., Peserico, A., & Alaibac, M. (2012). Erythroderma in the era of biological therapies. *European Journal of Dermatology, 22*(2), 167–71.

CHAPTER 10

MICROALGAE AND THEIR USES AS NUTRACEUTICALS IN PSORIASIS

DEEPTI DWIVEDI,[1] SATYA PRAKASH SINGH,[1] AJAY KUMAR SHUKLA,[1] SHAILENDRA KUMAR,[2] and MANISH KUMAR[3]

[1]Institute of Pharmacy, Dr. Ram Manohar Lohia Avadh University, Ayodhya, Uttar Pradesh, India

[2]Institute of Microbiology, Dr. Ram Manohar Lohia Avadh University, Ayodhya, Uttar Pradesh, India

[3]Department of Pharmacy, Madhav University, Pindwara, Rajasthan, India

ABSTRACT

The skin serves as the body's first line of protection against pathogens and other pollutants in the environment. Reactive oxygen species (ROS), which cause the skin to become inflamed, are continually present in the body. One of the most common skin conditions with prominent indications of inflammation is psoriasis. Patients with psoriasis disorders experience a number of difficulties due to ineffective and unsuitable therapy. Gene mutations are the main contributors to the psoriasis condition. A wide range of environmental factors, including physical trauma, pharmaceutical reactions, infection, psychological stress, obesity, smoking, and alcohol, can cause it. Psoriatic lesions can develop in previously healthy-looking skin as a result of physical trauma such as excoriation, tattoos, burns, or animal or insect bites. Lithium, beta-blockers, antimalarials, tetracyclines, and non-steroidal anti-inflammatory drugs are the most frequently reported pharmaceuticals to induce psoriasis. Several substances have also been associated with the start and severity of psoriasis. Microalgae are particularly beneficial in the treatment and management of skin conditions like psoriasis. The ability of microalgae to biosynthesize putative secondary metabolites with anti-psoriasis potential has been discovered by numerous researchers. The potential of microalgae and their bioactive chemicals to treat skin issues such as infections, inflammation, and psoriasis is discussed in this chapter.

10.1 INTRODUCTION

Psoriasis is an inflammatory skin disease that affects 0.5% to 1% of children and 2 to 3% of the world's population (Villanova et al., 2003). Psoriasis disease is largely distributed and found in the 20–30 age group and less found in the 50–60 age group. The exact factors of psoriasis disease are unknown. Clinically, various factors have been reported that cause the possibility of psoriasis, such as genetic vulnerability, environmental triggers combined with skin barrier disturbance, and immunological dysfunction in the development of psoriasis. Plaque, guttate, pustular, inverse, and erythrodermic are all subtypes of the condition of psoriasis. About 85%–90% of people with psoriasis have some form of plaque psoriasis, which is the most prevalent type (Griffiths et al., 2003). As a result of the physical and psychological suffering that psoriasis causes, patients' well-being is often negatively impacted. Individuals with psoriasis typically feel guilty about their condition, which makes them feel even more inferior about themselves. Interpersonal connections, sexual well-being, and intimacy have been reported to be affected by psoriasis (De Korte et al., 2004). In the workplace, people with psoriasis may face discrimination or have trouble finding a job because of the disease's stigmatizing effect. In the United States, psoriasis-related complications cause several deaths each year. Inflammatory bowel disease (IBD) and psoriatic arthritis are common physical co-morbidities of people with psoriasis and other chronic skin conditions (Van Den Bogaard et al., 2014).

10.2 POTENTIAL CAUSES/TRIGGERS OF PSORIASIS

10.2.1 GENES

According to genetic studies, psoriasis patients have a variety of immunological and skin barrier-related gene variants (Kimball et al., 2008). Psoriasis effects have been about 70% in monozygotic twins and 20% in dizygotic twins according to earlier studies of psoriasis incidence (Love et al., 2011). In families where one or both parents have psoriasis, the odds of their offspring getting it are 20%; in those with both parents, the odds are 60% (Jordan et al., 2012).

10.2.2 PSORIASIS

The first known PSORS locus was found on chromosome 6p at a place called PSORS1. The location of a psoriasis hereditary gene had been established. However, the gene's identity is yet unclear. The most likely PSORS1 gene is HLA-C, situated in the Class I area of the major histocompatibility complex (MHC). In this sensitive area of the genome, one of the most common and robust disease loci, HLA-Cw6, is encoded.

Haplotypes of people with the genetic mutation known as HLA-Cw0602 are 20 times more likely to develop the disease than those who don't have it (Bowcock et al., 2005; Lowes et al., 2014; Elder et al., 2006). So far, it is uncertain whether or not the HLA-C and HLA-Cw6 genes play any function in psoriasis development. In addition, HLA-C is only responsible for half of the family clustering in psoriasis, according to researchers. Only two gene mutations (IL36RN and CARD14) have been found to cause psoriasis independently by altering the skin and immune system, despite over 30 genetic variants enhancing the likelihood of acquiring the disease (Lowes et al., 2013).

10.2.2.1 PSORS2/CARD14 MUTATIONS

PSORS2 was found on chromosome 17q25 (Pearce et al., 2006; Armstrong et al., 2014) using genome-wide linkage scanning and family association mapping. A gain-of-function mutation in CARD14 has just been discovered in patients with familial psoriasis. Psoriatic individuals had a higher level of CARD14 mRNA and a 2.7-fold increase in the number of missense mutations in the CARD14 gene (Tomfohrde et al., 1994). An elevated level of NF-kappa B results in an uptick in the expression of several critical mediators. It is associated with the development of plaque psoriasis, such as CCL20, CXCL8, and IL-1F9 (Hrehorów et al., 2012). The psoriatic cascade is thought to be triggered by an extra environmental factor as well (Di Meglio et al., 2011).

10.2.2.2 IL36RN MUTATIONS

In addition to IL-1F9, the anti-inflammatory IL-36Ra protein encoded by IL36RN is a natural IL36R antagonist. The IL-36 family members are significantly uncontrolled in psoriasis, according to research. The IL-1 family includes the IL-36 stimulating cytokines (IL-36, IL-36, and IL-36), which bind to and activate IL-36R and NF-k. Loss of active protein due to IL-36 stimulating cytokine mutated IL-36Ra causes unrestricted pro-inflammatory effects. As seen in pustular psoriasis, a lack of IL-36Ra causes excessive neutrophil accumulation. A high concentration of IL-36Ra was found in patients with psoriasis Vulgaris, suggesting that it may reduce the activity of the agonist (Ayala-Fontánez et al., 2016).

10.2.3 SNPS

SNPs are single-nucleotide polymorphisms (SNPs) that occur in greater than 1% of people. It is common for SNPs to be detected in non-coding sections of DNA. Extensive genome-wide association studies (GWAS) have evaluated the frequencies of tens of thousands of distinct SNPs in psoriasis sufferers and healthy controls using high-throughput technology and statistical approaches. Psoriasis-related GWAS SNPs are connected with the IL-23/IL-17 axis. Recently, an SNP at the IL23 gene has been reported of functional significance because of its response gradient to T cell stimulation by IL-23 in normal and psoriasis patients. (Mallon et al., 1999) The findings were validated by a subsequent meta-GWAS analysis, which found 15 additional SNPs in psoriasis patients and controls (Muhr et al., 2011; Lowes et al., 2013). SNPs in the JAK-STAT pathway, T helper (Th)1 and Th17 cell regulation, and leukocyte adhesion were among the many immunological processes linked to psoriasis pathogenesis by these studies, including keratinocyte differentiation and proliferation, T cell proliferation, natural killer (NK) cell proliferation, cytokines, and other responses (Ayala-Fontánez et al., 2016).

10.2.4 PSORIASIS CAN BE TRIGGERED BY A VARIETY OF ENVIRONMENTAL FACTORS

Environmental factors such as physical trauma, pharmacological reactions, infection, and modifiable variables such as psychological stress, obesity, smoking, and alcohol have been associated with the development and worsening of psoriasis.

10.2.4.1 PHYSICAL TRAUMA

Heinrich Koebner first identified a psoriasis trigger and aggravating factor in 1872. A direct cutaneous injury such as excoriation, tattoos, burns, or animal or insect bites can cause psoriatic lesions in previously normal-looking skin. It was found similar to the damage site, which is morphologically known as an isomorphic response. Psoriasis sufferers are more likely to experience the Koebner response than those with other skin conditions, such as vitiligo and lichen planus. Between 24% and 51% of those with psoriasis have a Koebner response. The start of psoriasis after an accident can take anywhere from three days to two years, and it may be affected by seasonal variations (more frequently in winter) and the severity of the disease (pre-existing and stable psoriasis), as well as the genetics of the patient (Denadai et al., 2013).

10.2.4.2 DRUG-INDUCED PSORIASIS

Several drugs have been linked to the onset and worsening of psoriasis. Examples are lithium, beta-blockers, antimalarials, tetracyclines, and non-steroidal anti-inflammatory medicines, which are the most commonly reported pharmaceuticals to cause psoriasis (Ladizinski et al., 2013; Kalayciyan et al., 2007; Malhotra et al., 2008; Gupta et al., 1997). Several drugs, including TNF inhibitors, IL-6R blockers, IFN inhibitors (alpha, beta, gamma), and the TLR7 agonist imiquimod, have been linked to an increased risk of psoriasis development or worsening (Ayala-Fontánez et al., 2016; Tsankov et al., 2000; Tsankov et al., 1988; Basavaraj et al., 2010; Denadai et al., 2013; Fry et al., 2007; Grasland et al., 2013). ACE inhibitors, calcium channel blockers, and IL-2 are just a few of the drugs that have been linked to an increased risk of psoriasis flare-ups (Laurent et al., 2010).

10.2.4.3 INFECTIONS

According to extensive research, children are particularly susceptible to developing psoriasis as a result of infections. Through both the skin and the throat, *Streptococcus pyogenes* can cause initial guttate psoriasis (Cohen et al., 2001). Chronic psoriasis can be exacerbated by streptococcal throat infections. Patients with psoriasis are also more likely to suffer from sore throats than those without the condition. Exacerbation of psoriasis has also been related to gut and/or skin colonization of *Staphylococcus aureus* and

Candida albicans. Researchers have also shown a link between *Helicobacter pylori* infection status and illness severity. These microorganisms have been described as prospective candidates for activating T cells and contributing to psoriasis development through an aberrant immunological response, given the link between these infections and psoriasis (Sigurdardottir et al., 2013).

10.2.4.4 STRESS

Psoriasis can be exacerbated by psychological stress because it alters the immune system. Psoriasis aggravation may be caused by elevated levels of stress hormones due to activation of the hypothalamus-pituitary-adrenal axis, according to numerous studies (Baker et al., 2006; Fry et al., 2007; Kono et al., 2001). The hypothalamus-pituitary-adrenal axis' corticotrophin-releasing hormone (CRH) is a crucial player in coordinating systemic stress responses and controlling the inflammatory response. It has been established that CRH and CRH-receptor 1 maintain the skin's local homeostasis, and in psoriasis, CRH is significantly elevated (Sayeed et al., 1999). Although CRH's effects on the skin are currently unknown, it is probably stimulating the synthesis of IL-6 or IL-11 in the keratinocytes of people with psoriasis, which could lead to a worsening of the condition (Fry et al., 2007).

10.2.4.5 ALCOHOL AND SMOKING

Drinking alcohol and psoriasis appear to be linked, although the relationship is complicated. Psoriasis is more common in persons who drink excessively, according to research. Alcohol intake has also been linked to an increased incidence of psoriasis in a recent meta-analysis of case-control studies. According to epidemiological studies, patients with moderate to severe psoriasis are more likely to develop alcohol-related disorders, which may lead to death (Zbytek et al., 2005; Kim et al., 2007; Zbytek et al., 2002). However, the mechanism by which alcohol triggers psoriasis is still unknown. Biological factors TGF-beta TGF B beta-6 and IFN-beta production are directly stimulated by 0.05% ethanol *in vitro*. It has been seen to activate T cells and produce keratinocyte hyperproliferation. The ethanol and acetone stimulated non-tumorigenic human keratinocyte proliferation *in vitro* (Adamzik et al., 2013). Smoking has been shown to increase a person's risk of developing psoriasis. Previous studies have indicated a substantial link between smoking and an increased risk of psoriasis. Psoriasis can be more common in women than men, according to one study; former and current smokers were more likely to get the condition than those who never smoked. SNP genetic variations in the genome-wide psoriasis-associated loci CMD1 and TNIP/ANXA6 increase the risk of psoriasis when combined with smoking and alcohol consumption, according to a new study (Farkas et al., 2010).

10.2.4.6 OBESITY

Obesity has also been linked to an increased chance of developing psoriasis. It has been found that there is a link between obesity and greater severity of psoriasis, although the mechanism is not understood. The adipocyte-derived cytokines leptin and resistin may be involved in the pathway. In previous studies, psoriasis patients have elevated leptin and resistin levels. This level can be induced due to IL-8, TNF-α, and IL-1 among the proinflammatory cytokines. Leptin can trigger the production of the EGF family member AREG, which has been proven *in vitro* to enhance keratinocyte proliferation and inflammatory hyperplasia in transgenic mice that overexpress dermal leptin by using an ex vivo organotypic culture method. Additional research is required to better understand the impact of obesity and weight loss on psoriasis (Naldi et al., 2005).

10.3 TREATMENT STRATEGIES

In modern treatment strategies for psoriasis, various medicines and treatment systems are used. Commonly, people are focusing on allopathic as well as other systems of medicine such as naturopathy. The combination of naturopathy systems with Ayurveda, Yoga, Unani, Siddha, and Homeopathy systems are used for the treatment of psoriasis. Nutraceuticals are also very popular among people for the treatment of various complicated diseases, where patients take nutraceuticals as drugs for the treatment and management of the disease. In the formulation of nutraceuticals, various microalgae are used due to their therapeutic potential properties. There are many types of microalgae, including eukaryotic photoautotrophic protists and prokaryotic cyanobacteria, which are all part of the microalgae family (sometimes called blue-green algae). More than half of the world's photosynthetic activity is generated by these bacteria, found practically everywhere (Hunter-Cevera et al., 1996). (1). These microalgae provide the source of the food chain for more than 70% of the world's biomass (2). Small lagoons on marginal land can grow microalgae photosynthetically using solar power and carbon dioxide as a carbon source. Compared to open ponds, the production efficiency of ponds with plastic tubes can be up to seven times higher (Schnepf et al., 1995; Singh, Gu et al., 2010). (3). Microalgae organelles such as chloroplasts, which are intracellular structures used for their photosynthesis, are considered in the literature under molecular biology study (Gibbs, 2010). (4). But there is still some dispute over classifying algae according to the taxonomic hierarchy (Bold et al., 2010) (5). Based on pigment composition, storage profile, and diversity of ultrastructural traits, algae are categorized into more than a dozen types. Recently, families of the major algal groups and their links to other taxonomic groupings have been determined using various molecular techniques (Hecht et al., 1993) (6). Blue-green algae (BGA), also known as cyanobacteria, are organisms that have a genetic relationship with a wide variety of bacteria. The chloroplasts of some higher algae and plants are also thought to be derived from BGA (4). Green algae are closely related to higher plants on the other end of the spectrum. These microalgae organisms have traits somewhere between prokaryotes and eukaryotes, like flagellates and euglenoids (7). Mesokaryotes in this family may be more closely related to slime molds and red algae. The molecular phylogenetic study shows that algae are highly variable at the molecular level. Algae have a wide range of phylogenetic diversity (Fowden et al., 1998) (Figure 10.1).

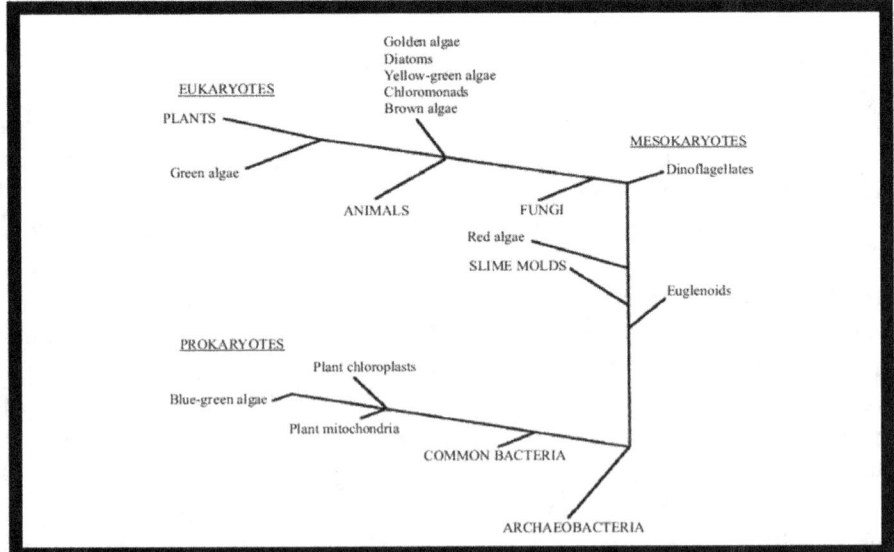

FIGURE 10.1 The study of ribosomal RNA sequences yields a phylogenic scheme.

10.4 DIVERSITY OF MICROALGAE

Microalgae constitute a large and unexplored resource. According to the scientific literature, microalgae are estimated to number between 200,000 to several million species, compared to roughly 250,000 species of larger plants (Norton et al., 1998). Their near-ubiquitous distribution in the biosphere reveals their genetic and phenotypic diversity. The Great Salt Lake in Utah, USA, and the Dead Sea in Israel are examples of places where green microalgae grow in freshwater as well as seawater. Microalgae can also grow in strange places like sloth and polar bear fur, rich humus soil, dry sand, boulders, and snowfields. Microalgae are easily available everywhere on Earth, even under the harshest conditions, such as on urban building walls, biotic crusts in scorching deserts, Antarctic snow, and the air at elevations of more than 2,000 meters. These are typically small (between 5 and 50 millimeters in diameter) cells. Microalgae species are found in huge numbers and are usually found in the form of black, green, red, or brown coloration. Microalgae can be described as either free-living or attached to other organisms, such as lichens (Sharma et al., 1996).

10.5 MICROBIOTA IN PSORIASIS

There are a variety of microorganisms living on the skin since it is a barrier that is also in direct contact with the outside environment. One square centimeter of skin is home to an estimated 1 million distinct bacterial species. The skin's microbiota community is influenced by various factors, including age, genetics, immunological response, climate, and cleanliness. Differences in skin thickness, hair follicle density, and skin invasions all contribute to the diversity of microbial habitats in a given individual. To keep the skin safe from harmful and more pathogenic microbes, good symbiotic partnerships form, which in turn help to educate and prime the host's T cells. As a result, sickness has been linked to changes in the skin's microbial community. Psoriatic skin lesions and non-lesional skin exhibit distinct bacterial and fungal populations, according to 16S-based genomic sequencing (Zackheim et al., 1971). Comparing healthy and non-lesional skin to psoriatic lesional skin, researchers found that the bacterial variety was higher in the latter, including higher levels of *S. pyogenes* and *S. aureus* (Cao et al., 2014; Johnston et al., 2008; Nowlin et al., 1976; Pérez-Pérez et al., 2009). In psoriasis, there have been three studies on the skin microbiome utilizing biopsies and swabs. As far as biopsies were concerned, the most often encountered bacterial species were *Streptococcus* and *Corynebacteria*. Tongue infections have previously been linked to the development of psoriasis. Researchers Diluvio et al. examined the TCR-chain rearrangements in psoriatic skin lesions, blood, tonsils, and T cells from tonsils in their investigation. Clonal T cell expansions predominate in psoriatic lesions, according to fractions, suggesting that *Streptococcus tonsillitis* and psoriasis inflammation are connected. Toxic *S. pyogenes* infections, according to scientists, stimulate and select tonsillar T cells for migration to the skin, where they are reactivated and expanded, aiding in the development of psoriatic skin lesions. Long-term remission of psoriatic skin irritation following tonsillectomy supported this mechanism. The study has a limited sample size (n=3). It is necessary to perform an investigation into the findings' significance (Baroni et al., 2006).

People with psoriasis have also been found to have different fungal compositions. Research suggests that Malassezia yeasts are likely to trigger the aggravation and induction of plaques in people who suffer from this condition. Ketoconazole medication has been found in multiple studies to improve scalp psoriasis. Because Malassezia yeasts are naturally occurring on the skin, it is critical to figure out what makes them aggravators of psoriasis (Paulino et al., 2006).

Candida species is another commensal yeast species linked to psoriasis. The oral cavity and the lesional skin of psoriasis patients have been found to have a significantly greater prevalence of *Candida* species. Candida toxins and super-antigens have also been linked to exacerbating psoriasis by stimulating T cells and keratinocyte cytokine secretion. Among Candida species, *C. albicans* is the most frequent in the mouth and on psoriasis-infected skin. *C. albicans* is a common commensal yeast that can induce various disorders when exposed to certain factors (Taheri Sarvtin et al., 2014; Waldman et al., 2001; Macias et al., 2011). Even though the microbiome has been demonstrated to be different between those with a skin condition and those without one, a relationship between the microbiome and the condition has yet to be found. The skin microbiome is also known to vary in dry, moist, and sebaceous areas, although it is unknown how this diversity can affect the development of psoriasis (Rosenberg et al., 1982).

10.6 MICROALGAE'S ANTI-INFLAMMATORY SKIN DISEASES PROTECTIVE EFFECTS

Microalgae have anti-inflammatory capabilities. Their extracts can stop pro-inflammatory cells from being produced and suppress the expression of inflammatory genes. For example, bioactive chemicals derived from microalgae can modify enzyme activity, influence cell activity, and NOS production, and target critical signaling pathways like NF-κB and MAPKs. Both of these routes play a significant role in producing numerous inflammatory mediators. The anti-inflammatory bioactive chemicals in algae, such as omega-3 polyunsaturated fatty acids (n-3 PUFA) and chlorophyll a, may make algae extract helpful in treating chronic inflammation-related metabolic illnesses like cardiovascular disease. Using lipopolysaccharide-stimulated human THP-1 macrophages, the anti-inflammatory activity of lipid extracts from four red seaweed species *(Porphyra dioica, Palmaria palmata, Chondrus crispus)* and one microalga species (*Pavlova lutheri*) was investigated here. It included 34% to 42% of the total fat as n-3 PUFA and 5–7% of the crude extract as pigments, including chlorophyll-a, beta-carotene, and fucoxanthin, respectively. Pretreatment of THP-1 cells with lipid extracts from *P. palmata* and *P. lutheri* reduced the production of the pro-inflammatory cytokines interleukin (IL)-6 and IL-8, respectively. The lipid extracts reduced the expression of 14 pro-inflammatory genes (TLR1, TLR2, TLR4, TLR8, TRAF5, TRAF6, TNFSF18, IL6R, IL23, CCR1, CCR4, CCL17, STAT3, and MAP3K1) in a quantitative gene expression analysis of genes associated with the inflammatory signaling pathway. The lipid extracts suppressed Toll-like receptors, chemokines, and nuclear factor kappa-light-chain-enhancer of activated B cells (NF-κB) signaling molecules.

This study shows that lipid extracts from *P. palmitate, P. dioica*, and the *C. Crispus* plant reduce LPS-induced inflammation in human macrophages. The anti-inflammatory properties of algal lipid extracts should be studied further in treating metabolic illnesses associated with chronic inflammation (Robertson et al., 2015) (Table 10.1).

10.7 CONCLUSION

Protect yourself from pathogens and pollutants that can harm your skin because they contain free radicals or reactive oxygen species. These reactive oxygen species (ROS) are always present in the body and can cause the skin to swell and become inflamed. Numerous studies have linked ROS to a wide range of inflammatory skin conditions. Patients with skin diseases face various challenges in ensuring they receive the best possible treatment for their condition. Elevated levels of ROS in the body result in oxidative stress, which disrupts normal cellular functions and leads to various forms of cell damage. During ROS-induced oxidative stress, multiple signaling pathways have significant effects. A naturally derived antioxidant from microalgae has

TABLE 10.1 THP-1 Macrophages Treated with Algal Lipid Extracts Followed by Exposure to Lipo Polysaccharide (LPS) to Examine the Effect on Gene Expression

Extract	Gene Symbol	Name	Fold Change	Gene Description and Function
P. lutheri	TLR8	Toll-like receptor 8	−3.33	PAMP recognition and activation of innate immunity. Mediates cytokine production through activation of NF-κB
	TLR1	Toll-like receptor 1	−4.16	Interacts with TLR2 for immune activation through PAMP recognition
	TRAF5	TNF receptor-associated factor 5	−2.69	Mediates signal transduction of the TNF receptor family. Mediates NF-Kb and JNK activation
	MAP3K1	Mitogen-acticated protein kinase1	−2.63	Activation protain kinase signal transduction cascade such as the ERK and JNK kinase pathways and NF-Kb pathway
	PTGER1	Prostaglandin E receptor1	+2.58	Encodes a receptor for PGE2. Down-regulates COX2 and hence resolve inflammation
P. palmata	TLR8	Toll-like receptor 8	−2.91	PAMP recognition and activation of innate immunity. Mediates cytokine production through of NF-κB
	TLR1	Toll-like receptor 1	−3.99	Interacts with TLR2 for immune activation through PAMP recognition
	TRAF5	TNF receptor-associated factor 5	−2.73	Mediates signal transduction of the TNF receptor family. Mediates NF-Kb and JNK activation
	NOS2	Nitric oxide synthase 2	+2.83	Encode nitric oxide synthase which mediates tumoricidal and bactericidal actions in macrophages
P. dioica	CCR1	Chemokine (C-C motif) receptor 1	−3.46	Acts as a receptor for chemokines such as MIP-1α and MCP-3 which assist in immune cell recruitment
	TLR8	Toll-like receptor 8	−3.29	PAMP recognition and activation of innate immunity. Mediates cytokine production through activation of NF-κB
	TLR2	Toll-like receptor 2	−4.25	Interacts with TLR2 for PAMP recognition leading to NF-κB and JNK activation
	TLR1	Toll-like receptor 1	−2.5	Interact with TLR2 for immune activation through PAMP recognition
	TRAF5	TNF receptor-associated factor 5	−3.37	Mediates signal transduction of the TNF receptor family. Mediates NF-Kb and JNK activation
	TNFSF18	TNF (ligand)-superfamily, member 18	−2.93	Regulate T-cell activation by lowering the threshold for T-cell activation

TABLE 10.1 (Continued)

Extract	Gene Symbol	Name	Fold Change	Gene Description and Function
	TRAF6	TNF receptor-associated factor 6	−2.99	Mediates signal transduction form TNF receptor and Toll/IL-1 receptor
	MAP3K1	Mitogen-acticated protein 3kinase1	−3.63	Activates protein kinase signal transduce ERK and JNK kinase pathway and NF-κB pathway
	STAT3	Signal transducer and activator of transcription 3	−3.56	Activated by cytokines to create transcription factors that form part of JAK-STAT signaling cascade
	CCR5	Chemokine (C-Cmotif) receptor 5	−2.72	Chemokine receptor, expressed in macrophages involved in immune cell recruitment
	TLR4	Toll-like receptor 4	−4.44	PAMP recognition and activation of inflammatory cascade. Specifically recognizes LPS
	IL6R	Interleukin 6 receptor	−2.54	Binds with low affinity to the inflammatory cytokine IL-6 regulating immune response and acute phase reactions
	PTGER1	Prostaglandin E receptor1	+2.7	Encode a receptor for PGE2. Down-regulates COX2 and hence resolves inflammation
C. crispus	IL23	Interleukin 23	−4.19	Activates STAT4 and stimulates production of IFNγ Associated with autoimmune inflammation and tumorigenesis
	TLR8	Toll-like receptor 8	−2.59	PAMP recognition and activation of innate immunity. Mediates cytokine production through activation of NF-κB
	CCL17	Chemokine (C-C motif) ligand 17	−3.33	Encode a cytokine that is a chemotactic factor for T-lymphocytes. Recruitment and activation of mature T-cells
	TLR1	Toll-like receptor 1	−3.25	Interacts with TLR2 for immune activation through PAMP recognition
	TRAF5	TNF receptor-associated factor 5	−2.76	Mediates signal transduction of the TNF receptor family. Mediates NF-κB and JNK activation
	TRAF6	TNF receptor-associated factor 6	−304	Mediates signal transduction of the TNF receptor

been identified for use in combating the increasing prevalence of inflammatory skin disorders. The anti-inflammatory and antioxidant properties of bioactive compounds extracted from microalgae have been demonstrated in previous studies. These compounds reduce inflammation and alter gene expression related to inflammation. Bioactive chemicals derived from microalgae modify enzyme activity, regulate cellular functions, and target important inflammation-related signaling pathways.

KEYWORDS

- corticotrophin-releasing hormone
- genome-wide association studies
- inflammatory bowel disease
- major histocompatibility complex
- reactive oxygen species
- single-nucleotide polymorphisms

REFERENCES

Adamzik, K., McAleer, M. A., & Kirby, B. (2013). Alcohol and psoriasis: Sobering thoughts. *Clinical and Experimental Dermatology, 38*(8), 819–822.

Alekseyenko, A. V., Perez-Perez, G. I., De Souza, A., Strober, B., Gao, Z., Bihan, M., & Blaser, M. J. (2013). Community differentiation of the cutaneous microbiota in psoriasis. *Microbiome, 1*(1), 1–7.

Armstrong, A. W., Gelfand, J. M., & Garg, A. (2014). Outcomes research in psoriasis and psoriatic arthritis using large databases and research networks: A report from the GRAPPA 2013 Annual Meeting. *The Journal of Rheumatology, 41*(6), 1233–1236.

Armstrong, A. W., Harskamp, C. T., & Armstrong, E. J. (2012). The association between psoriasis and obesity: A systematic review and meta-analysis of observational studies. *Nutrition & Diabetes, 2*(12), e54.

Ayala-Fontánez, N., Soler, D. C., & McCormick, T. S. (2016). Current knowledge of psoriasis and autoimmune diseases. *Psoriasis (Auckland, NZ), 6*, 7–32.

Baker, B. S., Laman, J. D., Powles, A., van der Fits, L., Voerman, J. S., Melief, M. J., & Fry, L. (2006). Peptidoglycan and peptidoglycan-specific Th1 cells in psoriatic skin lesions. *The Journal of Pathology, 209*(2), 174–181.

Baker, B. S., Powles, A., & Fry, L. (2006). Peptidoglycan: A major aetiological factor for psoriasis? *Trends in Immunology, 27*(12), 545–551.

Baroni, A., Orlando, M., Donnarumma, G., Farro, P., Iovene, M. R., Tufano, M. A., & Buommino, E. (2006). Toll-like receptor 2 (TLR2) mediates intracellular signaling in human keratinocytes in response to Malassezia furfur. *Archives of dermatological research, 297*(7), 280–288.

Baroni, A., Paoletti, I., Ruocco, E., Agozzino, M., Tufano, M. A., & Donnarumma, G. (2004). Possible role of Malassezia furfur in psoriasis: modulation of TGF-β1, integrin, and HSP70 expression in human keratinocytes and the skin of psoriasis-affected patients. *Journal of Cutaneous Pathology, 31*(1), 35–42.

Basavaraj, K. H., Ashok, N. M., Rashmi, R., & Praveen, T. K. (2010). The role of drugs in the induction and/or exacerbation of psoriasis. *International Journal of Dermatology, 49*(12), 1351–1361.

Bold, H. C., & Wynne, M. J. (1985). *Introduction to the Algae*. Prentice Hall, Inc. New Jersey. 720, 573–574.

Bowcock, A. M. (2005). The genetics of psoriasis and autoimmunity. *Annual Review of Genomics and Human Genetics, 6*, 93–122.

Broady, P. A. (1996). Diversity, distribution, and dispersal of Antarctic terrestrial algae. *Biodiversity & Conservation, 5*(11), 1307–1335.

Bunse, T., & Mahrle, G. (1996). Soluble Pityrosporum-derived chemoattractant for polymorphonuclear leukocytes of psoriatic patients. *Acta Dermato-Venereologica, 76*(1), 10–12.

Campanati, A., Ganzetti, G., Martina, E., Giannoni, M., Gesuita, R., Bendia, E., Giuliodori, K., Sandroni, L., & Offidani, A. (2015). Helicobacter pylori infection in psoriasis: Results of a clinical study and review of the literature. *International Journal of Dermatology, 54*(5), e109–e114.

Campuzano-Maya, G. (2011). Cure of alopecia areata after eradication of Helicobacter pylori: A new association? *World Journal of Gastroenterology, 17*(26), 3165–3166.

Cao, L. Y., Soler, D. C., Debanne, S. M., Grozdev, I., Rodriguez, M. E., Feig, R. L., & McCormick, T. S. (2014). Psoriasis and cardiovascular risk factors: Increased serum myeloperoxidase and corresponding immunocellular overexpression by Cd11b+ CD68+ macrophages in skin lesions. *American Journal of Translational Research, 6*(1), 16.

Chapman, B. P., & Moynihan, J. (2009). The brain–skin connection: Role of psychosocial factors and neuropeptides in psoriasis. *Expert Review of Clinical Immunology, 5*(6), 623–627.

Chiller, K., Selkin, B. A., & Murakawa, G. J. (2001). Skin microflora and bacterial infections of the skin. *Journal of Investigative Dermatology Symposium Proceedings, 6*(3), 170–174.

Cogen, A. L., Nizet, V., & Gallo, R. L. (2008). Skin microbiota: A source of disease or defense? *British Journal of Dermatology, 158*(3), 442–455.

Cohen, A. D., Kagen, M., Friger, M., & Halevy, S. (2001). Calcium channel blockers intake and psoriasis: A case-control study. *Acta Dermato-Venereologica, 81*(5), 347–349.

De Korte, J., Mombers, F. M., Bos, J. D., & Sprangers, M. A. (2004). Quality of life in patients with psoriasis: A systematic literature review. *Journal of Investigative Dermatology Symposium Proceedings, 9*(2), 140–147. Elsevier.

Denadai, R., Teixeira, F. V., Steinwurz, F., Romiti, R., & Saad-Hossne, R. (2013). Induction or exacerbation of psoriatic lesions during anti-TNF-α therapy for inflammatory bowel disease: A systematic literature review based on 222 cases. *Journal of Crohn's and Colitis, 7*(7), 517–524.

Di Meglio, P., Di Cesare, A., Laggner, U., Chu, C. C., Napolitano, L., Villanova, F., Tosi, I., Capon, F., Trembath, R. C., Peris, K., & Nestle, F. O. (2011). The IL23R R381Q gene variant protects against immune-mediated diseases by impairing IL-23-induced Th17 effector response in humans. *PLOS ONE, 6*(2), e17160.

Diluvio, L., Vollmer, S., Besgen, P., Ellwart, J. W., Chimenti, S., & Prinz, J. C. (2006). Identical TCR β-chain rearrangements in streptococcal angina and skin lesions of patients with psoriasis vulgaris. *The Journal of Immunology, 176*(11), 7104–7111.

Duffin, K. C., & Krueger, G. G. (2009). Genetic variations in cytokines and cytokine receptors associated with psoriasis were found by genome-wide association. *Journal of Investigative Dermatology, 129*(4), 827–833.

Elder, J. T. (2006). PSORS1: Linking genetics and immunology. *Journal of Investigative Dermatology, 126*(6), 1205–1206.

Elewski, B. (1990). Does Pityrosporum ovale have a role in psoriasis? *Archives of Dermatology, 126*(8), 1111–1112.

Fahlén, A., Engstrand, L., Baker, B. S., Powles, A., & Fry, L. (2012). Comparison of bacterial microbiota in skin biopsies from normal and psoriatic skin. *Archives of dermatological research, 304*(1), 15–22.

Farkas, A., & Kemény, L. (2010). Psoriasis and alcohol: Is cutaneous ethanol one of the missing links? *British Journal of Dermatology, 162*(4), 711–716.

Farr, P. M., Marks, J., Krause, L. B., & Shuster, S. (1985). Response of scalp psoriasis to oral ketoconazole. *The Lancet, 326*(8461), 921–922.

Feldman, S. R., Fleischer, A. B. Jr., Reboussin, D. M., Rapp, S. R., Bradham, D. D., Exum, M. L., & Clark, A. R. (1997). The economic impact of psoriasis increases with psoriasis severity. *Journal of the American Academy of Dermatology, 37*(4), 564–569.

Feldman, S. R., Malakouti, M., & Koo, J. Y. (2014). Social impact of the burden of psoriasis: Effects on patients and practice. *Dermatology Online Journal, 20*(8), 1–5.

Flechtner, V. R. (2007). North American desert microbiotic soil crust communities. In *Algae and Cyanobacteria in Extreme Environments* (pp. 537–551). Springer, Dordrecht.

Fowden, A. L., Li, J., & Forhead, A. J. (1998). Glucocorticoids and the preparation for life after birth: Are there long-term consequences of life insurance? *Proceedings of the Nutrition Society, 57*(1), 113–122.

Fredricks, D. N. (2001). Microbial ecology of human skin in health and disease. *Journal of Investigative Dermatology Symposium Proceedings, 6*(3), 167–169.

Fry, L., & Baker, B. S. (2007). Triggering psoriasis: The role of infections and medications. *Clinics in Dermatology, 25*(6), 606–615.

Fry, L., Baker, B. S., Powles, A. V., & Fahlen, A. (2013). Is chronic plaque psoriasis triggered by microbiota in the skin? *British Journal of Dermatology, 169*(1), 47–52.

Fry, L., Baker, B. S., Powles, A. V., Fahlen, A., & Engstrand, L. (2007). Psoriasis—A possible candidate for vaccination. *Autoimmunity Reviews, 6*(5), 286–289.

Gao, Z., Tseng, C. H., Strober, B. E., Pei, Z., & Blaser, M. J. (2008). Substantial alterations of the cutaneous bacterial biota in psoriatic lesions. *PloS One, 3*(7), e2719.

Gelfand, J. M., & Yeung, H. (2012). Metabolic syndrome in patients with psoriatic disease. *The Journal of Rheumatology Supplement, 89*, 24–28.

Gibbs, S. P. (1992). The evolution of algal chloroplasts. In *Origins of Plastids* (pp. 107–121). Springer, Boston, MA.

Grasland, A., Mahé, E., Raynaud, E., & Mahé, I. (2013). Psoriasis onset with tocilizumab. *Joint Bone Spine, 80*(5), 541–542.

Grice, E. A., Kong, H. H., Conlan, S., Deming, C. B., Davis, J., Young, A. C., & Green, E. D. (2009). Topographical and temporal diversity of the human skin microbiome. *Science, 324*(5931), 1190–1192.

Grice, E. A., Kong, H. H., Renaud, G., Young, A. C., Bouffard, G. G., Blakesley, R. W., & Segre, J. A. (2008). A diversity profile of the human skin microbiota. *Genome Research, 18*(7), 1043–1050.

Griffiths, C. E., & Barker, J. N. (2007). Pathogenesis and clinical features of psoriasis. *The Lancet, 370*(9583), 263–271.

Gupta, A. K., Sibbald, R. G., Knowles, S. R., Lynde, C. W., & Shear, N. H. (1997). Terbinafine therapy may be associated with the development of psoriasis de novo or its exacerbation: Four case reports and a review of drug-induced psoriasis. *Journal of the American Academy of Dermatology, 36*(5), 858–862.

Hayes, J., & Koo, J. (2010). Psoriasis: Depression, anxiety, smoking, and drinking habits. *Dermatologic Therapy, 23*(2), 174–180.

Hecht, J. (1993). Animals and fungi are closer than anyone expected. *New Scientist, 138*(1877), 16.

Helms, C., Cao, L., Krueger, J. G., Wijsman, E. M., Chamian, F., Gordon, D., Heffernan, M., Daw, J. A., Robarge, J., Ott, J., & Kwok, P. Y. (2003). A putative RUNX1 binding site variant between SLC9A3R1 and NAT9 is associated with susceptibility to psoriasis. *Nature Genetics, 35*(4), 349–356.

Higgins, E. (2000). Alcohol, smoking and psoriasis. *Clinical and Experimental Dermatology, 25*(2), 107–110.

Hrehorów, E., Salomon, J., Matusiak, L., Reich, A., & Szepietowski, J. C. (2012). Patients with psoriasis feel stigmatized. *Acta Dermato-Venereologica, 92*(1), 67–72.

Hunter-Cevera, J. C., & Belt, A. (Eds.). (1996). *Maintaining Cultures for Biotechnology and Industry*. 1st Edition, Elsevier. pp. 263. ISBN: 9780123619464.

Jin, Y., Yang, S., Zhang, F., Kong, Y., Xiao, F., Hou, Y., & Zhang, X. (2009). Combined effects of HLA-Cw6 and cigarette smoking in psoriasis vulgaris: A hospital-based case-control study in China. *Journal of the European Academy of Dermatology and Venereology, 23*(2), 132–137.

Johnston, A., Arnadottir, S., Gudjonsson, J. E., Aphale, A., Sigmarsdottir, A. A., Gunnarsson, S. I., & Valdimarsson, H. (2008). Obesity in psoriasis: Leptin and resistin as mediators of cutaneous inflammation. *British Journal of Dermatology, 159*(2), 342–350.

Johnston, A., Xing, X., Guzman, A. M., Riblett, M., Loyd, C. M., Ward, N. L., Wohn, C., Prens, E. P., Wang, F., Maier, L. E., & Kang, S. (2011). IL-1F5, -F6, -F8, and -F9: A novel IL-1 family signaling system that is active in psoriasis and promotes keratinocyte antimicrobial peptide expression. *The Journal of Immunology, 186*(4), 2613–2622.

Jordan, C. T., Cao, L., Roberson, E. D., Duan, S., Helms, C. A., Nair, R. P., Duffin, K. C., Stuart, P. E., Goldgar, D., Hayashi, G., & Olfson, E. H. (2012). Rare and common variants in CARD14, encoding an epidermal regulator of NF-kappaB, in psoriasis. *The American Journal of Human Genetics, 90*(5), 796–808.

Jordan, C. T., Cao, L., Roberson, E. D., Pierson, K. C., Yang, C. F., Joyce, C. E., Ryan, C., Duan, S., Helms, C. A., Liu, Y., & Chen, Y. (2012). PSORS2 is due to mutations in CARD14. *The American Journal of Human Genetics, 90*(5), 784–795.

Kalayciyan, A., Aydemir, E. H., & Kotogyan, A. (2007). Experimental Koebner phenomenon in patients with psoriasis. *Dermatology, 215*(2), 114–117.

Khadhim, M. M., & Ali, A. I. (2019). Inheritance of HLA-C and pro-inflammatory cytokines polymorphism in association with family history in Type-I psoriasis. *Biochem. Cell. Arch. 19*(1), 1181–1187.

Kim, J. E., Cho, D. H., Kim, H. S., Kim, H. J., Lee, J. Y., Cho, B. K., & Park, H. J. (2007). Expression of the corticotropin-releasing hormone–proopiomelanocortin axis in the various clinical types of psoriasis. *Experimental Dermatology, 16*(2), 104–109.

Kimball, A. B., Gladman, D., Gelfand, J. M., Gordon, K., Horn, E. J., Korman, N. J., Korver, G., Krueger, G. G., Strober, B. E., Lebwohl, M. G., & Foundation, N. P. (2008). National Psoriasis Foundation clinical consensus on psoriasis comorbidities and recommendations for screening. *Journal of the American Academy of Dermatology, 58*(6), 1031–1042.

Kimball, A. B., Jacobson, C., Weiss, S., Vreeland, M. G., & Wu, Y. (2005). The psychosocial burden of psoriasis. *American Journal of Clinical Dermatology, 6*(6), 383–392.

Kono, M., Nagata, H., Umemura, S., Kawana, S., & Osamura, R. Y. (2001). In situ expression of corticotropin-releasing hormone (CRH) and proopiomelanocortin (POMC) genes in human skin. *The FASEB Journal, 15*(12), 2297–2299.

Kwok, P. Y., & Chen, X. (2003). Detection of single nucleotide polymorphisms. *Current Issues in Molecular Biology, 5*(2), 43–60.

Ladizinski, B., Lee, K. C., Wilmer, E., Alavi, A., Mistry, N., & Sibbald, R. G. (2013). A review of the clinical variants and the management of psoriasis. *Advances in Skin & Wound Care, 26*(6), 271–284.

Laurent, S., Le Parc, J. M., Clérici, T., & Bréban, M. (2010). Onset of psoriasis following treatment with tocilizumab. *The British Journal of Dermatology, 163*(6), 1364–1365.

Lee, R. E., Gaspari, A. A., Lotze, M. T., Chang, A. E., & Rosenberg, S. A. (1988). Interleukin 2 and psoriasis. *Archives of Dermatology, 124*(12), 1811–1815.

Lober, C. W., Belew, P. W., Rosenberg, E. W., & Bale, G. (1982). Patch tests with killed sonicated microflora in patients with psoriasis. *Archives of dermatology, 118*(5), 322–325.

Love, T. J., Qureshi, A. A., Karlson, E. W., Gelfand, J. M., & Choi, H. K. (2011). Prevalence of the metabolic syndrome in psoriasis: Results from the National Health and Nutrition Examination Survey, 2003-2006. *Archives of Dermatology, 147*(4), 419–424.

Lowes, M. A., Russell, C. B., Martin, D. A., Towne, J. E., & Krueger, J. G. (2013). The IL-23/T17 pathogenic axis in psoriasis is amplified by keratinocyte responses. *Trends in Immunology, 34*(4), 174–181.

Lowes, M. A., Suárez-Fariñas, M., & Krueger, J. G. (2014). Immunology of psoriasis. *Annual Review of Immunology, 32*, 227–255.

Macias, E. S., Pereira, F. A., Rietkerk, W., & Safai, B. (2011). Superantigens in dermatology. *Journal of the American Academy of Dermatology, 64*(3), 455–472.

Malhotra, S. K., & Mehta, V. (2008). Role of stressful life events in induction or exacerbation of psoriasis and chronic urticaria. *Indian Journal of Dermatology, Venereology & Leprology, 74*(6), 594–599.

Mallon, E., Newson, R., & Bunker, C. B. (1999). HLA-Cw6 and the genetic predisposition to psoriasis: A meta-analysis of published serologic studies. *Journal of Investigative Dermatology, 113*(4), 693–695.

Muhr, P., Zeitvogel, J., Heitland, I., Werfel, T., & Wittmann, M. (2011). Expression of interleukin (IL)-1 family members upon stimulation with IL-17 differs in keratinocytes derived from patients with psoriasis and healthy donors. *British Journal of Dermatology, 165*(1), 189–193.

Naldi, L., Chatenoud, L., Linder, D., Fortina, A. B., Peserico, A., Virgili, A. R., & Schena, D. (2005). Cigarette smoking, body mass index, and stressful life events as risk factors for psoriasis: Results from an Italian case-control study. *Journal of Investigative Dermatology, 125*(1), 61–67.

Naldi, L., Peli, L., Parazzini, F., Carrel, C. F., & Psoriasis Study Group of the Italian Group for Epidemiological Research in Dermatology. (2001). Family history of psoriasis, stressful life events, and recent infectious disease are risk factors for a first episode of acute guttate psoriasis: Results of a case-control study. *Journal of the American Academy of Dermatology, 44*(3), 433–438.

Norrlind, R. (1954). A case of psoriasis pustulosa after an angina tonsillaris. *Acta Dermato-Venereologica, 34*(1–2), 122–123.

Norton, T. A., Melkonian, M., & Andersen, R. A. (1996). Algal biodiversity. *Phycologia., 35*, 308–326.

Nowlin, N., & Solomon, H. (1976). Weight loss and psoriasis. *Archives of Dermatology, 112*(10), 1465.

Parisi, R., Symmons, D. P., Griffiths, C. E., & Ashcroft, D. M. (2013). Global epidemiology of psoriasis: A systematic review of incidence and prevalence. *Journal of Investigative Dermatology, 133*(2), 377–385.

Paulino, L. C., Tseng, C. H., & Blaser, M. J. (2008). Analysis of Malassezia microbiota in healthy superficial human skin and psoriatic lesions by multiplex real-time PCR. *FEMS yeast research, 8*(3), 460–471.

Paulino, L. C., Tseng, C. H., Strober, B. E., & Blaser, M. J. (2006). Molecular analysis of fungal microbiota in samples from healthy human skin and psoriatic lesions. *Journal of Clinical Microbiology, 44*(8), 2933–2941.

Pearce, D. J., Lucas, J., Wood, B., Chen, J., Balkrishnan, R., & Feldman, S. R. (2006). Death from psoriasis: Representative US data. *Journal of Dermatological Treatment, 17*(5), 302–303.

Pérez-Pérez, L., Allegue, F., Caeiro, J. L., & Zulaica, J. M. (2009). Severe psoriasis, morbid obesity, and bariatric surgery. *Clinical and Experimental Dermatology, 34*(7), e421–e422.

Prohic, A. (2003). Identification of Malassezia species isolated from scalp skin of patients with psoriasis and healthy subjects. *Acta Dermatovenerol Croat, 11*(1), 10–16.

Radmer, R. J. (1996, April). Algal diversity and commercial algal products. *BioScience, 46*(4), 263–270.

Raychaudhuri, S. K., Maverakis, E., & Raychaudhuri, S. P. (2014). Diagnosis and classification of psoriasis. *Autoimmunity Reviews, 13*(4–5), 490–495.

Rindi, F., Allali, H. A., Lam, D. W., & López-Bautista, J. M. (2009). An overview of the biodiversity and biogeography of terrestrial green algae. *Biodiversity Hotspots, 1*, 125.

Robertson, R. C., Guihéneuf, F., Bahar, B., Schmid, M., Stengel, D. B., Fitzgerald, G. F., & Stanton, C. (2015). The anti-inflammatory effect of algae-derived lipid extracts on lipopolysaccharide (LPS)-stimulated human THP-1 macrophages. *Marine Drugs, 13*(8), 5402–5424.

Rosenberg, E. W., & Belew, P. W. (1982). Improvement of psoriasis of the scalp with ketoconazole. *Archives of Dermatology, 118*(6), 370–371.

Sagi, L., & Trau, H. (2011). The Koebner phenomenon. *Clinics in Dermatology, 29*(2), 231–236.

Schnepf, E., Starr, R. C., & Wiessner, W. (1995). *Algae, Environment, and Human Affairs*. Biopress, pp. 256. ISBN: 9780948737305.

Sharma, N. K., Rai, A. K., Singh, S., & Brown, R. M. Jr. (2007). Airborne algae: Their present status and relevance. *Journal of Phycology, 43*(4), 615–627.

Sigurdardottir, S. L., Thorleifsdottir, R. H., Valdimarsson, H., & Johnston, A. (2013). The association of sore throat and psoriasis might be explained by histologically distinctive tonsils and increased expression of skin-homing molecules by tonsil T cells. *Clinical & Experimental Immunology, 174*(1), 139–151.

Sigurdardottir, S. L., Thorleifsdottir, R. H., Valdimarsson, H., & Johnston, A. (2013). The role of the palatine tonsils in the pathogenesis and treatment of psoriasis. *British Journal of Dermatology, 168*(2), 237–242.

Singh, J., & Gu, S. (2010). Commercialization potential of microalgae for biofuel production. *Renewable and Sustainable Energy Reviews, 14*(9), 2596–2610.

Slominski, A. T., Botchkarev, V., Choudhry, M., Fazal, N., Fechner, K., Furkert, J., Krause, E., Roloff, B., Sayeed, M., Wei, E., & Zbytek, B. (1999). Cutaneous expression of CRH and CRH-R: Is there a "skin stress response system?" *Annals of the New York Academy of Sciences, 885*(1), 287–311.

Steinwurz, F., Denadai, R., Saad-Hossne, R., Queiroz, M. L., Teixeira, F. V., & Romiti, R. (2012). Infliximab-induced psoriasis during therapy for Crohn's disease. *Journal of Crohn's and Colitis, 6*(5), 610–616.

Sterry, W., Strober, B. E., Menter, A., & International Psoriasis Council. (2007). Obesity in psoriasis: The metabolic, clinical and therapeutic implications. Report of an interdisciplinary conference and review. *British Journal of Dermatology, 157*(4), 649–655.

Stuart, P., Malick, F., Nair, R. P., Henseler, T., Lim, H. W., Jenisch, S., Voorhees, J., Christophers, E., & Elder, J. T. (2002). Analysis of phenotypic variation in psoriasis as a function of age at onset and family history. *Archives of Dermatological Research, 294*(5), 207–213.

Su, O., Beycan, I., Ozkaya, D. B., & Senocak, M. (2012). Impact of Helicobacter pylori infection on severity of psoriasis and response to treatment. *European Journal of Dermatology, 22*(1), 117–120.

Taheri Sarvtin, M., Shokohi, T., Hajheydari, Z., Yazdani, J., & Hedayati, M. T. (2014). Evaluation of candidal colonization and specific humoral responses against Candida albicans in patients with psoriasis. *International Journal of Dermatology, 53*(12), e555–e560.

Takahata, Y., Sugita, T., Hiruma, M., & Muto, M. (2007). Quantitative analysis of Malassezia in the scale of patients with psoriasis using a real-time polymerase chain reaction assay. *British Journal of Dermatology, 157*(4), 670–673.

Thorleifsdottir, R. H., Sigurdardottir, S. L., Sigurgeirsson, B., Olafsson, J. H., Sigurdsson, M. I., Petersen, H., Arnadottir, S., Gudjonsson, J. E., Johnston, A., & Valdimarsson, H. (2012). Improvement of psoriasis after tonsillectomy is associated with a decrease in the frequency of circulating T cells that recognize streptococcal determinants and homologous skin determinants. *The Journal of Immunology, 188*(10), 5160–5165.

Tomfohrde, J., Silverman, A., Barnes, R., Fernandez-Vina, M. A., Young, M., Lory, D., Morris, L., Wuepper, K. D., Stastny, P., Menter, A., & Bowcock, A. (1994). Gene for familial psoriasis susceptibility mapped to the distal end of human chromosome 17q. *Science, 264*(5162), 1141–1145.

Tomi, N. S., Kränke, B., & Aberer, E. (2005). Staphylococcal toxins in patients with psoriasis, atopic dermatitis, and erythroderma, and healthy control subjects. *Journal of the American Academy of Dermatology, 53*(1), 67–72.

Tsankov, N. K., Vassileva, S. V., Lazarova, A. Z., Berowa, N. V., & Botev-Zlatov, N. (1988). Onset of psoriasis coincident with tetracycline therapy. *Australasian Journal of Dermatology, 29*(2), 111–112.

Tsankov, N., Angelova, I., & Kazandjieva, J. (2000). Drug-induced psoriasis. *American Journal of Clinical Dermatology, 1*(3), 159–165.

Tsoi, L. C., Spain, S. L., Knight, J., Ellinghaus, E., Stuart, P. E., Capon, F., Ding, J., Li, Y., Tejasvi, T., Gudjonsson, J. E., & Kang, H. M. (2012). The identification of 15 new psoriasis susceptibility loci highlights the role of innate immunity. *Nature Genetics, 44*(12), 1341–1348.

Van Den Bogaard, E. H., Tjabringa, G. S., Joosten, I., Vonk-Bergers, M., Van Rijssen, E., Tijssen, H. J., Erkens, M., Schalkwijk, J., & Koenen, H. J. (2014). Crosstalk between keratinocytes and T cells in a 3D microenvironment: A model to study inflammatory skin diseases. *Journal of Investigative Dermatology, 134*(3), 719–727.

Villanova, F., Di Meglio, P., & Nestle, F. O. (2013). Biomarkers in psoriasis and psoriatic arthritis. *Annals of the Rheumatic Diseases, 72*(Suppl 2), ii104–ii110.

Waldman, A., Gilhar, A., Duek, L., & Berdicevsky, I. (2001). Incidence of Candida in psoriasis–a study on the fungal flora of psoriatic patients. *Mycoses, 44*(3–4), 77–81.

Weigl, B. A. (2000). The significance of stress hormones (glucocorticoids, catecholamines) for eruptions and spontaneous remission phases in psoriasis. *International Journal of Dermatology, 39*(9), 678–688.

Wendling, D., Letho-Gyselinck, H., Guillot, X., & Prati, C. (2012). Psoriasis onset with tocilizumab treatment for rheumatoid arthritis. *The Journal of Rheumatology, 39*(3), 657.

Whyte, H. J., & Baughman, R. D. (1964). Acute guttate psoriasis and streptococcal infection. *Archives of Dermatology, 89*(3), 350–356.

Wolf, R., Tamir, A., & Brenner, S. (1990). Psoriasis related to angiotensin-converting enzyme inhibitors. *Dermatology, 181*(1), 51–53.

Yin, X. Y., Cheng, H., Wang, W. J., Wang, W. J., Fu, H. Y., Liu, L. H., & Zhang, X. J. (2013). TNIP1/ANXA6 and CSMD1 variants interacting with cigarette smoking, and alcohol intake affect the risk of psoriasis. *Journal of Dermatological Science, 70*(2), 94–98.

Zackheim, H. S., & Farber, E. M. (1971). Rapid weight reduction and psoriasis. *Archives of Dermatology, 103*(2), 136–140.

Zbytek, B., Mysliwski, A., Slominski, A., Wortsman, J., Wei, E. T., & Mysliwska, J. (2002). Corticotropin-releasing hormone affects cytokine production in human HaCaT keratinocytes. *Life Sciences, 70*(9), 1013–1021.

Zbytek, B., Pikula, M., Slominski, R. M., Mysliwski, A., Wei, E., Wortsman, J., & Slominski, A. T. (2005). Corticotropin-releasing hormone triggers differentiation in HaCaT keratinocytes. *British Journal of Dermatology, 152*(3), 474–480.

Zhu, K. J., Zhu, C. Y., & Fan, Y. M. (2012). Alcohol consumption and psoriatic risk: A meta-analysis of case-control studies. *The Journal of Dermatology, 39*(9), 770–773.

Zomorodian, K., Mirhendi, H., Tarazooie, B., Zeraati, H., Hallaji, Z., & Balighi, K. (2008). Distribution of Malassezia species in patients with psoriasis and healthy individuals in Tehran, Iran. *Journal of Cutaneous Pathology, 35*(11), 1027–1031.

CHAPTER 11

NUTRACEUTICALS AND PSORIASIS: RECENT SCIENTIFIC EVIDENCE IN CLINICAL TRIALS

ABHISH JADHAV,[1] MRUDULA BELE,[2] SAHEBRAO BORASTE,[3] ROHAN AHIRE,[1] EKNATH D. AHIRE,[1] MEENAKSHI JAISWAL,[4] RAJ K. KESERVANI,[5] and SWATI G. TALELE[6]

[1]Department of Pharmaceutics, MET's Institute of Pharmacy, Bhujbal Knowledge City, Adgaon, Nashik, Maharashtra, India

[2]Department of Pharmaceutics, N.D.M.V. P's College of Pharmacy, Nashik, Maharashtra, India

[3]Department of Pharmaceutics, Sir Dr. M. S. Gosavi College of Pharmaceutical Education and Research, Nashik, Maharashtra, India

[4]Assistant Professor, Department of Pharmacy, Guru Ghasidas Vishwavidyalaya (A Central University), Bilaspur, Chhattisgarh, India

[5]Associate Professor, Faculty of B. Pharmacy, CSM Group of Institutions, Prayagraj, Uttar Pradesh, India

[6]Department of Pharmaceutics, Sandip Institute of Pharmaceutical Sciences, Mahiravani, Nashik, Maharashtra, India

ABSTRACT

Psoriasis is an inflammatory skin condition caused by a persistent immunological response. Hyperproliferation of epidermal keratinocytes is related to an inflammatory cellular infiltration in both the dermis and the epidermis in psoriasis lesions. Despite recent evidence that nutrition may play a critical role in prevention and co-treatment, and despite patients' concerns about the ideal nutritional habits, clinical settings lack consensus on the nutritional techniques to be used. This chapter examines the impact of a number of nutritional therapies for people with psoriasis, including vitamins, extracts of herbs, phytochemicals, and dietary supplements. The goal of this review is to identify important nutraceuticals for better psoriasis control. The correct nutraceutical supplement can enhance a patient's quality of life and have a positive effect on their general health.

11.1 INTRODUCTION

Psoriasis is regarded as a severe, persistent, and unpredictably occurring skin condition that is linked to T-cell immunological dysfunction. An inflammatory condition called psoriasis is brought on by the inflammation of skin cells, which have a 10-fold higher rate of growth than normal cells. Despite the fact that the primary causes of psoriasis are unknown, it is thought to be a keratinocyte dysfunction (Barker et al., 1991). Psoriasis is a chronic inflammatory dermatological disease that frequently coexists with inflammatory arthritis (Liang et al., 2017). Psoriasis affects approximately 1.5 and 2.0% of the world's population, with more than 7.2 million persons in the United States alone (Porter et al., 2017). The most common type of the disease, psoriasis vulgaris, also referred to as plaque psoriasis, affects 85–90% of patients (Vickers et al., 2017). Recent breakthroughs in psoriasis pathogenesis have altered the illness's perception from a "skin disease" to a "T cell-mediated systemic disease" (Vickers et al., 2017). Various studies have described the cellular and molecular contributions to the hyperactive immune response over the years. T-cells, especially those with Th1 and Th17 polarization, have been observed to be abundant in psoriatic lesions (Fuentes-Duculan et al., 2017). The intensity and involvement of the skin determine whether the condition is mild or moderate to severe. Although the pathophysiology of psoriasis is unknown, activation of Th17-mediated immune responses in the skin has been characterized as a key component (Chandran et al., 2014). The skin generates flakes known as psoriatic plaques as a result of excessive and fast proliferation of epidermal cells. Due to the quick degradation process, the silvery-white plaques are caused by the accumulation and accelerated regeneration of skin in predilection areas. It is estimated that over 30% of psoriasis patients have a first- or second-degree family history of the illness. If both parents have psoriasis, the likelihood of an offspring is 41%, 14% if one parent has psoriasis, and 6% if any sibling has psoriasis (Lowe et al., 2018). Psoriasis is divided into distinct types depending on clinical characteristics such as plaque shape, redness, and location. The most prevalent variety of psoriasis is plaque psoriasis, which is defined by sharply circumscribed, round, or oval plaques that appear as raised, reddish lesions coated in dry silvery-white scales. Another type of psoriasis is pustular psoriasis, which is characterized by blisters surrounded by red skin. Guttate psoriasis, which is less scaly than plaque psoriasis and has smaller plaques, is the most prevalent kind of psoriasis seen in children and persons under the age of 30 (Lowe et al., 2018; Hasan et al., 2015).

The word 'psora' comes from the Greek word 'psora,' which means 'itch.' The tips of fingers, scalp, palms, soles, gluteus, toes, umbilicus, under the breast and genitals, elbows, sacrum, and knees are the most commonly affected areas. Psoriasis is a chronic condition with a tendency to relapse. Because psoriasis can lead to joint inflammation, it is associated with dandruff and some types of arthritis. Unfortunately, psoriasis is a disease that has been poorly treated in the past and is currently in search of effective treatment (Cowden et al., 2008). Topical medications, phototherapy, and oral and injectable pharmaceuticals are among the available treatments for psoriasis. Corticosteroids, topical retinoids, Anthralin, Calcineurin inhibitors, and other topical psoriasis medications are included in the treatment options. Topical corticosteroids are the first-line treatment available for psoriasis. However, prolonged or excessive use of potent corticosteroids may lead to skin thinning and eventual loss of effectiveness (Paul et al., 2011). Anthralin helps slow down skin cell proliferation, remove scales, and promote smoother skin. However, it can cause skin irritation and leave visible stains after use. Retinoids are vitamin A derivatives that can reduce inflammation; in severe cases of psoriasis, they can also be taken orally (Mrowietz et al., 2011).

Skin irritation is a typical side effect of retinoids, and they can also make you more sensitive to sunlight. Calcineurin inhibitors like Pimecrolimus and Tacrolimus act by reducing inflammation and accumulation of plaque. They are not suggested for long-term or chronic therapy due to their increased risk of lymphoma and skin cancer (Menter et al., 2007). Psoriasis is treated with ultraviolet light, either artificially or naturally, in a procedure known as phototherapy. One form of natural phototherapy involves exposing the skin to sunshine under regulated conditions. Psoriasis patients can also benefit from other innovative phototherapies, such as psoralen with UVA (PUVA), excimer laser, UVB, Narrow band UVB, and Goeckerman treatment. However, these treatments have a number of drawbacks, including the fact that prolonged exposure to the sun can worsen psoriatic symptoms and cause skin dryness, redness, itching, and damage (Cameron et al., 2002).

As a result, nutraceuticals (Keservani et al., 2010a, b, 2017, 2020) might be considered an auxiliary treatment for psoriasis management. Many psoriasis patients find that taking vitamins and dietary supplements might assist them in relieving discomfort and speeding up the healing process. The symptoms of psoriasis can be treated or lessened with the use of extracts or concentrates of dietary supplements, which are available in a range of dosage forms, including capsules, tablets, soft gelatin capsules, liquids, gels, and powders. In this chapter, we'll take a close look at some of the most popular nutraceuticals for psoriasis.

11.2 PATHOPHYSIOLOGY OF PSORIASIS

Psoriasis is thought to develop as a result of the body's overreaction and the acceleration of skin cell proliferation. It has been discovered that the genes that cause psoriasis can also control an individual's immune system reactions. Immune-mediated diseases like psoriasis, Type I Diabetes, and rheumatoid arthritis are caused by these genes (Mahajan et al., 2013).

For the pathophysiological progression of psoriasis, two basic hypotheses were proposed. According to the first hypothesis, psoriasis is caused by the uncontrolled development and reproduction of skin cells caused by a faulty epidermis and its keratinocytes. Skin cells mature and begin to shed from the skin's surface every 28–30 days, according to the natural cell growth cycle (Vickers et al., 2017).

Skin cells mature and transfer to the skin surface in 3–6 days in psoriasis, resulting in an overabundance of immature cells on the skin surface. Additionally, these cells create elevated red patches surrounded by dead cells, resulting in silvery scales or large white plaques seen in psoriasis (Weinstein et al., 1985). Another viewpoint regards psoriasis as an immune-mediated disease in which enhanced skin cell proliferation plays only a minor impact in the progression of the disease (Fuentes-Duculan et al., 2017). Immune-mediated psoriasis is caused by the body's immune system sending out erroneous signals. T-cells in the dermis, according to recent research, are primarily responsible for initiating and propagating immune-based inflammatory processes (Griffiths et al., 2007).

To respond with T-cells, Langerhans cells are hypothesized to travel from the epidermis to the regional lymph nodes. When an unknown antigen interacts with T-cells, it sends out co-stimulatory signals and activates the immune system, causing T-cell activation and the generation of cytokines. Activated T cells are released into the bloodstream and then returned to the skin. T-cell reactivation in the dermis and epidermis of the skin causes inflammation, hyperproliferation, and cell-mediated immune responses in psoriasis. Immunosuppressive drugs' ability to clear psoriasis plaques has also reinforced this immune-mediated theory. The immune system's role in psoriasis is still unknown, and psoriasis may be investigated further in naked mice lacking T-cells as an animal model, according to a new paper (Provost, 1981; ORTONNE, 1996; Pitzalis, 1996).

11.3 NUTRACEUTICALS FOR PSORIASIS

11.3.1 ALOE VERA

The Liliaceae family's Aloe barbadensis miller, also known as Aloe Vera (AV), is one of the most important therapeutic plants. The chemical composition consists of lignins, monosaccharides, amino acids, polysaccharides, anthraquinones, saponins, enzymes, minerals, and vitamins. It also contains salicylic acid and sterols. AV can address all skin conditions like dryness, peeling, irritation, and cracking. The chemical component of AV that aids in the treatment of psoriasis is lignin. The lignins have a penetrating mechanism that allows AV to penetrate deep into the epidermal layers (Surjushe et al., 2008). Herbal shampoos, lotions, gels, and organic extracts that maintain water retention in dry skin tissue, remove dead skin cells, and support the production of healthy skin are available to treat psoriasis. Because it acts as a digestive aid, internal cleanser, and anti-inflammatory, AV juice should be consumed on a regular basis. The most popular type of AV is a gel, which is beneficial in reducing psoriasis flakes' epidermal irritation (Vázquez et al., 1996). To determine the acceptability and efficacy of topically applied Aloe vera extract cream for psoriasis, Syed et al. undertook a double-blind, placebo-controlled clinical experiment. The cream was well tolerated by all of the patients for 16 weeks, with no side effects reported. Aloe vera extract cream treatment treated 25 out of 30 patients with considerable elimination of psoriatic plaques, compared to the placebo group. As a consequence, it was established that topically applied Aloe Vera cream is more effective than placebo (Syed et al., 1996).

Using a mouse tail model for psoriasis, Dhanabal et al. examined gel formulations of an ethanolic aloe vera extract for antipsoriatic effectiveness.

The extract generated considerable epidermal differentiation, which was comparable to the tazarotene (0.1%) gel used as a positive control (Dhanabal et al., 2012).

11.3.2 NEEM

The most widely utilized herb (Sharma et al., 2020; Rane et al., 2020a, b, c) in Ayurveda is neem, which is botanically known as Azadirachta indica and belongs to the Meliaceae family. Anti-inflammatory, antipyretic, antifungal, and antibacterial activities are all found in neem. It has a long history of being used to naturally clean blood, which makes it ideal for treating psoriasis (Brahmachari et al., 2004).

Neem oil is considered one of the safest, primary, and external treatments for psoriasis due to the presence of Azadirachtin, which penetrates deep layers to heal psoriasis. Psoriasis causes the skin to become extremely dry, and neem oil, which contains vitamin E and omega 6 and 9 fatty acids, moisturizes the skin and helps to reduce scales and dryness (Kumar et al., 2013). Nimbidin, an anti-inflammatory and anti-arthritic chemical found in neem, has been shown to have anti-inflammatory and anti-arthritic properties (Singh et al., 2014). Oral administration of neem is available in tablet and capsule form.

Using a topical regime of 5% coal tar and 3% salicylic acid, Pandey et al. conducted a double-blind clinical experiment to determine whether neem leaves' aqueous extract may benefit psoriasis vulgaris patients. After 12 weeks, patients receiving neem leaf extract considerably outperformed the placebo group in terms of their "Psoriasis area and severity index" (PASI) score (Pandey et al., 1994).

11.3.3 TURMERIC

In conventional Indian and Chinese medicine, turmeric is used to treat a variety of illnesses. Turmeric, scientifically known as *Curcuma longa*, is a member of the ginger family. Since ancient times, turmeric paste has been used for aesthetic purposes and to heal skin disorders. Curcumin, a key component of turmeric believed to be responsible for the majority of its therapeutic advantages, has a significant body of research behind it. It can be used to treat and prevent skin disorders like psoriasis and eczema. Curcumin inhibits nuclear factor kappa B, a protein family involved in psoriasis inflammation, and hence reduces inflammation. It has the ability to accelerate skin healing and regeneration, which can aid in psoriasis treatment.

It also protects the skin from oxidative stress by scavenging oxidizing reactive molecules and regulating detoxifying enzymes. Tumor necrosis factor-alpha and interleukin are two important proteins that play a role in the inflammatory phase of psoriasis as well as its spread. Curcumin prevents the activation of other metabolic pathways that could lead to disease progression by inhibiting the function of these proteins (Thangapazham et al., 2007; Gupta et al., 2013). The anti-inflammatory properties of curcumin gel were investigated in a mouse model of Imiquimod-induced psoriasis. Curcumin treatment reduced the inflammatory cytokines interleukin-23 (IL-23) and IL-17A; in addition, several inflammatory cytokines that contribute to the pathophysiology of psoriasis are also mentioned (Sun et al., 2013). Curcumin gel's anti-inflammatory activities were examined in a mouse model of Imiquimod-induced psoriasis. Curcumin treatment reduced interleukin-23 (IL-23)/IL-17A cytokine, as well as other inflammatory cytokines, which are important in the pathophysiology of psoriasis (Sun et al., 2013).

Turmeric microemulgel was given topically to plaque psoriasis patients in a 3-week clinical trial by Sarafian et al. When compared to the untreated group, the PASI score and quality of life metrics increased ($P<0.05$) in microemulgel-treated patients (Sarafian et al., 2015). To investigate the efficacy of curcumin for oral psoriasis treatment, Antiga et al. colleagues undertook a randomized, double-blind, placebo-controlled clinical trial. Curcumin has been proven to reduce IL-22 serum levels in patients with Psoriasis vulgaris (Bolivar-Telleria et al., 2018).

11.3.4 SOYABEAN

Barbadensis mill is a member of the *Fabaceae* plant family. Isoflavones are well-known phytoestrogens found in soybeans that are structurally similar to 17 beta-estradiol. The main isoflavone contained in soybeans is genistein, which has strong antioxidant and anti-inflammatory properties. Many Asian populations have safely taken large amounts of soybeans and genistein, and they contribute significantly to health promotion. By inhibiting NF-κB signaling, genistein has been discovered to have anti-proliferative effects. Genistein appears to lower the production and expression of proinflammatory biomarkers such as TNF-α, IL-6, IL-1, and IL-8, therefore modifying inflammatory responses (Avramidis et al., 2018; Wei et al., 2003). Genistein was discovered to lower acetylcholinesterase (AChE), which has an inhibitory effect on blood levels of angiotensin II, a proliferative and proinflammatory biomarker in a rat model (Xu et al., 2006). In the release of neutrophil elastase, genistein has also been shown to block a serine protease that is present in psoriatic lesions.

Shyong et al. discovered that topical genistein reduced skin thickness and cutaneous erythema in people with psoriasis caused by psoralen-ultraviolet A (PUVA) therapy in research. Combining genistein with PUVA therapy in psoriasis patients may improve therapeutic response while reducing complications (Shyong et al., 2002).

Ito et al. used glyteer, a delipidated soybean tar, topically on a psoriatic model in mice. In mice, glyteer inhibited epidermal mass and protein content. Furthermore, in psoriatic mice, glyteer decreased edema, and its anti-edema effect was comparable to that of betamethasone 17-valerate, indomethacin, and cyclosporine. According to these findings, soybeans may be effective for the therapy of psoriasis (Ito et al., 1992).

11.3.5 VITAMIN D

Ito et al. used glyteer, a delipidated soybean tar, topically on a psoriatic model in mice. In mice, glyteer inhibited epidermal mass and protein content. Moreover, in psoriatic mice, glyteer reduced edema, and its anti-edema effect was similar to that of betamethasone 17-valerate, indomethacin, and cyclosporine. These data suggested that soybeans might be useful in the treatment of psoriasis (Ito et al., 1992). As a result, it is the most commonly given vitamin for psoriasis treatment, either alone or in combination with other anti-psoriatic medications (Soleymani et al., 2015; Jabbar-Lopez et al., 2017). When vitamin D is produced in the skin, the duration and intensity of a psoriatic eruption are reduced. Mild to moderate psoriasis is treated with topical therapies containing synthetic forms of active vitamin D, such as tacalcitol or calcipotriene. It works by reducing local irritation and decreasing skin cell growth (Donțu et al., 2016).

In a double-blind, randomized clinical trial, Staberg et al. developed a novel vitamin D analog (MC903), which was subsequently evaluated in 10 patients with chronic plaque psoriasis in cream. Topical treatments comprising MC903 cream and placebo cream were compared for six weeks of therapy. The MC903 cream formulation eliminated the psoriatic lesions after 6 weeks of treatment, with no adverse drug responses. MC903 was discovered to have a strong influence on cell proliferation and differentiation while having no effect on calcium metabolism (Staberg et al., 1989).

11.3.6 OMEGA-3 FATTY ACIDS

In psoriasis, the amounts of arachidonic acid and leukotriene B4 in and around psoriatic plaques are higher. Because fish oil inhibits the production of leukotriene B4, it's been known for a long time that applying it topically to psoriatic skin areas will help with psoriasis symptoms (Maurice et al., 1987).

Around 25 psoriasis patients were given the option of applying fish oil or liquid paraffin to their psoriatic plaques on a daily basis for four weeks. Fish oil was clearly effective in reducing plaque thickness, erythema, and scaling. The plaque irritation was not relieved by fish oil treatment. Liquid paraffin treatment was shown to be successful in lowering erythema but was found to be ineffective in reducing scaling rate and had no discernible effect on plaque thickness or irritation. Patients liked both the liquid paraffin and the fish oil treatments; however, the latter was shown to be therapeutically superior to the paraffin treatment.

The marketed product available for treating psoriasis is fish oil soft-gelatin capsules (Escobar et al., 1992). Bittiner et al. conducted an 8-week clinical trial on 28 patients with chronic persistent psoriasis who were given fish oil capsules or placebo capsules daily along with a strict diet. The fish oil treatment group demonstrated a significant reduction in scaling, erythema, and itching, but the placebo group showed no improvement in psoriasis symptoms (Bittiner et al., 1988).

11.3.7 EVENING PRIMROSE OIL

Evening primrose oil's main ingredients are linoleic acid (LA) and gamma-linolenic acid (GLA), and its calming properties derive from an abundance of LA and GLA. In a few cases, it was used to treat psoriasis and other chronic skin disorders such as eczema, with encouraging outcomes.

Evening primrose oil is also thought to have a soothing influence on hormonal fluctuations. GLA and linoleic acid also aid in rehydrating and rejuvenating the skin and can help reduce the effects of aging (Ziboh et al., 2000). This essential oil also helps with psoriasis episodes by reducing dryness, itching, and scaliness, as well as increasing the natural production of prostaglandins, which helps reduce skin inflammation. Patients with skin diseases such as psoriasis have been found in studies to have a greater chance of getting cancer. This oil can help the body maintain the proper levels of LA and GLA. These findings are backed up by a double-blind, parallel trial undertaken by Oliwiecki et al. in plaque psoriasis patients who received a mixture of important fatty acids n-3 (marine oil) and n-6 (evening primrose oil) (Finlay et al., 1994). Evening primrose oil is available in pill form, oil form, and lotion form.

11.3.8 BLACK CUMIN

Nigella sativa Linn., a widely used medicinal plant, is a member of the Ranunculaceae family and is commonly referred to as black cumin. Thymoquinone, thymohydroquinone, dithymoquinone, thymol, carvacrol, and other active compounds are found in Nigella sativa. Because of its antibacterial, anti-inflammatory, anti-acne, antifungal, anticancer, and anti-psoriatic properties, it is commonly utilized for dermatological diseases (Vickers et al., 2007). The seeds are applied topically to skin breakouts and psoriasis patches to relieve general pain and increase patch size. Dwarampudi et al. conducted a study with an ethanolic extract of *Nigella sativa* seeds, which showed significant epidermal differentiation (71.36% ± 2.64) from its degree of orthokeratosis when compared to the placebo (17.30% ± 4.09) and had a similar effect to the positive control, Tazarotene gel. The ethanolic extract exhibits an IC_{50} of 239 µg/ml and shows anti-proliferative action. Therefore, this study supported its use as a traditional therapy for psoriasis with a reduction in comparative epidermal thickness to the control group (Dwarampudi et al., 2012).

Jawad et al. conducted a randomized clinical trial in 60 psoriatic patients to assess the efficacy and safety of *Nigella sativa* (NS) delivered orally and topically, using a PASI score and serum malondialdehyde as outcomes. Around 20 patients were given a 10% w/w topical NS ointment, 20 patients were given a 500 mg oral capsule of plain NS powder, and the remaining 20 patients were given a combination of ointment and capsule. When the PASI score was calculated, it was discovered that 65% of the ointment group had totally recovered from psoriatic lesions, whereas 50% of the oral administration group had been cured. Surprisingly, the combined therapy group has totally healed the lesions in 85% of patients (Ahmed Jawad et al., 2014).

11.3.9 BAKUCHI

Psoraliacorylifolia is a species of Psoralea. Linn is a member of the Fabaceae family and is used medicinally. Psoraliacorylifolia has traditionally been used in the treatment of a variety of ailments, including leprosy, leucoderma, and psoriasis. It also contains antioxidant, anti-inflammatory, antibacterial, anticancer, antifungal, and immunomodulatory properties. Psoralens, bakuchiol, bakuchalcone, isopsoralen, and volatile oils are all found in bakuchi. Psoralen is a photoactive furocoumarin that may absorb radiant energy and convert it to pyrimidine-based photoproducts. Psoralens photoactivation in the ultraviolet region of 200–320 nm slows DNA synthesis, preventing cell proliferation, and is thus beneficial in cutaneous illnesses such as psoriasis, mycosis fungoides, and vitiligo in humans (Chopra et al., 2013).

Ali et al. investigated Psoralea corylifolia oil, also known as babchi oil, in a microemulsion gel-based system for psoriasis treatment. A microemulsion-based formulation enhanced babchi oil penetration in the skin and demonstrated excellent *in-vivo* anti-inflammatory activity in a footpad edema model (Ali et al., 2008).

11.3.10 MILK THISTLE

Milk Thistle (*Silybum marianum*) is a plant native to Asia and North Africa that belongs to the Asteraceae family. The seeds of the Milk Thistle are used to treat psoriasis naturally. Silymarin is made up of three chemicals that help to prevent psoriasis: silicristin, silibinin, and silidianin. Silymarin is a powerful detoxifier and antioxidant that aids in the regeneration of damaged liver cells while also activating the immune system. All of Silymarin's characteristics are good for naturally combating psoriasis, hence milk thistle is thought to be efficient in the treatment of psoriasis. Psoriasis can be treated with a 150 mg dose of standardized milk thistle extract containing 70% Silymarin in tablet or capsule form (Bhattacharya et al., 2011; Sabir et al., 2014).

Khan et al. used Carbopol as a gelling agent to create a topical gel of Silymarin. It was tested for physicochemical and *in-vitro* drug release, and it was reported to release 96.30% of the medication within 3 hours. It was studied for primary skin irritation tests in healthy human volunteers after satisfactory *in vitro* parameters, and there was no indication of irritation at the end of 72 hours. In addition, the gel revealed that the lowest inhibitory concentration against Candida albicans was 5 mg/ml (Khan et al., 2014).

11.3.11 COAL TAR

Coal tar has long been used as a principal topical medication in dermatology to treat a variety of skin conditions, including psoriasis and eczema. Crude coal tar is made up of almost 10,000 different components, with a larger percentage of polycyclic aromatic hydrocarbons. It can be taken either alone or in conjunction with other drugs or phototherapy to treat persistent psoriasis. It slows down the proliferation of skin cells and rejuvenates the skin's look. Simultaneously, it may reduce psoriasis itching, scaling, and inflammation (Dimitrov et al., 2016; Dogra et al., 2010).

Coal tar is most usually sold as a solution (0.1 to 20%), which is mixed with additional substances like sulfur and salicylic acid to make creams, lotions, shampoos, and ointments. However, many studies have linked the long-term use of coal tar to an increased risk of cancer, therefore those who use or deal with coal tar should have frequent skin cancer screenings (Maughan et al., 1980; Pion et al., 1995).

Roelofzen and colleagues published a large cohort study with 13,200 psoriasis and eczema patients in which coal tar treatment was compared to dermatocorticosteroids, a reference medication, for 6 months. Surprisingly, there was no increase in the risk of non-skin malignancies or skin cancer after treatment with coal tar. As a result, the study (Roelofzen et al., 2010) suggested the safe use of coal tar in dermatological disorders. Furthermore, the United States Food and Drug Administration (FDA) has designated coal tar as "generally regarded as safe and effective" (GRASE) over-the-counter topical therapy for psoriasis and dandruff.

11.4 CONCLUSION

Psoriasis is a skin condition that can last a long time. There are various factors involved in the development of psoriasis, which makes finding a good solution challenging. Since psoriasis is an autoimmune disease, proper care is crucial beyond just medication. Additionally, longer treatment periods can lead to more medication side effects. Vitamins, herbal extracts, and nutritional supplements have shown promise in both preclinical and clinical studies, and are recommended as supplementary treatments for psoriasis. Therefore, patients may benefit from taking a single nutraceutical or a combination of nutraceuticals to help manage their psoriasis.

ACKNOWLEDGMENT

We, thank the MET's, Institute of Pharmacy, BKC, affiliated with Savitribai Phule Pune University, Nashik.

KEYWORDS

- acetylcholinesterase
- dermatologist
- environmental factors
- Food and Drug Administration
- gamma-linolenic acid
- generally regarded as safe and effective
- psoralen-ultraviolet A
- psoriasis

REFERENCES

Ahmed Jawad, H., IbraheemAzhar, Y., & Al-Hamdi Khalil, I. (2014). Evaluation of efficacy, safety and antioxidant effect of Nigella sativa in patients with psoriasis: A randomized clinical trial. *Journal of Clinical and Experimental Investigations, 5*(2), 186–193. Retrieved from: http://www.jceionline.org (accessed on 6 June 2024).

Ali, J., Akhtar, N., Sultana, Y., Baboota, S., & Ahuja, A. (2008). Antipsoriatic microemulsion gel formulations for topical drug delivery of babchi oil (Psoraleacorylifolia). *Methods and Findings in Experimental and Clinical Pharmacology, 30*(4), 277–285.

Avramidis, G., Krüger-Krasagakis, S., Krasagakis, K., Fragiadaki, I., Kokolakis, G., & Tosca, A. (2010). The role of endothelial cell apoptosis in the effect of etanercept in psoriasis. *British Journal of Dermatology, 163*(5), 928–934.

Barker, J. N. W. N. (1991). The pathophysiology of psoriasis. *The Lancet, 338*(8761), 227–230.

Bhattacharya, S. (2011). Phytotherapeutic properties of milk thistle seeds: An overview. *Journal of Advanced Pharmaceutical Education & Research, 1*, 69–79.

Bittiner, S. B., Cartwright, I., Tucker, W. F. G., & Bleehen, S. S. (1988). A double-blind, randomized, placebo-controlled trial of fish oil in psoriasis. *The Lancet, 331*(8582), 378–380.

Bolivar-Telleria, M., Turbay, C., Favarato, L., Carneiro, T., de Biasi, R. S., Fernandes, A. A. R., Santos, A., & Fernandes, P. (2018). Second-generation bioethanol from coconut husk. *BioMed Research International, 2018*, 1–20. https://doi.org/10.1155/2018/1234567.

Brahmachari, G. (2004). Neem—An omnipotent plant: A retrospection. *Chembiochem, 5*(4), 408–421.

Cameron, H., Dawe, R. S., Yule, S., Murphy, J., Ibbotson, S. H., & Ferguson, J. (2002). A randomized, observer-blinded trial of twice vs. three times weekly narrowband ultraviolet B phototherapy for chronic plaque psoriasis. *British Journal of Dermatology, 147*(5), 973–978.

Chandran, P., Netha, S., & Khan, S. S. (2014). Effect of humic acid on photocatalytic activity of ZnO nanoparticles. *Journal of Photochemistry and Photobiology B: Biology, 138*, 155–159.

Chattopadhyay, I., Biswas, K., Bandyopadhyay, U., & Banerjee, R. K. (2004). Turmeric and curcumin: Biological actions and medicinal applications. *Current Science, 87*(1), 44–53.

Chopra, B., Dhingra, A. K., & Dhar, K. L. (2013). Psoraleacorylifolia L. (Buguchi)—Folklore to modern evidence. *Fitoterapia, 90*, 44–56.

Cowden, A., & Voorhees, A. S. V. (2008). Introduction: History of psoriasis and psoriasis therapy. In *Treatment of Psoriasis* (pp. 1–9). Birkhäuser Basel.

Dhanabal, S. P., Priyanka Dwarampudi, L., Muruganantham, N., & Vadivelan, R. (2012). Evaluation of the antipsoriatic activity of Aloe vera leaf extract using a mouse tail model of psoriasis. *Phytotherapy Research, 26*(4), 617–619.

Dimitrov, M., Koleva, N., Obreshkova, D., & Petkova, V. (2016). The treatment of psoriasis–Approaches and advantages. *Comptes Rendus de l'Académie Bulgare des Sciences, 69*(4), 383–392.

Dogra, S., & Kaur, I. (2010). Childhood psoriasis. *Indian Journal of Dermatology, Venereology and Leprology, 76*(4), 357.

Donțu, N., Șalaru, V., & Șalaru, V. (2016). Removal of organic pollutants from wastewater by cyanobacteria. In *Cyanobacteria for Bioremediation of Wastewaters* (pp. 27–43). Springer, Cham.

Dwarampudi, L. P., Palaniswamy, D., & MurugananthamNithyanantham, P. S. (2012). Antipsoriatic activity and cytotoxicity of ethanolic extract of Nigella sativa seeds. *Pharmacognosy Magazine, 8*(32), 268.

Escobar, S. O., Achenbach, R., Iannantuono, R., & Torem, V. (1992). Topical fish oil in psoriasis—A controlled and blind study. *Clinical and Experimental Dermatology, 17*(3), 159–162.

Finlay, A. Y., & Khan, G. (1994). Dermatology Life Quality Index (DLQI)—A simple practical measure for routine clinical use. *Clinical and Experimental Dermatology, 19*(3), 210–216.

Fuentes-Duculan, J., Bonifacio, K. M., Hawkes, J. E., Kunjravia, N., Cueto, I., Li, X., Gonzalez, J., Garcet, S., & Krueger, J. G. (2017). Autoantigens ADAMTSL 5 and LL 37 are significantly upregulated in active psoriasis and localized with keratinocytes, dendritic cells, and other leukocytes. *Experimental Dermatology, 26*(11), 1075–1082.

Gisondi, P., Rossini, M., Di Cesare, A., Idolazzi, L., Farina, S., Beltrami, G., Peris, K., & Girolomoni, G. (2012). Vitamin D status in patients with chronic plaque psoriasis. *British Journal of Dermatology, 166*(3), 505–510.

Griffiths, C. E., & Barker, J. N. (2007). Pathogenesis and clinical features of psoriasis. *The Lancet, 370*(9583), 263–271.

Gupta, S. C., Patchva, S., & Aggarwal, B. B. (2013). Therapeutic roles of curcumin: Lessons learned from clinical trials. *The AAPS Journal, 15*(1), 195–218.

Hasan, M. A., Khan, M. A., Datta, A., Mazumder, M. H. H., & Hossain, M. U. (2015). A comprehensive immunoinformatic and target site study revealed the cornerstone of Chikungunya virus treatment. *Molecular Immunology, 65*(1), 189–204.

Hrenn, A., Steinbrecher, T., Labahn, A., Schwager, J., Schempp, C. M., & Merfort, I. (2006). Plant phenolics inhibit neutrophil elastase. *Planta Medica, 72*(12), 1127–1131.

Hwang, S. T., Nijsten, T., & Elder, J. T. (2017). Recent highlights in psoriasis research. *Journal of Investigative Dermatology, 137*(3), 550–556.

Ito, K., Namikawa, S., & Takeuchi, K. (1992). Effect of the dry distillation tar of delipidated soybean (Glyteer) on a psoriasic model in the mouse. *Nihon Yakurigakuzasshi. Folia Pharmacologica Japonica, 99*(1), 55–62.

Jabbar-Lopez, Z. K., Yiu, Z. Z., Ward, V., Exton, L. S., Mustapa, M. F. M., Samarasekera, E., Burden, A. D., Murphy, R., Owen, C. M., Parslew, R., & Venning, V. (2017). The author replies to a Letter to the editor in response to the recently published article, 'Quantitative evaluation of biologic therapy options for psoriasis: A systematic review and network meta-analyses. *Journal of Investigative Dermatology, 137*(12), 2644–2646.

Keservani, R. K., Kesharwani, R. K., Sharma, A. K., Vyas, N., & Chadoker, A. (2010b). Nutritional supplements: An overview. *International Journal of Current Pharmaceutical Review and Research, 1*(1), 59–75.

Keservani, R. K., Kesharwani, R. K., Vyas, N., Jain, S., Raghuvanshi, R., & Sharma, A. K. (2010a). Nutraceutical and functional food as future food: A review. *Der Pharmacia Lettre, 2*(1), 106–116.

Keservani, R. K., Sharma, A. K., & Kesharwani, R. K. (2017). An overview and therapeutic applications of nutraceutical and functional foods. In *Recent Advances in Drug Delivery Technology* (pp. 160–201). ISBN: 9781522507543.

Keservani, R. K., Sharma, A. K., & Kesharwani, R. K. (Eds.). (2020). *Nutraceuticals and Dietary Supplements: Applications in Health Improvement and Disease Management*, Apple Academic Press, CRC Press. pp. 1–344. ISBN: 9781771888738.

Kesharwani, R. K., & Misra, K. (2011). Prediction of the binding site for curcuminoids at human topoisomerase II α protein: An in-silico approach. *Current Science*, 100(7), 1060–1065.

Kesharwani, R. K., Singh, D. B., Singh, D. V., & Misra, K. (2018). Computational study of curcumin analogs by targeting DNA topoisomerase II: A structure-based drug designing approach. *Network Modeling Analysis in Health Informatics and Bioinformatics, 7*(1), 1–7.

Kesharwani, R. K., Srivastava, V., Singh, P., Rizvi, S. I., Adeppa, K., & Misra, K. (2015). A novel approach for overcoming drug resistance in breast cancer chemotherapy by targeting new synthetic curcumin analogs against aldehyde dehydrogenase 1 (ALDH1A1) and glycogen synthase kinase-3 β (GSK-3β). *Applied Biochemistry and Biotechnology, 176*(7), 1996–2017.

Khan, P. A., Thube, R., & Rab, R. A. (2014). Formulation development and evaluation of silymarin gel for psoriasis treatment. *Journal of Innovative Pharmacy and Biological Sciences, 1*(1), 21–26.

Kumar, V. S., & Navaratnam, V. (2013). Neem (*Azadirachta indica*): Prehistory to contemporary medicinal uses to humankind. *Asian Pacific Journal of Tropical Biomedicine, 3*(7), 505–514.

Liang, Y., Sarkar, M. K., Tsoi, L. C., & Gudjonsson, J. E. (2017). Psoriasis: A mixed autoimmune and autoinflammatory disease. *Current Opinion in Immunology, 49*, 1–8.

Lowe, A. J., Su, J. C., Allen, K. J., Abramson, M. J., Cranswick, N., Robertson, C. F., & Dharmage, S. C. (2018). A randomized trial of a barrier lipid replacement strategy for the prevention of atopic dermatitis and allergic sensitization: the PEBBLES pilot study. *British Journal of Dermatology*, *178*(1), e19–e21.

Mahajan, R., & Handa, S. (2013). Pathophysiology of psoriasis. *Indian Journal of Dermatology, Venereology & Leprology*, *79*, 1.

Maughan, W. Z., Muller, S. A., Perry, H. O., Pittelkow, M. R., & O'Brien, P. C. (1980). Incidence of skin cancers in patients with atopic dermatitis treated with coal tar: A 25-year follow-up study. *Journal of the American Academy of Dermatology*, *3*(6), 612–615.

Maurice, P. D. L., Allen, B. R., Barkley, A. S. J., Cockbill, S. R., Stammers, J., & Bather, P. C. (1987). The effects of dietary supplementation with fish oil in patients with psoriasis. *British Journal of Dermatology*, *117*(5), 599–606.

Menter, A., & Griffiths, C. E. (2007). Current and future management of psoriasis. *The Lancet*, *370*(9583), 272–284.

Mishra, H., Kesharwani, R. K., Singh, D. B., Tripathi, S., Dubey, S. K., & Misra, K. (2019). Computational simulation of inhibitory effects of curcumin, retinoic acid, and their conjugates on GSK-3 beta. *Network Modeling Analysis in Health Informatics and Bioinformatics*, *8*(1), 3.

Mrowietz, U., Kragballe, K., Reich, K., Spuls, P., Griffiths, C. E. M., Nast, A., Franke, J., Antoniou, C., Arenberger, P., Balieva, F., & Bylaite, M. (2011). Definition of treatment goals for moderate to severe psoriasis: A European consensus. *Archives of Dermatological Research*, *303*(1), 1–10.

Ortonne, J. P. (1996). Aetiology and pathogenesis of psoriasis. *British Journal of Dermatology*, *135*, 1–5.

Pandey, S. S., Jha, A. K., & Vineet, K. (1994). Aqueous extract of neem leaves in the treatment of Psoriasis vulgaris. *Indian Journal of Dermatology, Venereology and Leprology*, *60*(2), 63–67.

Paul, C., Gallini, A., Maza, A., Montaudié, H., Sbidian, E., Aractingi, S., Aubin, F., Bachelez, H., Cribier, B., Joly, P., & Jullien, D. (2011). Evidence-based recommendations on conventional systemic treatments in psoriasis: Systematic review and expert opinion of a panel of dermatologists. *Journal of the European Academy of Dermatology and Venereology*, *25*, 2–11.

Pavement Council. (n.d.). Food & Drug Administration (FDA) classification of coal tar. https://pctc.memberclicks.net/in-the-news (accessed on 6 June 2024).

Pion, I. A., Koenig, K. L., & Lim, H. W. (1995). Is dermatologic usage of coal tar carcinogenic? A review of the literature. *Dermatologic Surgery*, *21*(3), 227–231.

Pitzalis, C., Cauli, A., Pipitone, N., Smith, C., Barker, J., Marchesoni, A., Yanni, G., & Panayi, G. S. (1996). Cutaneous lymphocyte antigen-positive T lymphocytes preferentially migrate to the skin but not to the joint in psoriatic arthritis. *Arthritis & Rheumatism: Official Journal of the American College of Rheumatology*, *39*(1), 137–145.

Porter, M. L., Lockwood, S. J., & Kimball, A. B. (2017). Update on biologic safety for patients with psoriasis during pregnancy. *International Journal of Women's Dermatology*, *3*(1), 21–25.

Provost, T. T. (1981). Lupus band test. *International Journal of Dermatology*, *20*(7), 475–481.

Psoriasis Self-Management. (n.d.). Evening primrose oil for psoriasis. Retrieved from: https://psoriasisselfmanagement.com/natural-herbs-supplements/evening-primrose-oil-for-psoriasis/ (accessed on 6 June 2024).

Rane, B. R., Bharath, M. S., Patil, R. R., Keservani, R. K., & Jain, A. S. (2020b). Novel approaches in nutraceuticals. In R. K. Kesharwani, R. K. Keservani, & A. K. Sharma (Eds.), *Enhancing the Therapeutic Efficacy of Herbal Formulations through Novel Drug Delivery Systems* (pp. 241–266). IGI Global. ISBN: 9781799844532.

Rane, B. R., Patil, A. S., Keservani, R. K., & Jain, A. S. (2020a). Novel approaches in herbal formulation. In R. K. Kesharwani, R. K. Keservani, & A. K. Sharma (Eds.), *Enhancing the Therapeutic Efficacy of Herbal Formulations through Novel Drug Delivery Systems* (pp. 43–68). IGI Global. ISBN: 9781799844532.

Rane, B. R., Tadavi, S. A., & Keservani, R. K. (2020c). Naturopathy. In A. K. Sharma, R. K. Keservani, & S. P. Gautam (Eds.), *Herbal Product Development* (pp. 321–347). Apple Academic Press, CRC Press, Taylor & Francis Group. ISBN: 9781771888776.

Roelofzen, J. H., Aben, K. K., Oldenhof, U. T., Coenraads, P. J., Alkemade, H. A., Van De Kerkhof, P. C., Van Der Valk, P. G., & Kiemeney, L. A. (2010). No increased risk of cancer after coal tar treatment in patients with psoriasis or eczema. *Journal of Investigative Dermatology, 130*(4), 953–961.

Sabir, S., Arshad, M., Asif, S., & Chaudhari, S. K. (2014). An insight into the medicinal and therapeutic potential of *Silybum marianum* (L.) Gaertn. *International Journal of Biosciences, 4*(11), 104–115.

Sarafian, G., Afshar, M., Mansouri, P., Asgarpanah, J., Raoufinejad, K., & Rajabi, M. (2015). Topical turmeric microemulgel in the management of plaque psoriasis; a clinical evaluation. *Iranian Journal of Pharmaceutical Research: IJPR, 14*(3), 865.

Sharma, A. K., Keservani, R. K., & Gautam, S. P. (2020). *Herbal Product Development*. Apple Academic Press, CRC Press, Taylor & Francis Group. 1st Edition, pp. 376. ISBN: 9781003003182.

Shyong, E. Q., Lu, Y., Lazinsky, A., Saladi, R. N., Phelps, R. G., Austin, L. M., Lebwohl, M., & Wei, H. (2002). Effects of the isoflavone 4,' 5, 7-trihydroxy isoflavone (genistein) on psoralen plus ultraviolet A radiation (PUVA)-induced photodamage. *Carcinogenesis, 23*(2), 317–321.

Singh, D. B., Gupta, M. K., Kesharwani, R. K., & Misra, K. (2013a). Comparative docking and ADMET study of some curcumin derivatives and herbal congeners targeting β-amyloid. *Network Modeling Analysis in Health Informatics and Bioinformatics, 2*(1), 13–27.

Singh, D. V., Agarwal, S., Kesharwani, R. K., & Misra, K. (2013b). 3D QSAR and pharmacophore study of curcuminoids and curcumin analogs: Interaction with thioredoxin reductase. *Interdisciplinary Sciences: Computational Life Sciences, 5*(4), 286–295.

Singh, K. K., & Tripathy, S. (2014). Natural treatment alternative for psoriasis: A review on herbal resources. *Journal of Applied Pharmaceutical Science, 4*(11), 114–121.

Singh, P., Kesharwani, R. K., Misra, K., & Rizvi, S. I. (2015). The modulation of erythrocyte Na+/K+-ATPase activity by curcumin. *Journal of Advanced Research, 6*(6), 1023–1030.

Singh, P., Kesharwani, R. K., Misra, K., & Rizvi, S. I. (2016). Modulation of erythrocyte plasma membrane redox system activity by curcumin. *Biochemistry Research International*, 2016, Article ID 702039.

Soleymani, T., Hung, T., & Soung, J. (2015). The role of vitamin D in psoriasis: A review. *International Journal of Dermatology, 54*, 383–392.

Staberg, B., Roed-Petersen, J., & Menne, T. (1989). Efficacy of topical treatment in psoriasis with MC903, a new vitamin D analog. *Acta Dermato-Venereologica, 69*(2), 147–150.

Sun, J., Zhao, Y., & Hu, J. (2013). Curcumin inhibits imiquimod-induced psoriasis-like inflammation by inhibiting IL-1beta and IL-6 production in mice. *PloS One, 8*(6), e67078.

Surjushe, A., Vasani, R., & Saple, D. G. (2008). Properties, mechanism of action, and clinical uses of Aloe vera plant. *Indian Journal of Dermatology, 53*(4), 163–166.

Syed, T. A., Ahmad, S. A., Holt, A. H., Ahmad, S. A., Ahmad, S. H., Afzal, M., & Moore, J. (1996). Management of psoriasis with Aloe vera extract in a hydrophilic cream: A placebo-controlled, double-blind study. *Tropical Medicine and International Health, 1*(4), 505–509.

Thangapazham, R. L., Sharma, A., & Maheshwari, R. K. (2007). The beneficial role of curcumin in skin diseases. In R. A. Watson & V. R. Preedy (Eds.), *The Molecular Targets and Therapeutic Uses of Curcumin in Health and Disease* (pp. 343–357). Springer.

Upadhyaya, J., Kesharwani, R. K., & Misra, K. (2009). Metabolism, pharmacokinetics, and bioavailability of ascorbic acid; synergistic effect with tocopherols and curcumin. *Journal of Computational Intelligence in Bioinformatics, 2*(1), 77–84.

Vázquez, B., Avila, G., Segura, D., & Escalante, B. (1996). Anti-inflammatory activity of extracts from Aloe vera gel. *Journal of Ethnopharmacology, 55*(1), 69–75.

Vickers, N. J. (2017). Animal communication: When I'm calling you, will you answer too? *Current Biology, 27*(14), R713–R715.

Wei, H., Saladi, R., Lu, Y., Wang, Y., Palep, S. R., Moore, J., & Lebwohl, M. G. (2003). Isoflavone genistein: Photoprotection and clinical implications in dermatology. *The Journal of Nutrition, 133*(11), 3811S–3819S.

Weinstein, G. D., McCullough, J. L., & Ross, P. A. (1985). Cell kinetic basis for pathophysiology of psoriasis. *Journal of Investigative Dermatology, 85*(6), 579–583.

Xu, Y. Y., Yang, C., & Li, S. N. (2006). Effects of genistein on angiotensin-converting enzyme in rats. *Life Sciences, 79*(9), 828–837.

Ziboh, V. A., Miller, C. C., & Cho, Y. (2000). Metabolism of polyunsaturated fatty acids by skin epidermal enzymes: Generation of anti-inflammatory and antiproliferative metabolites. *The American Journal of Clinical Nutrition, 71*(1), 361s–366s.

CHAPTER 12

ROLE OF VITAMINS AND OILS IN THE TREATMENT OF PSORIASIS

AKSHADA ATUL BAKLIWAL,[1] VIJAY SHARAD CHUDIWAL,[2] SWATI GOKUL TALELE,[1] and GOKUL SHRAVAN TALELE[3]

[1]*Department of Pharmaceutics, Sandip Institute of Pharmaceutical Sciences, Mahiravani, Nashik, Maharashtra, India*

[2]*Research Scientist, Pune, Maharashtra, India*

[3]*Department of Pharmaceutical Chemistry, Matoshri College of Pharmacy, Eklahare, Nashik, Maharashtra, India*

AB1STRACT

Psoriasis is a constant incendiary skin illness. Immunological, hereditary, and natural variables, including diet, have an influence on the pathogenesis of psoriasis. Metabolic condition or its parts are regular co-morbidities in people with psoriasis. A difference in dietary patterns can work on the personal satisfaction of patients by easing skin sores and lessening the gamble of different illnesses. A low-energy diet is suggested for patients with an abundant body weight. People experiencing psoriasis ought to restrict the admission of immersed unsaturated fats and supplant them with polyunsaturated unsaturated fats from the omega-3 family, which make a calming difference. In diet treatment for people with psoriasis, the presentation of cell reinforcements like vitamin A, L-ascorbic acid, vitamin E, carotenoids, flavonoids, and selenium is critical. Vitamin D supplementation is likewise suggested. A few creators propose that elective eating regimens emphatically affect the course of psoriasis. These weight control plans include a without gluten diet, a vegan diet, and a Mediterranean eating regimen. Diet treatment for patients with psoriasis ought to likewise be custom-fitted to pharmacological treatment. For example, folic corrosive supplementation is presented in people taking methotrexate. The motivation behind this chapter is to talk about exhaustively the job of nutrients and oils for people with psoriasis.

12.1 INTRODUCTION

Psoriasis is perhaps the most well-known chronic skin disease (Vanderpuye-Orgle et al., 2015). As assessed by the World Health Organization (WHO), this dermatosis affects 0.09–11.43% of the global population, and the number of patients varies from 1.50% to 5.00% in developed countries (Villani et al., 2015). It consists of abnormal hyperplasia of keratinocytes (epidermal cells), which leads to the formation of psoriatic plaques (Menter et al., 2011). It is a chronic disease characterized by periods of spontaneous remission followed by relapses (Vanderpuye-Orgle et al., 2015). The disease affects the skin but is also a systemic disease (Menter et al., 2011). Immune disorders, which result in increased pro-inflammatory cytokine production, contribute to the pathogenesis of psoriasis. An increase in the activity of Th1, Th17, and Th22 lymphocytes leads to the production of pro-inflammatory factors in excessive amounts.

These elements include C-reactive protein (CRP), interleukins 1, 2, 6, 8, 12, 17, 22, 23 (IL), Interferon γ (IFN-γ), tumor necrosis factor (TNF-α), ceruloplasmin, α2-macroglobulin, α1-antitrypsin, and others. The grouping of these variables is expanded both during the intense period of psoriasis and disappearing (Smith et al., 2017). TNF-α assumes a vital part in the pathogenesis of psoriasis because of its invigorating impact on the multiplication of keratinocytes (Armstrong et al., 2017). Aside from immune issues, genetic and environmental factors also have an impact on the pathogenesis of the illness (Vanderpuye-Orgle et al., 2015). Among other things, a connection between the occurrence of psoriasis and genes in the HLA complex (specifically HLA-Cw6) has been illustrated. However, it is often the case that the disease never develops in individuals carrying psoriasis-related genes (Dogra et al., 2014).

The environmental factors that can lead to the appearance of psoriasis or worsening of lesions are as follows (Dogra et al., 2014):

- Actual elements (X-beams, subcutaneous and intradermal infusions, surgeries; inoculations, tattoos, bug chomps, scraped spots, consumes (counting burns from the sun), needle therapy, UV illumination);

- Substance factors (compound consumes, skin medicines, others);
- Skin sicknesses (rosacea, parasitic diseases, hypersensitive contact dermatitis);
- Contaminations (primarily streptococcal pharyngitis, viral diseases);
- Stress;
- Drugs (β-adrenolytic, angiotensin-changing over chemical inhibitors, lithium, terbinafine, nonsteroidal calming drugs, against malarial medications, antibiotic medications, fast withdrawal of fundamental corticosteroids);
- Diet;
- Tobacco smoking;
- Liquor utilization.

Regardless of various examinations, the etiopathogenesis of psoriasis has not been completely understood (Torma et al., 1998). It is perplexing and vague. The aforementioned factors (immunological, hereditary, and ecological) impact the development and severity of this dermatosis to varying degrees. Additionally, it is worth noting the association between psoriasis and other diseases (Schmitt et al., 1987). Psoriasis is a systemic disease often accompanied by other conditions, such as metabolic syndrome and cardiovascular diseases (Saurat, 1999). The fact that individuals suffering from psoriasis live an average of five years less compared to healthy individuals. The most common causes of death in patients with psoriasis include thromboembolic events and myocardial infarction (Siegenthaler et al., 1986). The chronic inflammatory process is the mechanism that links psoriasis with its comorbidities (Babina et al., 2017).

12.2 METABOLIC SYNDROME

Metabolic disorder and its parts, which incorporate stomach stoutness, atherogenic dyslipidemia, insulin obstruction, disabled glucose resilience or type 2 diabetes, and hypertension, are noticed more as often as possible in people with psoriasis than in the general populace (Hirayama et al., 2008; Van Zander et al., 2005). Certain individuals likewise consider the accompanying as a real part of the side effects: hyperhomocysteinemia, expanded convergence of procoagulant factors, microalbuminuria, and non-alcoholic fatty liver disease (Lebwohl et al., 2005; Guenther, 2002).

In a population-based cross-sectional study by Langan et al. (Mehta et al., 2011), 34% of people with psoriasis and 26% of the benchmark group had metabolic disorders. A positive relationship between the occurrence of metabolic conditions and the severity (determined by the BSA-Body Surface Area marker) was also observed. In the focused-on group, the metabolic condition was diagnosed in 32% of patients with mild psoriasis, 36% of those with moderate psoriasis, and as many as 40% of those with a severe form of dermatosis (Mehta et al., 2011). Therefore, metabolic conditions are more likely to affect patients with moderate to severe psoriasis, especially patients who developed the disease at a young age (Mehta et al., 2011).

Supportive of fiery cytokines as well as Th1 and Th17 lymphocytes play a significant role in psoriasis. Levels of cytokines, for example, IL-6, TNF-α, angiogenic elements, and gripatoms are raised in corpulence psoriasis and ischemic coronary illness. What's more, these incendiary go-betweens have been displayed to impact fat statement, insulin activity, and lipid digestion. Accordingly, constant aggravation in psoriasis might incline toward diabetes, atherosclerosis, and corpulence. On the other hand, incendiary go-betweens, whose creation goes with metabolic issues, may start the appearance of psoriatic injuries or worsen existing psoriatic side effects (Dogra et al., 2013). In patients with psoriasis, TNF-α is found in blood serum and skin sores, while it is missing in sound skin. TNF-α is additionally discharged in adipocytes and plays a part in the advancement of insulin obstruction. Furthermore, the presence of TNF-α prompts an increment in the concentration of free unsaturated fats and fatty oils in the blood, which might cause atherogenic dyslipidemia (Lee et al., 2009). IL-6, found in high concentrations in psoriatic injuries, also assumes a significant role in metabolic issues. Its production is multiple times higher in visceral fat tissue than in subcutaneous fat tissue and connects with the chance of developing type 2 diabetes. In addition, elevated IL-6 levels are also found in patients with unhealthy coronary artery disease (Lee et al., 2009) (Table 12.1).

TABLE 12.1 Sources of Some Antioxidants

Antioxidants	Sources
Vitamin A	Fish fat, liver, cheese, eggs, butter, carotenoids.
Vitamin C	Raw vegetables and fruits.
Vitamin E	Vegetable oils, nuts, sunflower seeds, wheat germ.
Carotenoids	Vegetables with orange, yellow, and green color, carrots, tomato, spinach.
Flavonoids	Tomatoes, peppers, onions, citrus fruits, apples, grapes, green tea, coca.
Selenium	Meat, fish, whole grains, dairy products, mushrooms.

12.3 USE OF SEAWEED IN PSORIASIS

The human microbiota is a climate rich in microorganisms that impact protein, starch, and lipid digestion, immune system development, and body homeostasis. The largest microbiota resource in the human body is the intestine. In the literature, many studies show a link between digestive dysbiosis and the development of diseases with an extraintestinal location, such as multiple sclerosis, type 1 diabetes, systemic lupus erythematosus, or psoriasis. Significant differences have been observed between the gut microbiota of psoriasis patients and that of the healthy population, suggesting a potential influence of gut dysbiosis on the development of psoriasis. Several reports demonstrate a connection between dietary modifications, microbiota composition, and immunostimulatory effects. Probiotic microorganisms are commonly found in fermented dairy products, such as kefir and yogurt, as well as in pickled vegetables. Recent studies indicate a beneficial effect of probiotic supplementation in patients with psoriasis. Polysaccharides, which are components of dietary fiber, exhibit prebiotic impacts, gainfully changing the digestive microflora. Concentrates by Takahashi et al. Furthermore, different reports demonstrate that fucoidan, a sulfated polysaccharide viewed in the cell walls of brown seaweed, shows anticoagulant, anticancer, immunomodulatory, and apoptosis-initiating effects. Fucoidan has also been found to positively affect the digestive barrier and the composition of the bacterial flora, as well as improve the course of psoriasis. Likewise, marine kelp is a sustainable source of bioactive lipids with high concentrations of omega-3 unsaturated fats and vitamin D3, whose beneficial effects in psoriasis patients have been observed previously. The application of seaweed directly to the patient's skin also makes a beneficial impact on the course of dermatosis. In a study by Grether-Beck et al., it was shown that Blue Lagoon kelp extract has a positive effect on the skin, influences the expression levels of mRNAs relevant for melanin synthesis, and reduces imbalance in skin pigmentation.

12.4 ESPRESSO AND PSORIASIS

Espresso is perhaps the most consumed beverage, regardless of geographical location. According to statistics, only water and tea are more frequently consumed beverages. Importantly, espresso is a pharmacologically active liquid. There are many biologically active substances in its composition.

These include carbohydrates, lipids, nitrogenous compounds, minerals, vitamins, phenolic compounds, lactones, diterpenes, antioxidants, alkaloids, and caffeine, which make up about 1% of the total composition of espresso. This substance exhibits various beneficial actions. It has been shown to reduce the migration of monocytes and neutrophils, lower blood glucose levels, have an anti-inflammatory and immunosuppressive effect, and protect against neurodegeneration. The most studied component of espresso is caffeine. Its action involves inhibition of Th1/Th2 cell proliferation, inhibition of the release of pro-inflammatory cytokines (IL-1, IL-6, IL-11, TNF-alpha), and promotion of the release of anti-inflammatory markers such as IL-4, IL-10, and adiponectin. Additionally, it inhibits cyclin adenosine monophosphate (cAMP) phosphodiesterase, which acts as an immunomodulator, stimulates the release of anti-inflammatory cytokines, and acts as an adenosine receptor antagonist. Hall et al. argue that the anti-inflammatory effects of espresso are linked to the presence of substances called polyphenols in its structure. A gathering of these mixtures, particularly chlorogenic acid and its metabolites, show strong inhibitory effects on proinflammatory cytokines, while caffeic acid reduces nitrite levels and inhibits inflammatory responses. The arabinogalactan proteins present in coffee create an immunosuppressive effect, stimulating splenocytes and peritoneal macrophages, resulting in a reduction in skin inflammation and decreasing the severity of allergic reactions. Research on the use of coffee in the treatment or management of psoriasis is inconclusive. Zampelas et al. speculated that coffee consumption increases the body's inflammatory process, which may negatively interact with psoriasis severity. A study conducted by this research group showed that regular coffee consumption increased IL-6, CRP, and TNF-alpha levels, which correlated with the clinical severity of psoriasis symptoms. However, it is important to note that this study associated high coffee consumption (>200 mg/day) with psoriasis severity. Contrary to the norm, Li et al. demonstrated that coffee improved the effectiveness of the pharmacological treatment of psoriasis, especially when methotrexate or sulfasalazine was used. Interestingly, decaffeinated coffee influenced the risk of developing psoriasis. A similar report additionally evaluated the relationship between caffeine consumption and the risk of developing psoriasis. It was shown that the risk of psoriasis was moderately associated with an increase in caffeine intake, although this finding was not statistically significant in cigarette smokers. It should be noted here that this study had a significant limitation: the effects of caffeine from various sources, including caffeinated drinks and highly processed foods, were assessed, which may have influenced the conclusions drawn. Studies by Sharif et al. and Hall et al. have shown that regular coffee consumption increases the levels of anti-inflammatory factors and reduces the production of proinflammatory factors (especially TNF-alpha), which is important in reducing the severity of psoriasis. Recent studies indicate that the effect of coffee is dose-dependent. Moderate regular coffee consumption (up to 3 cups per day) alleviates psoriasis symptoms and creates an anti-inflammatory effect, while higher coffee consumption (especially >4 cups of coffee per day) worsens clinical symptoms of psoriasis, which is associated with an increase in pro-inflammatory substances.

12.5 VITAMIN A

Vitamin A derivatives known as retinoids have been used for many years both topically and orally. The main retinoid mechanism is the antiproliferative effects and promotion of epithelial differentiation. They effectively inhibit the hyperproliferation of keratinocytes and normalize the abnormal differentiation seen in psoriasis (Dogra et al., 2014). However, studies have revealed a paradox in psoriatic lesions where there is a higher level of retinoic acid within the lesions due to a change in vitamin A metabolism, yet retinoid treatment is effective in such lesions. The increased level of retinoic acid is caused by elevated levels of inflammatory cytokines found in psoriasis, particularly interferon gamma (IFN-γ) (Torma et al., 1998). To unravel the paradox, an oral form of vitamin A, acitretin, has been studied resulting in several proposed mechanisms. These include the downregulation of inflammatory cytokines, induction of alternative binding proteins, and modulation of vitamin A metabolism through synthetic rather than endogenous retinoids. Retinoids also have an inhibitory effect on cutaneous mast cells (Babina et al., 2017). In psoriasis, mast cells, key cellular mediators of cytokine expression and propagation of lesions, are considered activated and present in greater numbers in the papillary dermis (Haryima et al., 2008). Cancer prevention properties of vitamin A and its derivatives have also been implicated in its effectiveness on psoriatic plaques (Van et al., 2005; Lebwohl et al., 2005). Tazarotene, an effective form of retinoid, demonstrates efficacy in the treatment of plaque psoriasis and has been shown to be non-inferior to steroid creams in palmoplantar psoriasis (Guenther, 2002; Mehta et al., 2011). Acitretin has been used as monotherapy and in combination treatment for various types of psoriasis. In a study using escalating doses of acitretin alone in severe chronic plaque psoriasis, more than half of patients achieved a

54–76% reduction in Psoriasis Area Severity Index (PASI) score in 12 weeks with 35–50 mg/day dosing (Dogra et al., 2013). Although monotherapy is effective, it can be safely used in combination with other treatments, particularly UVB therapy (Lee et al., 2009; Kopp et al., 2004). Several studies have indicated a vitamin A deficiency in patients with psoriasis. In a large study adjusting for age, race, gender, nutrient intake, smoking status, and BMI, the precursor for vitamin A, carotenoid, was found to be reduced in the skin of psoriasis patients compared to those without the disease (Lima et al., 2011). A study by Majewski et al. looked at the baseline levels of vitamin A and found a decrease in all psoriasis patients compared to controls. Additionally, the study found that levels associated with disease severity were lower in more active disease (Majewski et al., 1989). Further research is needed to clarify the relationship between vitamin A levels and supplementation in the management of psoriasis.

12.6 VITAMIN D

The efficacy of vitamin D in psoriasis depends on its hindrance of keratinocyte multiplication because of genome-mediated impacts and induction of keratinocyte differentiation by increasing intracellular calcium levels (Barrea et al., 2017; Soleymani et al., 2015). Vitamin D also exerts anti-inflammatory effects by inhibiting the production of various inflammatory cytokines through direct inhibition of T cells and T regulatory cell activation. More specifically, vitamin D has been found to downregulate toll-like receptor (TLR) expression, key initiators of the inflammatory cascade, and cell proteins implicated in the pathogenesis of psoriasis (Sadeghi et al., 2006). One study showed an increase in TLR2-induced production of cytokines in vitamin D-deficient patients with levels <50 nmol/L. After normalization to >100 nmol/L through supplementation, TLR2-dependent production of cytokines was significantly reduced (Ojaimi et al., 2013). The physiological mechanism by which TLRs exert their inflammatory activity is through the recognition of microbe-related molecular patterns. Upon activation, TLRs initiate a signaling cascade that culminates in increased activity of nuclear factor kappa-B (NF-κB) among other proteins. NF-κB is a crucial protein responsible for signaling the production of tumor necrosis factor-alpha (TNF-α) and other pro-inflammatory interleukins (Akira et al., 2004). Specifically, TLR2 and TLR4 have been shown to play a significant role in psoriasis and other cutaneous infection processes. In a study examining the expression of TLRs in cutaneous diseases, TLR2 and

TLR4 were found to be disproportionately expressed in psoriasis-affected epidermis (Panzer et al., 2014). The identification of increased expression of TLRs and their contribution to psoriasis is supported by various studies demonstrating the role of different receptors in psoriasis, including increased epidermal TLR2 expression (Curry et al., 2003; Kondelkova et al., 2014). Another study indicated that TLR2 and TLR4 polymorphisms were found to increase patient susceptibility to psoriasis vulgaris (Shi et al., 2016). Allen et al. demonstrated a high density of TLR2 within upper dermal vessels in psoriatic plaques, supporting a fundamental immune response (Allen et al., 2016). Effective vitamin D analogs are the mainstays of treatment following steroid or vitamin A treatment failure in psoriasis. Several studies concluded that both calcitriol and calcipotriol were equally effective as betamethasone dipropionate and were also effective as monotherapy. Combination treatment with topical steroids has a synergistic effect and is commonly used in practice. The short-term adverse effect of topical vitamin D is minimal if present and consists of only minor facial dermatitis. No calcium level alterations were found in any studies (Kragballe et al., 1991; Van et al., 1989; Kragballe et al., 1988). Long-term safety and efficacy studies have also demonstrated efficacy and an excellent safety profile for topical tacalcitol (Miyachi et al., 2002). While effective types of vitamin D have demonstrated success, oral vitamin D supplementation should be considered in cases with significant body surface area involvement. Several studies have shown that oral vitamin D supplementation and vitamin D analogs have positive clinical responses and maintain a similar safety profile to effective forms. Although patients did not experience adverse effects, the risk of hypercalcemia and bone demineralization is theoretically possible (Van et al., 2002). While vitamin deficiency is supported in the literature, an older study found that affected fibroblasts within psoriatic lesions are moderately resistant to activated forms of vitamin D *in vitro*. This discovery may support the efficacy of active vitamin D administered at higher concentrations than those found in endogenous vitamin D. The study could also address a mechanism for functional deficiency in patients with otherwise normal vitamin D levels (Holick et al., 1989).

12.7 VITAMIN E

Vitamin E is a significant cutaneous, non-enzymatic antioxidant, scavenging free radicals generated through a variety of mechanisms leading to skin pathology. Vitamin E is also anti-inflammatory as demonstrated in various animal models. Only two forms of vitamin E exist in the body: α-tocopherol and γ-tocopherol. Both are present in abundance within the stratum corneum after their release by sebaceous glands. The increased concentration of vitamin E within the stratum corneum preserves the integrity and barrier function of the skin while protecting the outermost cutaneous layer from oxidation. Supplementation of vitamin E, orally or intravenously, has been shown to reach the peripheral areas of the skin and does so within approximately two weeks of supplementation. The diet eliminated all processed foods and sugars; the dietary supplementation included 29.1 mg of α-tocopherol, 2.6 mg of other natural tocopherols, and >35 additional vitamins, minerals, and amino acids. The patient experienced complete symptom reduction within six months.

Not many investigations exist deciding vitamin E levels in psoriasis patients. A new report tracked down a decline in intraepidermal levels of vitamin E, coenzyme Q10, and selenium in both psoriasis and atopic dermatitis. While this might uphold a possible by and large deficiency, foundational vitamin E deficiency in psoriasis still can't seem to be displayed in the writing. Because of the extraordinary act of vitamin E testing and intriguing finding of deficiency in everyone, testing vitamin E levels is uncommon. Further exploration is shown to decide whether a deficiency exists in psoriasis (Finamor et al., 2013).

12.8 VITAMIN K

Vitamin K is classified into three sorts: K1, K2, and K3. K1 is responsible for the creation of coagulation factors and plays a role in vessel calcification homeostasis. K3, menadione, prevents deficiency as a catalyst cofactor. K2, menaquinone, impacts bone health, modifies calcification in the cardiovascular system, and limits inflammation among its various effects in different tissues, making it a target for research in autoimmunity. Vitamin K reduces inflammation through a variety of pathways. Several *in vitro* studies have shown that vitamin K2 inhibits the production of prostaglandins and important pro-inflammatory cytokines including IL-1, IL-6, and TNF-α. Research is also lacking in vitamin K deficiency in psoriasis. Deficiency data would support its role in disease management. While some evidence exists, further research on the effects of vitamin K and possible deficiency in psoriasis is needed (Morimoto et al., 1986).

12.9 ALTERNATIVE DIETS IN THE TREATMENT OF PSORIASIS

12.9.1 GLUTEN-FREE DIET

Asymptomatic celiac disease is noticed more often in patients with psoriasis compared to everyone. A meta-analysis of the relationship between psoriasis and celiac disease concluded that patients with this dermatosis have an approximately three-fold increased risk of celiac disease. Meanwhile, the risk of psoriasis in patients with celiac disease is higher than in the general population. In celiac disease, inflammation of the small intestine mucosa and gastrointestinal villous atrophy occurs due to consuming gluten-containing cereals (wheat, rye, barley, oats, triticale), leading to absorption issues. Moreover, upon returning to a regular diet containing gluten, a worsening of psoriatic lesions was observed. However, in patients without present antibodies, no improvement in lesions was noted. Initiating a gluten-free diet in patients with psoriasis may be controversial, and further research is needed to understand the role of this dietary approach comprehensively.

12.9.2 VEGETARIAN DIET

Some authors point out the positive effect of a vegetarian diet on the course of the infection in patients with psoriasis. The diet consists of giving up meat products while increasing the intake of vegetables, fruits, legumes, nuts, and grain products. As a result, the diet is low in saturated, trans, and arachidonic acid and high in antioxidants and omega-3 fatty acids (Perez et al., 1996).

Additionally, a vegetarian diet may help balance potassium deficiencies. An increase in potassium intake may lead to an increase in cortisol synthesis, which creates an anti-inflammatory effect. It is known that a diet rich in vegetables and fruit may significantly contribute to improving the clinical condition of individuals suffering from psoriasis.

12.9.3 MEDITERRANEAN DIET

The Mediterranean eating regimen is characterized by a high consumption of vegetables, cereals, legumes, fish, fruit, and nuts. Extra virgin olive oil is the main source of fat in this diet. It is recommended to consume small amounts of wine with meals. The intake of meat, dairy products, and eggs is limited. Animal fats such as butter, cream, and lard are excluded from this diet. The Mediterranean diet is associated with the prevention of metabolic, cardiovascular, and chronic inflammatory diseases. The health-promoting properties of this diet are linked to the high consumption of:

- Items with cell reinforcement and calming impacts (natural products, vegetables, red wine, normal spices);
- Unsaturated fats (fish, olive oil, nuts);
- Items that are a wellspring of dietary fiber; and
- Items that are a wellspring of nutrients and minerals.

12.9.4 KETOGENIC DIET

Despite adipocytokine levels, muscle versus fat, body weight, and glycemic values, soaked unsaturated fat admission is a critical exacerbator of psoriasis. A ketogenic diet based on increased fat intake (75–80% kcal from fat, 5–10% kcal from carbohydrates, and 15–25% kcal from protein) increases ketone bodies, may have anti-inflammatory effects, and lowers blood glucose levels. The high content of medium-chain fatty acids (MCT) with a stronger anti-inflammatory effect compared to long-chain fatty acids (LCT), as well as the anti-angiogenic nature and the high amount of omega-3 unsaturated fats, make the ketogenic diet a potentially beneficial nutritional intervention in patients with psoriasis.

12.10 DIET THERAPY AND THE USE OF MEDICINES

Nutrition of patients with psoriasis ought to also be customized to their treatment. The use of methotrexate contributes to an increase in the concentration of toxic homocysteine and reduces the blood level of folic acid. Additionally, deficiencies of this nutrient are also associated with increased homocysteine levels. Supplementation with folic acid, generally in the amount of 10–15 mg/week, should be introduced in patients taking methotrexate. Supplementation strategies vary, but the vitamins should always be administered at least 12 or 24 hours (according to different reports) after taking methotrexate due to the risk of a decrease in the effectiveness of the medication. This is possible because methotrexate is required once every week. It should be remembered that the bioavailability of folic acid decreases when it is taken with a meal. Supplementation of this nutrient in people taking methotrexate can also help alleviate other adverse reactions associated with the bone marrow, gastrointestinal tract, and liver, caused by the medication. It should also be noted that methotrexate may cause nausea, which in turn is a common cause of loss of appetite in patients and may contribute to the development of deficiencies of certain nutrients. Therefore, it is necessary to include a good diet, providing all the necessary components in the proper amounts. (Millsop et al., 2014).

Cyclosporine A might increase the risk of hypertension. In one study, patients starting treatment with this medication followed a low-sodium diet, followed by a high-sodium diet. After four months of treatment with a low-sodium diet, blood pressure did not increase, but in the subsequent period, when patients followed a high-sodium diet, there was a significant increase in both systolic and diastolic pressure.

Combining cyclosporine with grapefruit juice results in an increase in the drug's bioavailability by up to 60%. Therefore, patients taking this medication should avoid grapefruit juice, grapefruit, and other citrus fruits. (Tremezaygues et al., 2011).

Vitamin A derivatives are also used in psoriasis. It should be noted that this may lead to hypervitaminosis, especially in patients who choose to use additional supplementation of this vitamin and consume many products rich in vitamin A. Retinoids can also cause elevated cholesterol and triglyceride levels in blood serum. Therefore, it is recommended to consume foods rich in polyunsaturated fatty acids from the omega-3 family and to limit the intake of simple sugars and alcohol (Morimoto et al., 1985).

12.11 CONCLUSION

Unfortunately, no particular wholesome treatment regimens for psoriasis have been laid out yet. Be that as it may, various investigations confirm the positive outcome of the utilization or elimination of the supplements and food items mentioned previously. When planning the diet of patients with psoriasis, one should also consider co-morbidities and implement measures to prevent the diseases to which these individuals are susceptible. The diet for patients with psoriasis should be adjusted and personalized to each individual patient. Patients should avoid alcohol, animal fats, red meat, simple sugars, and highly processed foods. A variety of vegetables and fruits, which are a source of antioxidants, as well as vegetable oils, nuts, and marine fish providing unsaturated fats from the omega-3 family, should be consumed. They should choose whole grain cereal products and increase the intake of vegetables. At times, patients should consider a gluten-free diet and vitamin D supplementation. A diet that is properly chosen and consistently followed by the patient can have a positive impact not only on the course of psoriasis and the prognosis but also on comorbidities.

Vitamin A and D have mounting proof for existing deficiencies in psoriasis patients. These nutrients are backbones of treatment which uphold a system of deficiency in the infection process. A few examinations have exhibited clear pathways for sickness improvement at the cell level with effective oral treatments. Vitamin E has also shown efficacy at the cell level, yet needs research supporting a deficiency in psoriasis. The current vitamin K research involves a cell, anti-inflammatory pathway that embroils its role in psoriasis management. Further exploration is required on vitamin K to determine the potential benefit of supplementation in psoriasis patients. The ideal health profile and minimal cost of fat-soluble nutrient supplementation give significant potential benefits expected to lay out the role and significance of deficiencies of fat-soluble nutrients and nutrient supplementation to be considered additionally as a supportive treatment.

KEYWORDS

- cyclin adenosine monophosphate
- interferon gamma
- long-chain fatty acids
- medium-chain fatty acids
- nutrition
- psoriasis
- psoriasis area severity index

REFERENCES

Akira, S., & Takeda, K. (2004). Toll-like receptor signaling. *Nature Reviews Immunology, 4*(7), 499–511.

Allen, H. B., Miller, B., Durkin, J., & Joshi, S. G. (2016). Psoriasis: A sequela of streptococcal infection similar to acute rheumatic fever. *Clinical Microbiology, 5*(3), 2.

Armstrong, A. W., Koning, J. W., Rowse, S., Tan, H., Mamolo, C., et al. (2017). Initiation, switching, and cessation of psoriasis treatments among patients with moderate to severe psoriasis in the United States. *Clinical Drug Investigation, 37*(6), 493–501.

Babina, M., Artuc, M., Guhl, S., & Zuberbier, T. (2017). Retinoic acid negatively impacts the proliferation and MCTC-specific attributes of human skin-derived mast cells but reinforces allergic stimulability. Zhang, G. (Ed.). *International Journal of Molecular Sciences, 18*(3), 525.

Barrea, L., Savanelli, M. C., Di Somma, C., Napolitano, M., Megna, M., et al. (2017). Vitamin A and its role in psoriasis: An overview of the dermatologist and nutritionist. *Reviews in Endocrine & Metabolic Disorders, 18*(2), 195–205.

Curry, J. L., Qin, J. Z., Bonish, B., Carrick, R., Bacon, P., et al. (2003). Innate immune-related receptors in normal and psoriatic skin. *Archives of Pathology & Laboratory Medicine, 127*(2), 178–186.

Dogra, S. S., Jain, A., & Kanwar, A. J. (2013). Efficacy and safety of acitretin in three fixed doses of 25, 35 and 50 mg in adult patients with severe plaque-type psoriasis: a randomized, double-blind, parallel-group, dose-ranging study. *Journal of the European Academy of Dermatology and Venereology, 27*(3), e305–e311.

Dogra, S., & Yadav, S. (2014). Acitretin in psoriasis: an evolving scenario. *International Journal of Dermatology, 53*(5), 525–538.

Finamor, D. C., Sinigaglia-Coimbra, R., Neves, L. C., Gutierrez, M., Silva, J. J., Torres, L. D., et al. (2013). A pilot study assessing the effect of prolonged administration of high daily doses of vitamin D on the clinical course of vitiligo1 and psoriasis. *Dermato-Endocrinology, 5*(2), 222–234.

Guenther, L. C. (2002). Topical tazarotene therapy for psoriasis, acne vulgaris, and photoaging. *Skin Therapy Letter, 7*(6), 1–4.

Harvima, I. T., Nilsson, G., Suttle, M. M., & Naukkarinen, A. (2008). Is there a role for mast cells in psoriasis? *Archives of Dermatological Research, 300*(8), 461–478.

Holick, M. F., Pochi, P., & Bhawan, J. (1989). Topically applied and orally administered 1,25-dihydroxy-Vitamin D3 is a novel, safe, effective therapy for the treatment of psoriasis: a three-year experience with histologic analysis. *Journal of Investigative Dermatology, 92*(4), 446.

Kondelkova, K., Krejsek, J., Borska, L., Fiala, Z., Hamakova, K., et al. (2014). Membrane and soluble Toll-like receptor 2 in patients with psoriasis treated by Goeckerman therapy. *International Journal of Dermatology, 53*(4), e512–e517.

Kopp, T., Karlhofer, F., Szepfalusi, Z., Schneeberger, A., Stingl, G., et al. (2004). Successful use of acitretin in conjunction with narrowband ultraviolet B phototherapy in a child with severe pustular psoriasis, von Zumbusch type. *British Journal of Dermatology, 151*(4), 912–916.

Kragballe, K., Beck, H. I., & Sogaard, H. (1988). Improvement of psoriasis by topical Vitamin D3 analogue (MC 903) in a double-blind study. *British Journal of Dermatology, 119*(2), 223–230.

Kragballe, K., Gjertsen, B. T., De Hoop, D., Karlsmark, T., van de Kerkhof, P. C., et al. (1991). Double-blind, right/left comparison of calcipotriol and betamethasone valerate in treatment of psoriasis vulgaris. *The Lancet, 337*(8742), 193–196.

Lebwohl, M., Ting, P. T., & Koo, J. Y. (2005). Psoriasis treatment: Traditional therapy. *Annals of the Rheumatic Diseases, 64*(suppl 2), 83–86.

Lee, C. S., & Li, K. (2009). A review of acitretin for the treatment of psoriasis. *Expert Opinion on Drug Safety, 8*(6), 769–779.

Lima, X. T., & Kimball, A. B. (2011). Skin carotenoid levels in adult patients with psoriasis. *Journal of the European Academy of Dermatology and Venereology, 25*(8), 945–949.

Majewski, S., Janik, P., Langner, A., Glinska-Ferenz, M., Swietochowska, B., et al. (1989). Decreased levels of vitamin A in the serum of patients with psoriasis. *Archives of Dermatological Research, 280*(8), 499–501.

Mehta, B. H., & Amladi, S. T. (2011). Evaluation of topical 0.1% tazarotene cream in the treatment of palmoplantar psoriasis: An observer-blinded randomized controlled study. *Indian Journal of Dermatology, 56*(1), 40–43.

Menter, A., Korman, N. J., Elmets, C. A., Feldman, S. R., American Academy of Dermatology Work Group, et al. (2011). Guidelines of care for the management of psoriasis and psoriatic arthritis: section 6. Guidelines of care for the treatment of psoriasis and psoriatic arthritis: case-based presentations and evidence-based conclusions. *Journal of the American Academy of Dermatology, 65*(1), 137–174.

Millsop, J. W., Bhatia, B. K., Debbaneh, M., Koo, J., Liao, W., et al. (2014). Diet and psoriasis, part III: Role of nutritional supplements. *Journal of the American Academy of Dermatology, 71*(3), 561–569.

Miyachi, Y., Ohkawara, A., & Ohkido, M. (2002). Long-term safety and efficacy of high-concentration (20 μg/g) tacalcitol ointment in psoriasis vulgaris. *European Journal of Dermatology, 12*(5), 463–468.

Morimoto, S., & Kumahara, Y. (1985). A patient with psoriasis was cured by 1αhydroxyvitamin D3. *Medical Journal of Osaka University, 35*, 51–54.

Morimoto, S., Yoshikawa, K., Kozuka, T., Kitano, Y., & Imanaka, S., et al. (1986). An open study of vitamin D3 treatment in psoriasis vulgaris. *British Journal of Dermatology, 115*(4), 421–429.

Ojaimi, S., Skinner, N. A., Strauss, B. J., Sundararajan, V., Woolley, I., et al. (2013). Vitamin D deficiency impacts on the expression of toll-like receptor-2 and cytokine profile: a pilot study. *Journal of Translational Medicine, 11*(1), 176.

Panzer, R. R., Blobel, C., Folster-Holst, R., & Proksch, E. (2014). TLR2 and TLR4 expression in atopic dermatitis, contact dermatitis and psoriasis. *Experimental Dermatology, 23*(5), 364–366.

Perez, A., Raab, R., Chen, T. C., Turner, A., Holick, M. F., et al. (1996). Safety and efficacy of oral calcitriol (1,25-dihydroxyvitamin D3) for the treatment of psoriasis. *British Journal of Dermatology, 134*(6), 1070–1078.

Sadeghi, K., Wessner, B., Laggner, U., Ploder, M., Tamandl, D., et al. (2006). Vitamin D3 down-regulates monocyte TLR expression and triggers hyporesponsiveness to pathogen-associated molecular patterns. *European Journal of Immunology, 36*(2), 361–370.

Saurat, J. H. (1999). Retinoids and psoriasis: Novel issues in retinoid pharmacology and implications for psoriasis treatment. *Journal of the American Academy of Dermatology, 41*(2), S2–S6.

Schmitt, A., Hauser, C., Didierjean, L., Mérot, Y., Dayer, J. M., et al. (1987). Systemic administration of etretin increases epidermal interleukin-1 in the rat. *British Journal of Dermatology, 116*(5), 615–622.

Shi, G., Wang, T., Li, S., Cheng, Y., Sheng, P., et al. (2016). TLR2 and TLR4 polymorphisms in Southern Chinese Psoriasis Vulgaris patients. *Journal of Dermatological Science, 83*(2), 145–147.

Siegenthaler, G., & Saurat, J. H. (1986). Therapy with synthetic retinoid (Ro 10-1670) etretin increases the cellular retinoic acid-binding protein in nonlesional psoriatic skin. *Journal of Investigative Dermatology, 87*(1), 122–124.

Smith, J., Cline, A., & Feldman, S. R. (2017). Advances in Psoriasis. *Southern Medical Journal, 110*(2), 65–75.

Soleymani, T. T., Hung, T., & Soung, J. (2015). The role of vitamin D in psoriasis: A review. *International Journal of Dermatology, 54*(4), 383–392.

Törmä, H., Rollman, O., & Vahlquist, A. (1998). Interferon-γ increases retinoic acid and 3,4-didehydroretinoic acid concentrations in cultured keratinocytes: A clue to the abnormal vitamin A metabolism in psoriatic skin. *Journal of Investigative Dermatology, 110*(4), 551.

Tremezaygues, L., & Reichrath, J. (2011). Vitamin D analogs in the treatment of psoriasis: Where are we standing and where will we be going? *Dermato-Endocrinology, 3*(3), 180–186.

Van de Kerkhof, P. C. M., Van Bokhoven, M., Zultak, M., & Czarnetzki, B. M. (1989). A double-blind study of topical 1,25-dihydroxy-Vitamin D3 in psoriasis. *British Journal of Dermatology, 120*(5), 661–664.

Van de Kerkhof, P. C., Berth-Jones, J., Griffiths, C. E., Harrison, P. V., Hönigsmann, H., et al. (2002). Long-term efficacy and safety of tacalcitol ointment in patients with chronic plaque psoriasis. *British Journal of Dermatology, 146*(3), 414–422.

Van Zander, J., & Orlow, S. J. (2005). Efficacy and safety of oral retinoids in psoriasis. *Expert Opinion on Drug Safety, 4*(1), 129–138.

Vanderpuye-Orgle, J., Zhao, Y., Lu, J., Shrestha, A., Sexton, A., et al. (2015). Evaluating the economic burden of psoriasis in the United States. *Journal of the American Academy of Dermatology, 72*(5), 961–967.

Villani, A. P., Rouzaud, M., Sevrain, M., Barnetche, T., Paul, C., et al. (2015). Prevalence of undiagnosed psoriatic arthritis among psoriasis patients: Systematic review and meta-analysis. *Journal of the American Academy of Dermatology, 73*(2), 242–248.

CHAPTER 13

NUTRACEUTICALS AS A NON-PHARMACOLOGICAL APPROACH FOR PSORIASIS

ROHIT[1] and PANKAJ KUMAR[2]

[1]Department of Pharmacy Practice, ISF College of Pharmacy, Moga, Punjab, India

[2]Professor, Department of Pharmacology, Adesh Institute of Pharmacy and Biomedical Science, Adesh University, Bathinda, Punjab, India

ABSTRACT

Psoriasis is a chronic skin condition characterized by the premature death of skin cells, most noticeably on the skin's surface. Accumulated dead skin causes scaling and red, itchy spots. While several treatments have shown promise in alleviating the symptoms of psoriasis, a permanent solution remains elusive. Moreover, poor treatment outcomes and medication toxicity make these approaches uncomfortable for treating psoriasis. The focus of research into potential treatments for this illness has shifted to nutraceuticals, of which only a small number have been recorded thus far. Nutritional supplements, vitamins, herbal extracts, and phytochemicals are all covered. The purpose of this analysis was to focus attention on useful nutraceuticals for enhanced management of psoriasis. Including the right nutraceuticals in a patient's treatment plan has the potential to enhance their quality of life and affect the disease state as a whole.

13.1 INTRODUCTION

Common sites of psoriasis manifestation include the scalp, elbows, and knees. It causes red, itchy, and scaly patches to appear. Psoriasis is a chronic, rapidly worsening disease for which there is no treatment. When psoriasis is present, skin cells may proliferate up to 10 times more rapidly than normal. The affected areas become red, scratchy, and covered with white scales. Psoriasis cannot be transmitted from person to person. Even members of the same family aren't immune to it. Psoriasis often appears in the early adult years. Most individuals are only affected in a small number of locations. Psoriasis, in its extreme forms, may cover large regions of the body. The patches might heal and return at various times during a person's life. Though prevalence varies by area, this ailment affects around 2% of the world's population. While the prevalence is lower in people of Asian and certain African origin, it may reach as high as 11% in people of Caucasian and Scandinavian heritage (Naldi, 2004). There is a wide variety of psoriasis. Increased skin lesions, scaly erythematous (red) plaques, acanthosis (epidermal hyperproliferation), parakeratosis (abnormal keratinocyte differentiation), and inflammatory cell infiltration, especially in the scalp, elbows, and knees, are hallmarks of psoriasis, which is strongly associated with environmental and genetic factors (Campalani & Barker, 2005). Psoriasis has an unknown etiology, but a number of shared pathophysiological events have been identified. These include an altered immune response (immunological dysfunction), an increased inflammatory response, an overabundance of plasmacytoid dendritic cells, and a hyperproliferation of keratinocytes (dermal cells). Psoriasis is an autoimmune disorder characterized by a significant and prolonged inflammatory response mediated by cytokines/chemokines (IL-23, 22, 17A, 1 and TNF) that are produced by numerous immune cells, in particular T cells, and dermal cells (Bowcock, 2005).

Clinical severity of lesions, percentage of affected body surface area, and patient quality of life are used to classify psoriatic patients into two groups: mild and moderate to severe. It is possible to treat mild to severe psoriasis using topical glucocorticoids, vitamin D analogs, and phototherapy (O'Neill & Feldman, 2010). Psoriasis with moderate to severe severity often needs systemic treatment. Psoriasis treatments available topically include corticosteroids, topical retinoids, Anthralin, and Calcineurin inhibitors, among others. When treating psoriasis, topical corticosteroids are typically the first line of defense (Robinson et al., 2012). However, potent corticosteroids may induce skin thinning and ultimately fail if used for an extended period of time or in excess. Additionally, calcineurin inhibitors like Pimecrolimus and Tacrolimus are used to reduce inflammation and plaque formation. Due to the high risk of developing lymphoma and skin cancer, they should not be used for prolonged or continuous treatment. Second, UV light, either naturally occurring or artificially produced, may be used in a therapy known as phototherapy. Phototherapy is an easy and all-natural treatment that involves exposing the skin to a certain quantity of sunlight. In the treatment of psoriasis, novel phototherapies include psoralen plus ultraviolet A (PUVA), Excimer laser, UVB phototherapy, Narrowband UVB phototherapy, and Goeckerman therapy (Elmets et al., 2019). However, there are a few downsides to these treatments that should be taken into account. For example, prolonged sun exposure may make psoriatic symptoms worse by increasing skin dryness, redness, irritation, and even damage.

Psoriasis symptoms may be managed and treated with the use of nutraceuticals (Keservani et al., 2010a, b, 2017, 2020). Vitamins and nutritional supplements are well known to help individuals with psoriasis with inflammation reduction and skin clearing. Psoriasis sufferers may get relief from their symptoms by taking dietary supplement extracts or concentrates in the form of a tablet, capsule, soft gelatin capsule, liquid, gel, or powder (Lebwohl & Ali, 2001).

13.2 PSORIASIS

The great dermatological enigma, psoriasis has been there since Hippocrates' day and is one of the oldest illnesses known to man. Modern therapy restores hope for successful recovery, in contrast to the gloomy days when the stigma was widespread and individuals were shunned. A wide range of biological agents have joined the traditional arsenic and boiling viper in today's medicinal toolkit (Henseler & Christophers, 1995). Disease preventive and treatment programs have benefited greatly from epidemiological studies. Psoriasis comes in a few different flavors:

1. **Psoriasis Vulgaris:** Chronic plaque psoriasis accounts for almost 90% of all instances of psoriasis vulgaris. Plaques that are red, itchy, and coated with silvery scales are classic clinical manifestations. When the plaques coalesce, they may spread across large areas of skin. Common locations include the head, the extensor surfaces of the limbs, and the trunk (Griffiths et al., 2007).

2. **Inverse Psoriasis:** Clinically, inverted psoriasis, also called flexural psoriasis, manifests as intertriginous zones of slightly erosive erythematous plaques and patches (Syed & Khachemoune, 2011).

3. **Guttate Psoriasis:** Plaques of psoriasis are red and raised and appear suddenly. Infections with group A streptococcus bacteria are a typical trigger. When they reach adulthood, around a third of those who were born with guttate psoriasis will develop plaque psoriasis (Chalmers et al., 2001).

4. **Pustular Psoriasis:** It is characterized by the development of many, harmless papules that eventually merge into larger plaques. Psoriasis with pustules may appear in either a localized or systemic pattern. Two regional forms of psoriasis have been recognized: psoriasis pustulosa palmoplantar (PPP) and acrodermatitis continua of Hallopeau. While PPP is localized to the palms and soles, ACS affects the nail apparatus at the very tips of the fingers and toes. The hands and feet are impacted by both. Generalized pustular psoriasis is acute and rapidly progressive, characterized by widespread redness and subocular pustules and sometimes accompanied by systemic symptoms (Gooderham et al., 2019).

5. **Erythrodermic Psoriasis:** It is an acute skin disorder that causes more than 90% of the body's surface to look erythematous and inflamed. Erythroderma may appear as a complication of any kind of psoriasis and hence requires prompt medical intervention (Singh et al., 2016) (Figure 13.1).

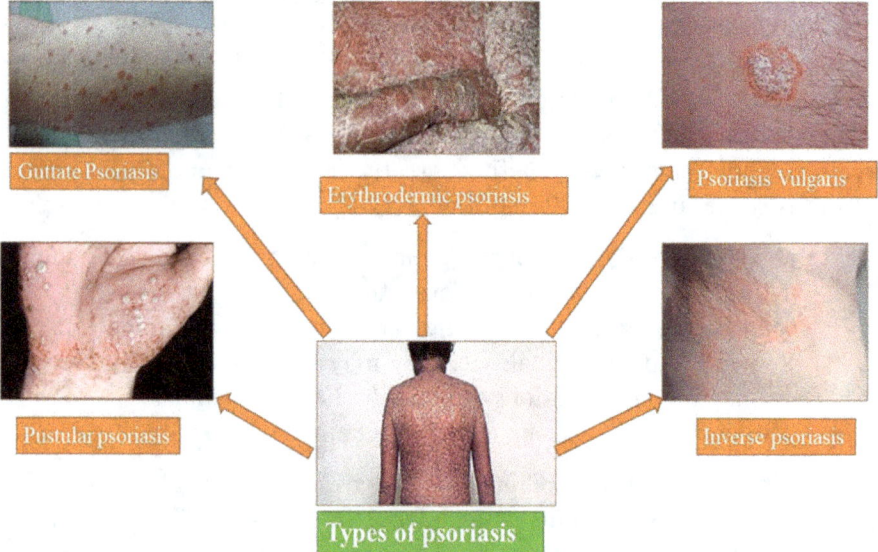

FIGURE 13.1 The types of psoriasis are based on symptoms.

13.3 EPIDEMIOLOGY

Psoriasis affects between 0.5 and 5% of the population. According to reports, Norway's rate is 4.2%, while Italy's is 2.8%. Population-based studies have revealed prevalence rates of 0.47% in China, 0.34% in Japan, 2.84% in Denmark, and 2.53% in Germany (Burden, 1997). Studies conducted in clinical settings have shown an even greater frequency; as many as 8% of individuals suffer from psoriasis. Statistics from Norway suggest that young women have a higher incidence of psoriasis than males of the same age. Similarly, psoriasis appeared early in life among women in this community. Psoriasis was more common in males than females in the majority of previous studies.

13.4 PATHOPHYSIOLOGY OF PSORIASIS

Psoriasis is an inflammatory skin condition that has several potential causes, including genetics, the environment, and an aberrant immune response. Roughly 2% of people have psoriasis, but due to advances in research and treatment options, that number is decreasing (Smith & Barker, 2006). In addition to skin-resident immune cells and essential signaling pathways, recent advancements in biological treatment have shown the crucial role of tumor necrosis factor, interleukin (IL)-23p19, and the IL-17A axis in the pathogenesis of psoriasis. Rashes from psoriasis are caused not only by IL-17-producing T helper 17 cells but also by innate lymphocyte cell (ILC)3, which responds to antimicrobial peptides produced by activated keratinocytes and inflammatory cytokines. Elevated levels of ILC3s are seen in blood, psoriatic rash, and even non-rash areas of psoriatic skin. Heart disease, metabolic syndrome, inflammatory, and metabolic syndrome disorders are all highly associated with severe psoriasis. Psoriatic gut enterobacteria are similar to those seen in people with diabetes, suggesting a possible relationship between the two diseases in terms of pathogenesis (Polak et al., 2021).

13.5 NUTRACEUTICALS

The phrase "Nutraceutical" was first used in 1989 by Dr. Stephen De Felice, who invented it by fusing the terms "Nutrition" and "Pharmaceutical." An example of this would be a food or food additive that has therapeutic or preventative health benefits (Santini & Novellino, 2018). Nutraceuticals may also refer to natural functional/medical foods or bioactive phytochemicals that have health-promoting, disease-preventing, or therapeutic properties. These nutraceuticals often include the recommended daily allowance of vitamins, fats, proteins, carbohydrates, minerals, or other crucial substances, with the exact proportions chosen for each product (El Sohaimy, 2012). Commonly used interchangeably, the phrases "nutraceuticals," "functional" "medical" foods, and "dietary supplements" all contribute to confusion. For instance, although both healthy food and functional food highlight the need for eating for optimal health, functional food is a broader term that promotes foods with distinct or powerful purposes. Vitamins, minerals, herbs and botanicals, amino acids, and other dietary supplements are intended to complement the diet by increasing the total dietary intake of these elements and have more clearly defined health responsibilities (Brown, 2017). Nutraceuticals focus more of a focus on the desired results of these products, such as illness prevention or treatment, while dietary supplements are not designed to treat or cure disease. Nutritional treatment utilizes a wide variety of nutraceuticals, the efficacy of which is predicated on extensive study into their chemical composition, biological mechanisms, clinical efficacy, and quality assurance. Most modern nutraceuticals are now recognized as essential nutrients, but many details about their use, including dosage, drug-drug interactions, nutraceutical-nutraceutical interactions, and effects on certain populations, remain unclear.

Preclinical and clinical studies support the use of nutraceuticals such as vitamins, herbal extracts (Sharma et al., 2020; Rane et al., 2020a, b, c), and nutritional supplements as an auxiliary therapy for psoriasis. Limited effectiveness and possible adverse effects have rendered pharmacological therapies for psoriasis, including biologic medications, ineffectual so far. Furthermore, individual variations in patients' reactions to treatments (Miroddi et al., 2015) should be considered. As an added caution, anti-psoriatic systemic drugs are associated with a higher likelihood of renal function decline, hypertension, and nephrotoxicity. Therefore, psoriatic patients are more likely to use phytomedicine as a complementary therapy, as they search for safer and more acceptable options. Some possible treatments for psoriasis include aloe vera, turmeric, neem, soy, vitamin D, fish oil, evening primrose oil, black cumin, bakuchi, milk thistle, and coal tar (Raychaudhuri et al., 2017).

13.5.1 ANNUM CAPSICUM FOR PSORIASIS

A large, evergreen shrub that blooms with solitary, off-white flowers and has many branches. The mature fruit resembles a berry and may be either green, yellow, or red. Capsaicin, which is found in the plant, reduces the inflammation and irritation caused by psoriasis. Plaque reduction with topical use of dry leaf pastes Psoriasis (Rout et al., 2017).

13.5.2 PONGAMIA PINNATA FOR PSORIASIS

Pongamia pinnata, a member of the Leguminosae family, is a somewhat glabrous, semi-evergreen tree that has a short bole and spreading crown with grayish-green or brown bark. The imparipinnate, alternating leaves have 5–7 elliptical, opposite leaflets. This tree is known as Karanja in Hindi, Indian Beech and Derris indica in English, and Hongae in Kannada. *P. pinnata* is a tree native to India that is grown as an avenue tree in gardens for its ability to treat skin diseases. (Badole & Patil, 2014). These energized seeds are used to cure leukoderma. Pongamia seed oil has medicinal properties and is used to treat a variety of parasites, including insects, bacteria, and worms. *P. pinnata* is used in alternative medicinal practices like Ayurveda and Unani because of its anti-inflammatory, anti-plasmodial, anti-nociceptive, anti-hyperglycemic, anti-lipid peroxidation, anti-diarrheal, anti-ulcer, anti-hyper-ammonic, and antioxidant effects. Biodiesel is derived from its oil. It also has a sustainable, secure, and pollution-free alternative energy source.

13.5.3 ALOE VERA FOR PSORIASIS

Plants belonging to the *Liliaceae* family include *Aloe vera Linnaeus*, also known as *Aloe barbadensis* Miller. Many cosmetics and medicines use aloe vera because of its leaf pulp. The pulp is composed of cell walls, degenerated organelles, and viscous liquid that has been accumulated inside the cells (Miroddi et al., 2015). The biological properties of aloe are not fully known, despite the fact that a large body of research suggests that polysaccharide and glycoprotein fractions play an important role in their pharmacological activity. Approximately 98.5% of the pulp and 99.5% of the mucilage or gel are water, with the remaining 0.5–1% consisting of anthraquinones/anthrones, chromones, carbohydrates, minerals, enzymes, various water-soluble and fat-soluble vitamins, polysaccharides, proteins, phenolic compounds, and organic acids (Dhanabal et al., 2012). Aloe vera's chemical diversity may account for the plant's wide array of therapeutic uses. The chemical composition may alter from product to product due to the broad variety of processing processes used to manufacture preparations from the plant. As a result of its effects on macrophages, and lymphocytes, the production of nitric oxide and cytokines, and the stimulation of immature dendritic cell maturation, aloe vera exhibits immunomodulatory capabilities. It is possible that aloe's capacity to influence the immune response is due to its effect on secondary humoral immunity, which it enhances, and cell-mediated immunity, which it dampens. Moreover, its anti-inflammatory, anti-pain, and anti-nociceptive activities were discussed. Psoriasis may be treated using a variety of aloe vera products, such as herbal shampoos, lotions, gels, and organic extracts, all of which help restore moisture to dry skin, clear away any lingering dead skin cells, and promote new skin cell development. In addition to its many other health benefits, aloe vera juice is excellent as a digestive aid, internal purifier, and anti-inflammatory when used on a regular basis. (Grundmann, 2012). Common aloe vera comes in the form of a gel, which is excellent for soothing the skin inflammation brought on by psoriasis flakes. Dhanabal et al. investigated the efficacy of a gel formulation of ethanolic Aloe Vera extract in treating psoriasis of the mouse tail. Significant epidermal differentiation occurred as a result of the extract, which was on par with that produced by the tazarotene (0.1%) gel serving as the gold standard positive control. Results from the study by Choonhakarn et al. suggested that aloe vera therapy was more effective than 0.1% TA cream in alleviating psoriasis symptoms. (Miroddi et al., 2015).

13.5.4 AZADIRACHTA INDICA FOR PSORIASIS

The *Meliaceae* family includes *Azadirachta indica* (Neem). All parts of this tree are useful, and some of them even have healing properties. Chickenpox lowered malaria fever, different foot fungus, termite prevention, neuromuscular pain relief, and skin diseases like leprosy and psoriasis are just some of the ailments that neem leaves may help with. The neem seed cake has both pesticide and fertilizing properties (Bharade et al., 2019). The bark and roots of the neem tree may be used to keep dogs free of fleas and ticks; they can also be used to treat a wide variety of human illnesses, including diabetes, HIV, cancer, heart disease, herpes, allergies, ulcers, hepatitis, and more. There are several medicinal uses for neem, including its analgesic, anthelminthic, hypoglycemic, antibacterial, immunomodulator, antiulcer, antifungal, antihyperglycemic, anti-inflammatory, antiviral, antimalarial, diuretic, and antipyretic qualities (Smith et al., 2009). Its natural blood-cleansing function has long been recognized, and this has made it a valuable tool in the fight against psoriasis. Neem oil is considered the main external therapy for psoriasis due to the presence of Azadirachtin, which may penetrate deep layers to cure the disease. In psoriasis, the skin gets very dry, but using Neem oil, which is rich in vitamin E and omega 6 and 9 fatty acids, helps hydrate the skin and reduces scales and dryness. As an anti-inflammatory and anti-arthritic, neem's active component nimbidin is a welcome discovery (Naik et al., 2014). Neem is available in tablet and capsule forms for oral administration. Pandey et al. conducted double-blind clinical research to evaluate the efficacy of neem leaves aqueous extract in psoriasis vulgaris patients who were on a topical regimen of 5% coal tar and 3% salicylic acid (Raut & Wairkar, 2018). Patients who were given neem leaf extract had a considerably lower 'Psoriasis area and severity index' (PASI) score after 12 weeks than those who were given a placebo.

13.5.5 TURMERIC FOR PSORIASIS

Curcuma longa, more often known as turmeric, is a brilliant yellow plant that has been used for centuries in cuisine, dye, cosmetics, and medicine (Vyas et al., 2010; Kesharwani et al., 2015, 2018; Mishra et al., 2019; Singh et al., 2013a, b, 2015, 2016; Upadhyaya et al., 2009; Kesharwani & Misra, 2011). Curcumin (diferuloylmethane), the active component of turmeric, was first identified and characterized in 1910 (Himesh et al., 2011). It has been shown to offer a variety of health benefits, including the ability to treat psychological disorders and inflammation, germs, and cancer. It has been claimed to have antibacterial and anti-inflammatory properties when used topically, making it useful as a paste for treating skin eruptions and infections. Modulation of signal transduction and receptor phosphorylation during epidermal proliferation by ATP-phosphorylase b phosphotransferase (PhK). PhK activity is elevated in psoriatic skin, which has been associated with epidermal hyperproliferation and accelerated migration of inflammatory cells (Heng et al., 2000). The most common treatments for psoriasis include topical steroid creams, vitamin D-based medications, retinoids, immunosuppressants, and ultraviolet radiation. Around 40 males between the ages of 40 and 80 participated in a study that found a topical alcoholic gel formulation of 1% curcumin improved psoriasis, as measured by a significant decrease in PhK activity compared to untreated psoriasis. These results were comparable to those seen with a topical vitamin D3 analog. Results from this research suggest that curcumin may help speed up the healing process for psoriatic disease by decreasing PhK levels. Curcuminoid C3 Complex® pills (4.5 g curcumin per day) were used in another trial lasting 16 weeks (Vaughn et al., 2016). The Physicians Global Assessment, the PASI, and safety measures were used to evaluate the efficacy of the study's interventions. If a patient's score on the Physicians Global Assessment increased by 54% or more, we deemed them to be a "responder." Intent-to-treat analysis revealed that just one of the eight participants responded to the study. Their PASI increased by 75%, shared by these two responders (Met a PASI 75). Both the small size of the sample and the lack of a placebo group were limitations of the research. Additionally, it protects the skin from oxidative stress by scavenging oxidative reactive species and influencing detoxifying enzymes. Key proteins such as tumor necrosis factor-alpha and interleukin have a role in psoriasis inflammation and progression. As a result of curcumin's ability to severely suppress the function of these proteins, other biochemical pathways that may contribute to disease development are not stimulated. To determine whether or not curcumin is effective as an oral therapy for psoriasis, Antiga and coworkers conducted a randomized, double-blind, placebo-controlled clinical trial (Zeng et al., 2017). Serum levels of IL-22 are decreased in *Psoriasis vulgaris* patients who take curcumin. Patients with plaque psoriasis were given Turmeric microemulgel to apply topically for three weeks in a clinical trial conducted by Sarafian et al. Patients who were given microemulgels had a higher PASI score and better quality of life indicators than the control group ($P<0.05$) (Sarafian et al., 2015).

13.5.6 SOYABEAN FOR PSORIASIS

A member of the Fabaceae family, soybeans are a legume. The predominant phytoestrogens in soybean are isoflavones, which are structurally similar to 17 beta-estradiol. Soybeans contain an isoflavone called genistein, which has potent anti-inflammatory and antioxidant effects. Numerous Asian communities have benefited greatly from the safe, massive use of soybeans and genistein. Genistein inhibits proliferation in laboratory settings by disrupting nuclear factor kappa B (NF-κB) signaling. Immunological studies have shown that genistein inhibits the production and activation of proinflammatory cytokines such as tumor necrosis factor-alpha, interleukin 6 (IL-6), interleukin 1 (IL-1β), and interleukin 8 (IL-8) (Avramidis et al., 2010). Genistein's inhibitory impact on blood levels of angiotensin II, a proliferative and proinflammatory biomarker, was studied in a rat model for its capacity to decrease acetylcholinesterase (ACE). In a similar vein, genistein has been demonstrated to reduce the activity of neutrophil elastase, a serine protease that is present in psoriatic lesions. Psoriasis treatment including genistein may therefore warrant more study. Researchers Shyong et al. reported that when applied topically to people with psoriasis, psoralen-ultraviolet A (PUVA) treatment decreased skin thickness and cutaneous erythema. Psoriasis patients who combine Genistein with PUVA treatment may have fewer side effects and a better therapeutic response (Shyong et al., 2002). Ito et al. examined Glyteer, a collection of soybean tar, in a mouse model of psoriasis. In mice, glyteer treatment reduced both the thickness of the epidermis and the amount of protein it contained. Glyteer's anti-edema effectiveness was equivalent to that of betamethasone 17-valerate, indomethacin, and cyclosporine, all of which were effective in reducing edema in psoriatic mice. Based on these results, soybean could be useful in treating psoriasis (Ito et al., 1992).

13.5.7 FISH OIL FOR PSORIASIS

Omega-3 polyunsaturated fatty acids (ω-3 PUFAs) are found in fish oil and have been demonstrated to enhance blood lipids. These fatty acids include docosahexaenoic acid (DHA), docosapentaenoic acid (DPA), and eicosapentaenoic acid (EPA). Fish oil's key components have anti-inflammatory effects and aid in the immune system and metabolic regulation. As an added bonus, psoriasis is associated with a host of health problems, many of which may be mitigated with the help of omega-3 PUFAs (Maurice et al., 1987). Fish oil and its contents may be a viable therapeutic option given the relevance of inflammation in the genesis of psoriasis and its related comorbidities. Fish oil was originally studied as a possible therapy for psoriasis in a randomized controlled experiment that was published in January 1988. However, the results of this study showed no improvement in psoriasis symptoms. In contrast, the clinical study had 25 psoriasis patients randomly assigned to either liquid paraffin or fish oil, with both groups applying the treatment to their psoriatic plaques daily for 4 weeks while wearing an occlusive bandage for 6 hours. Plaque thickness, erythema, and scaling were all noticeably improved by fish oil. Fish oil therapy, however, did not reduce plaque inflammation (Escobar et al., 1992). While liquid paraffin treatment did help reduce erythema, it was much less effective than fish oil in decreasing scaling rate and had no noticeable effect on plaque thickness or discomfort. In spite of positive patient feedback for both liquid paraffin and fish oil treatments, the latter was ultimately deemed more effective. Bittiner et al. delivered fish oil capsules or placebo capsules daily with a controlled diet to 28 patients with chronic persistent psoriasis for 8 weeks in a clinical study (Bittiner et al., 1988). Psoriasis symptoms improved significantly in the fish oil therapy group while showing no improvement in the placebo group.

13.5.8 EVENING PRIMROSE OIL FOR PSORIASIS

It is the high concentration of linoleic acid (LA) and gamma-linolenic acid (GLA) in evening primrose oil that is responsible for its sedative effects. In a small number of instances, it showed promise in treating psoriasis and other chronic skin conditions including eczema. Researchers have shown that evening primrose oil has a calming effect on women experiencing hormonal swings (Ziboh et al., 2000). GLA and linoleic acid both help restore moisture and heal damage to the skin, which helps slow the aging process. Psoriasis symptoms, including dryness, itching, and scaliness, are all alleviated by this essential oil, and the condition's inflammatory response is naturally moderated by an increase in prostaglandin synthesis. Natural low amounts of gamma linoleic acid have been found in patients with skin illnesses including psoriasis and eczema. This oil may aid in keeping your body's LA and GLA levels steady. Positive effects of co-administration of n-3 (marine oil) and n-6 (evening primrose oil) essential fatty acids in plaque psoriasis were demonstrated in a double-blind, parallel experiment, which supports these results. You may get evening primrose oil in capsules, oil, and lotion (Oliwiecki & Burton, 1994).

13.5.9 NIGELLA SATIVA FOR PSORIASIS

A member of the *Ranunculaceae* family, *Nigella sativa* Linn., is more popularly known as black cumin due to its traditional usage as a medicinal plant. Nigella sativa contains several bioactive compounds, such as thymoquinone, dithymoquinone, thymohydroquinone, thymol, carvacrol, and others. Commonly used to treat a wide variety of skin conditions due to its anti-inflammatory, antibacterial, anti-acne, antifungal, anticarcinogenic, and antipsoriatic characteristics (Aljabre et al., 2015). The protein found in Nigella sativa seeds contains eight of the nine necessary amino acids, in addition to other nutrients including carbs, lipids, vitamins, minerals, and protein. The seeds are used as a topical treatment for eczema, psoriasis, and other skin conditions that cause itching, redness, and inflammation. In research using ethanolic extract of N. sativa seeds, Dwarampudi et al. showed a substantial response to the positive control, Tazarotene gel, and epidermal differentiation (71.36% ± 2.64) based on its degree of orthokeratosis compared to the placebo (17.30% ± 4.09) (Ahmed Jawad et al., 2014). An IC_{50} of 239 µg/ml was found for the ethanolic extract's anti-proliferative effects. This research supported its use as a conventional treatment for psoriasis due to a reduction in relative epidermal thickness compared to the control group.

Using PASI grade and serum malondialdehyde as outcomes, Jawad et al. performed a randomized clinical study on 60 psoriatic patients to evaluate the effectiveness and safety of Nigella sativa administered orally and topically (Ahmed Jawad et al., 2014). Around 40 participants were given a 10% w/w NS ointment, 40 were given a 500 mg dietary pill of plain NS powder, and the remaining 20 received both forms of NS. As measured by the PASI score, it was found that 65% of the ointment group and 50% of the oral group were completely free of psoriatic lesions. 85% of patients in the combination treatment group had complete lesion resolution, which is an impressive result.

13.5.10 GIVOTIA ROTTLERIFORMI FOR PSORIASIS

The *Givotia rottleriformis* tree is a moderately large member of the *Euphorbiaceae* family. Its bark and seeds are used to treat rheumatism, dandruff, and psoriasis in traditional medicine.

13.5.11 MOMORDICA CHARANTIA FOR PSORIASIS

The bitter gourd is a herbaceous vine that may grow up to five meters in length. The leaves are 3–7 lobes deep and 4–12 cm broad, and they are simple and alternate. Decoctions and infusions made from the plant are used to treat bacterial infections and a wide range of skin conditions including psoriasis, acne, and wounds. *Momordica charantia*, a member of the *Cucurbitaceae* family, is a popular Indian plant used for its antifungal, wound-healing, and anti-diabetic properties. The use of these plants in the form of decoctions, infusions, and tinctures has a long history of success in traditional medical practice for the treatment of skin diseases including psoriasis and leprosy (Grover & Yadav, 2004).

13.5.12 CROTALARIA JUNCEA FOR PSORIASIS

For its fiber, Indo-Pakistan cultivates sun hemp, a fast-growing crop. A tall annual with elliptic lanceolate leaves and terminal clusters of yellow flowers. Sunn hemp, or *Crotalaria juncea* Linn. (Leguminosae), is a plant utilized for food, fiber, and medicine by people of many cultural backgrounds. It has a wide distribution in the tropical and subtropical zones of India, Nepal, Sri Lanka, and southern Africa. Uses for *C. juncea* include those of a blood purifier, abortifacient, astringent, demulcent, emetic, and purgative, as well as those for treating anemia, impetigo, menorrhagia, and psoriasis (Chandrasekar & Sivagami, 2016).

13.5.13 SILYBUM MARIANUM FOR PSORIASIS

Milk Thistle, or *Silybum marianum*, is a member of the Asteraceae family and is used medicinally. In order to cure psoriasis naturally, people often turn to Milk Thistle seeds. Psoriasis-fighting silicristin, silibinin, and silidianin are all found in silymarin. Activating the immune system and promoting the regeneration of damaged liver cells are two of silymarin's many beneficial effects. Milk thistle is regarded to be efficient in the treatment of psoriasis due to the Silymarin it contains, which has characteristics that are helpful in naturally fighting psoriasis. Psoriasis may be treated with standardized milk thistle extract containing Silymarin (70%) in a tablet or pill containing 150 mg (Daniyal et al., 2019).

Khan et al. developed a Silymarin topical gel using Carbopol as a gelling ingredient in a synthetic synthesis. In physicochemical and *in-vitro* drug release tests, 96.30% of the medication was found to be released within three hours. After meeting the *in vitro* standards, it was tested for primary cutaneous irritation in healthy human volunteers; after 72 hours, there was no sign of irritation. In addition, the gel showed an inhibitory MIC of 5 mg/ml against *Candida albicans* (Dabholkar et al., 2021).

13.5.14 VITAMIN D3 FOR PSORIASIS

Cholecalciferol, or vitamin D3, helps the body absorb and use calcium. The liver receives cholecalciferol directly through circulation after it is absorbed via food, sunshine, or a dietary supplement. Multiple liver enzymes convert cholecalciferol to calcidiol, and finally, the kidneys convert calcitriol, the active form of calcium, from calcidiol (Gisondi et al., 2012). A healthy phosphate and calcium balance is regarded to be best for suppressing psoriasis infection, and calcitriol may help you achieve that. Psoriasis sufferers, particularly those living in colder climates, are at increased risk of vitamin D3 deficiency. Therefore, it is the vitamin that doctors recommend the most for treating psoriasis, either alone or in conjunction with other antipsoriatic medications. Psoriatic outbreaks are less severe and last less time when vitamin D is produced by the skin (Soleymani et al., 2015). Synthetic versions of active vitamin D, such as tacalcitol or calcipotriene, are used topically for moderate psoriasis. The new skin cell development and inflammation are inhibited locally. 10 people with persistent plaque psoriasis were given a cream containing a new vitamin D analog (MC903) developed by Staberg and colleagues. Over the course of six weeks, participants were randomly assigned to either receive an MC903 cream or a placebo cream. Psoriatic lesions were entirely eradicated after 6 weeks of topical treatment with the MC903 cream formulation without any adverse medication reactions (Staberg et al., 1989).

13.5.15 PSORALEA CORYLIFOLIA FOR PSORIASIS

There is a medicinal plant in the Fabaceae family called *Psoralea corylifolia* (Bakuchi) Linn. Because of its antioxidant, anti-inflammatory, antibacterial, anticancer, antifungal, and immunomodulatory properties, *Psoralea corylifolia* has been used for centuries to treat a wide range of conditions, including skin illnesses like leprosy, leukoderma, and psoriasis. Psoralens, bakuchiol, bakuchalcone, iso-psoralen, and volatile oils make up bakuchi. In order to produce photoproducts containing pyrimidine bases, radiant light is absorbed by the photoactive furocoumarin psoralen. Treatment of dermatological diseases including psoriasis, mycosis fungoides, and vitiligo in humans may benefit from photoactivation of psoralens at ultraviolet wavelengths of 200–320 nm since this reduces cell growth. Ali et al. looked into treating psoriasis using a microemulsion gel containing Babchi oil, extracted from the *Psoralea corylifolia* plant. There was talk that a microemulsion-based formulation would let Babchi oil penetrate the skin better and that it would have remarkable *in-vivo* anti-inflammatory effects in a footpad edema model (Kumar et al., 2019).

13.5.16 CALENDULA OFFICINALIS FOR PSORIASIS

The herbaceous perennial *Calendula officinalis* has oblong-lanceolate leaves that are hairy on both sides and have entire, sometimes wavy, or weakly serrated edges. A member of the daisy family, *Calendula officinalis* (Family: Compositae) is a popular Indian plant used for its antifungal, wound-healing, and anti-diabetic properties, among others. The use of these plants in the form of decoctions, infusions, and tinctures has a long history of success in traditional medical practice for the treatment of skin diseases including psoriasis and leprosy (Chandrasekar & Sivagami, 2016) (Figure 13.2).

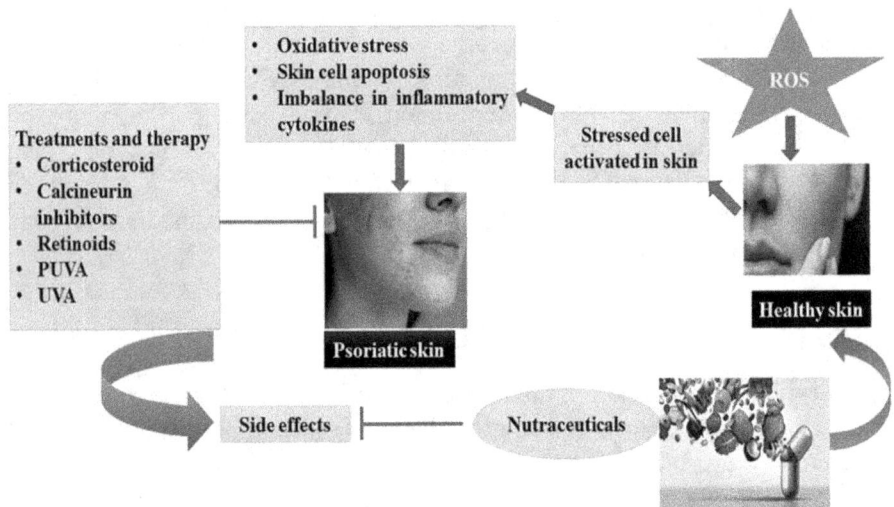

FIGURE 13.2 Pathways and management of psoriasis.

13.6 COMORBIDITIES

A common complication of psoriasis is psoriatic arthritis. In 1818, Alibert noticed that psoriasis patients often had inflammatory joint sickness, and he linked the two conditions. The inflammatory bowel diseases Crohn's disease and ulcerative colitis both have relapse forms. Prevalence estimates sit between 0.1% and 3.0%. Similar to psoriasis, the most common time for symptoms to appear is between the ages of 20 and 40. Psoriasis patients are 7 times more likely to develop Crohn's disease compared to healthy people. More women than men had a connection between psoriasis and being overweight, diabetic, or having a heart attack. Naldi et al., who conducted case-control research on people with psoriasis, found that obesity was a significant factor among their patients. Long-term systemic therapy-related comorbidities (e.g., methotrexate or cyclosporin) have been the subject of substantial research elsewhere. Long-term psoralen-UV-A therapy has also been linked to serious side effects, such as an increased risk of skin cancer. Patients treated with TNF-blocking antibodies over extended periods of time have shown some intriguing improvements. Nearly 50 individuals with severe psoriasis flare-ups or psoriatic disease onsets have been detected using current therapy options (infliximab, etanercept, and adalimumab). The majority of persons with PPP have lesions that look like plaques, although around half of those with PPP also have PsA. Almost half of these reports come from people being treated for RA, while the other half come from people with ulcerative colitis. Rheumatoid arthritis (RA) patients account for nearly half of these observations, while those with ulcerative colitis and CD account for the other half.

13.7 CONCLUSION

The skin ailment psoriasis lasts a long time and is quite annoying. Several factors in the pathophysiology of psoriasis make it difficult to find a good treatment option. Due to the autoimmune nature of psoriasis, it is essential to focus on management rather than treatment. In addition, reports of adverse drug reactions seem to be more common among patients who have been on their current medicine for an extended period of time. It is advised as an adjuvant therapy for psoriasis that nutraceuticals, which include vitamins, herbal extracts, and nutritional supplements, be used. Therefore, patients may use either alone or in conjunction with nutraceuticals to improve the efficacy of treatment for psoriasis.

KEYWORDS

- acetylcholinesterase
- herbal extracts
- interleukin
- nuclear factor kappa B
- nutritional supplements
- phosphotransferase
- phytochemicals

REFERENCES

Ahmed Jawad, H., Ibraheem Azhar, Y., & Al-Hamdi Khalil, I. (2014). Evaluation of efficacy, safety and antioxidant effect of Nigella sativa in patients with psoriasis: A randomized clinical trial. *Journal of Clinical and Experimental Investigations, 5*(2), 186–193.

Aljabre, S. H., Alakloby, O. M., & Randhawa, M. A. (2015). Dermatological effects of Nigella sativa. *Journal of Dermatology & Dermatologic Surgery, 19*, 92–98.

Avramidis, G., Krüger-Krasagakis, S., Krasagakis, K., Fragiadaki, I., Kokolakis, G., & Tosca, A. (2010). The role of endothelial cell apoptosis in the effect of etanercept in psoriasis. *British Journal of Dermatology, 163*(4), 928–934.

Badole, S. L., & Patil, K. Y. (2014). *Pongamia pinnata* (Linn.) Pierre and inflammation. In *Polyphenols in Human Health and Disease* (pp. 463–465). Academic Press.

Bharade, S., Gupta, N., Jain, S., Kapoor, V., & Rajpoot, D. S. (2019). Development of microemulsion gel based topical delivery of salicylic acid and neem oil for the management of psoriasis. *Journal of Drug Delivery and Therapeutics, 9*(2), 186–191.

Bittiner, S., Cartwright, I., Tucker, W., & Bleehen, S. (1988). A double-blind, randomized, placebo-controlled trial of fish oil in psoriasis. *The Lancet, 331*(8582), 378–380.

Bowcock, A. M. (2005). The genetics of psoriasis and autoimmunity. *Annual Review of Genomics and Human Genetics, 6*, 93–122.

Brown, A. C. (2017). An overview of herb and dietary supplement efficacy, safety, and government regulations in the United States with suggested improvements. Part 1 of 5 series. *Food and Chemical Toxicology, 107*, 449–471.

Burden, A. D. (1997). Molecular Genetics of Psoriasis. (Doctoral dissertation, The University of Manchester, United Kingdom). pp. 1–20.

Campalani, E., & Barker, J. (2005). The clinical genetics of psoriasis. *Current Genomics, 6*(1), 51–60.

Chalmers, R., O'Sullivan, T., Owen, C. M., & Griffiths, C. (2001). A systematic review of treatments for guttate psoriasis. *British Journal of Dermatology, 145*(6), 891–894.

Chandrasekar, R., & Sivagami, B. (2016). Alternative treatment for psoriasis – A review. *International Journal of Research and Development in Pharmacy and Life Sciences, 5*(5), 2188–2197.

Dabholkar, N., Rapalli, V. K., & Singhvi, G. (2021). Potential herbal constituents for psoriasis treatment as a protective and effective therapy. *Phytotherapy Research, 35*(5), 2429–2444.

Daniyal, M., Akram, M., Zainab, R., Munir, N., Shah, S. M. A., Liu, B., Wang, W., Riaz, M., & Jabeen, F. (2019). Progress and prospects in the management of psoriasis and developments in phyto-therapeutic modalities. *Dermatologic Therapy, 32*(6), e12866.

Dhanabal, S., Priyanka Dwarampudi, L., Muruganantham, N., & Vadivelan, R. (2012). Evaluation of the antipsoriatic activity of Aloe vera leaf extract using a mouse tail model of psoriasis. *Phytotherapy Research, 26*(4), 617–619.

El Sohaimy, S. (2012). Functional foods and nutraceuticals-modern approach to food science. *World Applied Sciences Journal, 20*(5), 691–708.

Elmets, C. A., Lim, H. W., Stoff, B., Connor, C., Cordoro, K. M., Lebwohl, M., Armstrong, A. W., Davis, D. M., Elewski, B. E., & Gelfand, J. M. (2019). Joint American Academy of Dermatology–National Psoriasis Foundation guidelines of care for the management and treatment of psoriasis with phototherapy. *Journal of the American Academy of Dermatology, 81*(3), 775–804.

Escobar, S., Achenbach, R., Iannantuono, R., & Torem, V. (1992). Topical fish oil in psoriasis—a controlled and blind study. *Clinical and Experimental Dermatology, 17*(3), 159–162.

Gisondi, P., Rossini, M., Di Cesare, A., Idolazzi, L., Farina, S., Beltrami, G., Peris, K., & Girolomoni, G. (2012). Vitamin D status in patients with chronic plaque psoriasis. *British Journal of Dermatology, 166*(3), 505–510.

Gooderham, M. J., Van Voorhees, A. S., & Lebwohl, M. G. (2019). An update on generalized pustular psoriasis. *Expert Review of Clinical Immunology, 15*(9), 907–919.

Griffiths, C., Christophers, E., Barker, J., Chalmers, R., Chimenti, S., Krueger, G., Leonardi, C., Menter, A., Ortonne, J. P., & Fry, L. (2007). A classification of psoriasis vulgaris according to phenotype. *British Journal of Dermatology, 156*(2), 258–262.

Grover, J., & Yadav, S. (2004). Pharmacological actions and potential uses of *Momordica charantia*: A review. *Journal of Ethnopharmacology, 93*, 123–132.

Grundmann, O. (2012). Aloe vera gel research review. *Natural Medicine Journal, 4*, 1–5.

Heng, M., Song, M., Harker, J., & Heng, M. (2000). Drug-induced suppression of phosphorylase kinase activity correlates with resolution of psoriasis as assessed by clinical, histological, and immunohistochemical parameters. *British Journal of Dermatology, 143*, 937–949.

Henseler, T., & Christophers, E. (1995). Disease concomitance in psoriasis. *Journal of the American Academy of Dermatology, 32*, 982–986.

Himesh, S., Sharan, P. S., Mishra, K., Govind, N., & Singhai, A. (2011). Qualitative and quantitative profile of curcumin from ethanolic extract of Curcuma longa. *International Research Journal of Pharmacy, 2*, 180–184.

Ito, K., Namikawa, S., & Takeuchi, K. (1992). Effect of the dry distillation tar of delipidated soybean (Glyteer) on a psoriasic model in the mouse (4). *Nihon Yakurigaku Zasshi. Folia Pharmacologica Japonica, 99*, 55–62.

Keservani, R. K., Kesharwani, R. K., Sharma, A. K., Vyas, N., & Chadoker, A. (2010b). Nutritional Supplements: An Overview. *International Journal of Current Pharmaceutical Review and Research, 1*(1), 59–75.

Keservani, R. K., Kesharwani, R. K., Vyas, N., Jain, S., Raghuvanshi, R., & Sharma, A. K. (2010a). Nutraceutical and functional food as future food: A review. *Der Pharmacia Lettre, 2*(1), 106–116.

Keservani, R. K., Sharma, A. K., & Kesharwani, R. K. (2017). An overview and therapeutic applications of nutraceutical and functional foods. In R. K. Keservani, A. K. Sharma, & R. K. Kesharwani (Eds.), *Recent Advances in Drug Delivery Technology* (pp. 160–201). CRC Press.

Keservani, R. K., Sharma, A. K., & Kesharwani, R. K. (Eds.). (2020). *Nutraceuticals and Dietary Supplements: Applications in Health Improvement and Disease Management*, Apple Academic Press, CRC Press. pp. 1–344. ISBN: 9781771888738.

Kesharwani, R. K., & Misra, K. (2011). Prediction of the binding site for curcuminoids at human topoisomerase II α protein; an in-silico approach. *Current Science, 101*(8), 1060–1065.

Kesharwani, R. K., Singh, D. B., Singh, D. V., & Misra, K. (2018). Computational study of curcumin analogs by targeting DNA topoisomerase II: A structure-based drug designing approach. *Network Modeling Analysis in Health Informatics and Bioinformatics, 7*(1), 1–7.

Kesharwani, R. K., Srivastava, V., Singh, P., Rizvi, S. I., Adeppa, K., & Misra, K. (2015). A novel approach for overcoming drug resistance in breast cancer chemotherapy by targeting new synthetic curcumin analogs against aldehyde dehydrogenase 1 (ALDH1A1) and glycogen synthase kinase-3 β (GSK-3β). *Applied Biochemistry and Biotechnology, 176*(7), 1996–2017.

Kumar, S., Singh, K. K., & Rao, R. (2019). Enhanced anti-psoriatic efficacy and regulation of oxidative stress of a novel topical babchi oil (*Psoralea corylifolia*) cyclodextrin-based nanogel in a mouse tail model. *Journal of Microencapsulation, 36*, 140–155.

Lebwohl, M., & Ali, S. (2001). Treatment of psoriasis. Part 2. Systemic therapies. *Journal of the American Academy of Dermatology, 45*, 649–664.

Maurice, P., Allen, B., Barkley, A., Cockbill, S., Stammers, J., & Bather, P. (1987). The effects of dietary supplementation with fish oil in patients with psoriasis. *British Journal of Dermatology, 117*, 599–606.

Miroddi, M., Navarra, M., Calapai, F., Mancari, F., Giofrè, S. V., Gangemi, S., & Calapai, G. (2015). Review of clinical pharmacology of Aloe vera L. in the treatment of psoriasis. *Phytotherapy Research, 29*, 648–655.

Mishra, H., Kesharwani, R. K., Singh, D. B., Tripathi, S., Dubey, S. K., & Misra, K. (2019). Computational simulation of inhibitory effects of curcumin, retinoic acid, and their conjugates on GSK-3 beta. *Network Modeling Analysis in Health Informatics and Bioinformatics, 8*(1), 3.

Naik, M. R., Bhattacharya, A., Behera, R., Agrawal, D., Dehury, S., & Kumar, S. (2014). Study of the anti-inflammatory effect of neem seed oil (*Azadirachta indica*) on infected albino rats. *Journal of Health Research and Reviews, 1*, 66.

Naldi, L. (2004). Epidemiology of psoriasis. *Current Drug Targets-Inflammation & Allergy, 3*, 121–128.

O'Neill, J. L., & Feldman, S. R. (2010). Vitamin D analogue-based therapies for psoriasis. *Drugs of Today (Barcelona, Spain: 1998), 46*, 351-360.

Oliwiecki, S., & Burton, J. (1994). Evening primrose oil and marine oil in the treatment of psoriasis. *Clinical and Experimental Dermatology, 19*, 127–129.

Polak, K., Bergler-Czop, B., Szczepanek, M., Wojciechowska, K., Frątczak, A., & Kiss, N. (2021). Psoriasis and gut microbiome—current state of art. *International Journal of Molecular Sciences, 22*, 4529.

Rane, B. R., Bharath, M. S., Patil, R. R., Keservani, R. K., & Jain, A. S. (2020). Novel Approaches in Nutraceuticals. In R. K. Keservani, R. K. Kesharwani, A. K. Sharma (Eds.), *Enhancing the Therapeutic Efficacy of Herbal Formulations through Novel Drug Delivery Systems* (pp. 241–266). IGI Global.

Rane, B. R., Patil, A. S., Keservani, R. K., & Jain, A. S. (2020a). Novel Approaches in Herbal Formulation. In R. K. Kesharwani, R. K. Keservani, & A. K. Sharma (Eds.), *Enhancing the Therapeutic Efficacy of Herbal Formulations Through Novel Drug Delivery Systems* (pp. 43–68). IGI Global. ISBN13: 9781799844532.

Rane, B. R., Tadavi, S. A., & Keservani, R. K. (2020c). Naturopathy. In A. K. Sharma & R. K. Keservani (Eds.), *Herbal Product Development* (pp. 321–347). Apple Academic Press, CRC Press, Taylor & Francis Group. ISBN: 9781771888776.

Raut, G., & Wairkar, S. (2018). Management of psoriasis with nutraceuticals: An update. *Complementary Therapies in Clinical Practice, 31*, 25–30.

Raychaudhuri, S. P., Raychaudhuri, S., & Bagchi, D. (2017). *Psoriasis and Psoriatic Arthritis: Pathophysiology, Therapeutic Intervention, and Complementary Medicine*. CRC Press. 1st Edition, pp. 370. ISBN: 9781315152912.

Robinson, A., van Voorhees, A. S., Hsu, S., Korman, N. J., Lebwohl, M. G., Bebo Jr, B. F., & Kalb, R. E. (2012). Treatment of pustular psoriasis: From the Medical Board of the National Psoriasis Foundation. *Journal of the American Academy of Dermatology, 67*, 279–288.

Rout, S. K., Tripathy, B. C., & Kar, B. R. (2017). Natural green alternatives to psoriasis treatment–A review. *Global Journal of Pharmacy & Pharmaceutical Sciences, 4*, 001–007.

Santini, A., & Novellino, E. (2018). Nutraceuticals-shedding light on the grey area between pharmaceuticals and food. *Expert Review of Clinical Pharmacology, 11*, 545–547.

Sarafian, G., Afshar, M., Mansouri, P., Asgarpanah, J., Raoufinejad, K., & Rajabi, M. (2015). Topical turmeric microemulgel in the management of plaque psoriasis; a clinical evaluation. *Iranian Journal of Pharmaceutical Research, 14*, 865.

Singh, D. B., Gupta, M. K., Kesharwani, R. K., & Misra, K. (2013a). Comparative docking and ADMET study of some curcumin derivatives and herbal congeners targeting β-amyloid. *Network Modeling Analysis in Health Informatics and Bioinformatics, 2*(1), 13–27.

Singh, D. V., Agarwal, S., Kesharwani, R. K., & Misra, K. (2013b). 3D QSAR and pharmacophore study of curcuminoids and curcumin analogs: Interaction with thioredoxin reductase. *Interdisciplinary Sciences: Computational Life Sciences, 5*(4), 286–295.

Singh, P., Kesharwani, R. K., Misra, K., & Rizvi, S. I. (2015). The modulation of erythrocyte Na+/K+-ATPase activity by curcumin. *Journal of Advanced Research, 6*(6), 1023–1030.

Singh, P., Kesharwani, R. K., Misra, K., & Rizvi, S. I. (2016). Modulation of erythrocyte plasma membrane redox system activity by curcumin. *Biochemistry Research International, 2016, Article ID 702039.*

Singh, R. K., Lee, K. M., Ucmak, D., Brodsky, M., Atanelov, Z., Farahnik, B., Abrouk, M., Nakamura, M., Zhu, T. H., & Liao, W. (2016). Erythrodermic psoriasis: Pathophysiology and current treatment perspectives. *Psoriasis (Auckland, NZ), 6*, 93.

Smith, C. H., & Barker, J. (2006). Psoriasis and its management. *BMJ, 333*, 380–384.

Smith, N., Weymann, A., Tausk, F. A., & Gelfand, J. M. (2009). Complementary and alternative medicine for psoriasis: A qualitative review of the clinical trial literature. *Journal of the American Academy of Dermatology, 61*, 841–856.

Soleymani, T., Hung, T., & Soung, J. (2015). The role of vitamin D in psoriasis: A review. *International Journal of Dermatology, 54*, 383–392.

Staberg, B., Roed-Petersen, J., & Menne, T. (1989). Efficacy of topical treatment in psoriasis with MC903, a new vitamin D analog. *Acta Dermato-Venereologica, 69*, 147–150.

Syed, Z. U., & Khachemoune, A. (2011). Inverse psoriasis. *American Journal of Clinical Dermatology, 12*, 143–146.

Upadhyaya, J., Kesharwani, R. K., & Misra, K. (2009). Metabolism, pharmacokinetics, and bioavailability of ascorbic acid; synergistic effect with tocopherols and curcumin. *J. ComputIntellBioinform, 2*(1), 77–84.

Vaughn, A. R., Branum, A., & Sivamani, R. K. (2016). Effects of turmeric (*Curcuma longa*) on skin health: A systematic review of the clinical evidence. *Phytotherapy Research, 30*, 1243–1264.

Vyas, N., Keservani, R. K., Nayak, A., Jain, S., & Singhal, M. (2010). Effect of *Tamarindus indica* and *Curcuma longa* on stress-induced alopecia. *Pharmacology online, 1*, 377–384.

Zeng, N., Ayyub, M., Sun, H., Wen, X., Xiang, P., & Gao, Z. (2017). Effects of physical activity on motor skills and cognitive development in early childhood: A systematic review. *BioMed Research International, 2017*, 1–13.

Ziboh, V. A., Miller, C. C., & Cho, Y. (2000). Metabolism of polyunsaturated fatty acids by skin epidermal enzymes: Generation of anti-inflammatory and antiproliferative metabolites. *The American Journal of Clinical Nutrition, 71*, 361s–366s.

CHAPTER 14

ROLE OF PROBIOTIC SUPPLEMENTS IN PSORIASIS

RUSHIKESH D. PATIL, SHWETA S. GEDAM, SWATI G. TALELE, LAXMIKANT B. BORSE, and ABHIJEET D. KULKARNI

Sandip Institute of Pharmaceutical Sciences, Nashik, Maharashtra, India

ABSTRACT

Psoriasis is a type of disease that reduces immunity and causes sickness, which can be dealt with using probiotics. In this research, probiotic strains that could or couldn't lower interleukin (IL)-17 levels were administered orally to imiquimod (IMQ)-induced psoriasis-like mice. The psoriasis-like pathological traits were improved by *Bifidobacterium* adolescentis CCFM667, B. breve CCFM1078, *Lacticaseibacillus paracasei* CCFM1074, and *Limosilactobacillus reuteri* CCFM1132, while B. animalis CCFM1148, L. paracasei CCFM1147, and L. reuteri CCFM10 did not show the same effect. The amount of short-chain fatty acids increased across all effective strains, which were negatively correlated with the levels of inflammatory cytokines. By analyzing 16S ribosomal RNA sequenced genes, a decrease in the diversity of intestinal microbiota in psoriasis-like mice was observed, but effective strains made some unique changes to the composition of intestinal microbiota compared to the ineffective strains. Recent research suggests that the inflammatory microenvironment shaped by bacterial products, migratory patterns of intestinal immune cells, and systemic cytokine release may also contribute to psoriasis. The diversity of intestinal microbiota in fecal samples of individuals with psoriasis is notably decreased, and a variety of digestive tract microorganisms are generally decreased in individuals with psoriasis and psoriatic arthritis. Therefore, altering the intestinal flora can be a potential treatment. Current research also indicates that it has positive benefits in improving the symptoms and pathological process of psoriasis by adjusting and enhancing the intestinal microbial community in psoriasis. Methods to improve the regulation of microbial communities include probiotics and fecal microbiota transplantation. Studies have shown that probiotics can reduce the psoriasis area and severity index of psoriasis patients, inhibit the inflammation level of psoriasis, and regulate immune cells.

14.1 INTRODUCTION

Psoriasis is a skin ailment with primary medical manifestations. Psoriasis was originally thought to be a disease of epidermal keratinocytes but is now considered one of the most common immune-mediated diseases (Grayson et al., 2018). The occurrence of psoriasis worldwide is about 2% but varies according to different regions (Christophers et al., 2001). Although psoriasis occurs at any age, its occurrence is highest between 18 and 39 years of age, or between 50 and 69 years of age (Parisi et al., 2013). Scales and erythema are two of the most prevalent medical symptoms of psoriasis, localized or widely distributed (Ferreli et al., 2018). According to the different medical manifestations of diseased skin, psoriasis is classified as pustular psoriasis, guttate psoriasis, inverse psoriasis, plaque-type psoriasis, and palmoplantar psoriasis (Griffiths et al., 2007). Although there have been a large number of studies on psoriasis, the pathogenesis of psoriasis is not fully understood. It has been shown these days that the pathogenesis of psoriasis isn't because of a single cause, and entails many aspects, along with genetic, immunological, environmental, and different factors (Greb et al., 2016). Additionally, psoriasis is an innate and adaptive immune system disorder in which keratinocytes, accessory cells, and Thymus cells play a vital role (Schn et al., 2019). Furthermore, keratinocytes are affected by the innate and adaptive immune system condition known as psoriasis, abnormalities arise throughout the development of psoriasis. Additionally, when an antigen is presented, the nuclear activation kappa-B signaling pathway, T helper (Th) cells population differentiation (specifically T-helper 17 cells), and IL-17 responses are improved (Greb et al., 2016; Diani et al., 2016). Recently, the interleukin (IL)-23/Th17 axis in psoriasis is receiving more attention. T helper cell 17 cells are differentiated by interleukin-23, and these cells eventually produce interleukin-22 and interleukin-17 (Pust et al., 2016). These inflammatory cytokines, specifically

IL-17, boost the development of psoriasis (Boehncke et al., 2015). Given the intricacy of psoriasis etiology, there aren't any strategies to cure it, and relapse occurs after stopping the medication. Biotechnology is currently the only approach for treating psoriasis and having positive safety. However, biological preparations are usually expensive. Many types of biologics, such as anti-IL-12/23p40 antibodies and IL-17 inhibitors, have been used to treat psoriasis (Kamata et al., 2018). The application of IL-17 inhibitors, such as secukinumab, ixekizumab, and brodalumab, has shown that IL-17 is a therapeutic target for psoriasis (Kamata et al., 2018). Therefore, it is predicted that probiotics will suppress the release of IL-17 and can be used to treat psoriasis. The gut microbiota population is in dynamic equilibrium with various functions, such as resistance to pathogen invasion, maintenance of gut homeostasis, metabolism of carbon and nitrogen, and nourishment of the host; therefore, human health is closely related to alterations in gut microbiota (Thursby et al., 2017; He et al., 2013; Dominguez-Bello et al., 2019). Additionally, the gut microbiota regulates immunity, the production of carbohydrate digestion products by the gut microbiota promotes thymus cell reprogramming to become regulatory T cells, and this in turn inhibits the differentiation of other T cells, including Th17 cells (Tyagi et al., 2018; Chen et al., 2019). Numerous studies have reported gut microbial issues in psoriasis patients, noting a significant decrease in gut microbial diversity (Hidalgo-Cantabrana et al., 2019; Scher et al., 2015). At the phylum level, the proportion of Firmicutes significantly increases while that of Bacteroidetes decreases significantly, leading to an increased Firmicutes/Bacteroidetes ratio; moreover, there is a positive correlation between this ratio and psoriasis severity (Cheng et al., 2018; Doaa et al., 2016). Akkermansia and *Ruminococcus* show a sharp decline in relative abundance at the genus level; these genera may produce short-chain fatty acids (SCFAs) which can lead to regulatory T cell differentiation or maintain intestinal homeostasis (Scher et al., 2015; Codoner et al., 2018). At the species level, the relative abundance of *Akkermansia muciniphila* and *Faecalibacterium prausnitzii* drastically decreased; each is referred to as a useful intestine microbiota (Codoner et al., 2018; Tan et al., 2018). Therefore, adjustments in intestine microbiota are essential for psoriasis development, and regulating intestine microbiota can be an opportunity remedy for psoriasis. Severe psoriasis has been associated with nutrient deficiency, due to the fact hyperproliferation and desquamation of the skin dermis will boost nutrient loss (Wolters et al., 2005). Besides this, reviews in the literature have validated that certain nutritional styles have anti-inflammatory effects, and hence have the impact of assuaging psoriasis (Barrae et al., 2020). Therefore, it is possible to improve psoriasis by adjusting the diet. Probiotics are described as living microorganisms that have a beneficial effect on the health of the host when ingested in sufficient quantities. Dairy products are a probiotic's primary food source. Additionally, probiotics improve the microbial equilibrium in the colon and have immunomodulatory effects (Cosme-Silva et al., 2020; Li et al., 2020). *Lactobacillus pentosus* GMNL-77 to imiquimod (IMQ)-induced psoriasis-like mice via intragastric administration, resulting in decreased pathological features in mice (Cheng et al., 2017). *L. sakei* proBio-65 extract to IMQ-induced psoriasis-like mice via topical application, which also led to decreased pathological features in mice (Rather et al., 2018). Although the mechanism is not spelled out, each study found that levels of IL-23/Th17 axis-associated inflammatory cytokines, including IL-23, IL-22, and IL-17, decreased following probiotic therapy. Therefore, we hypothesize that increasing the consumption of foods with anti-inflammatory probiotics can reduce psoriasis symptoms. In this study, probiotic strains that could or could not reduce IL-17 levels in different animal disease models, such as mice with rheumatoid arthritis, asthma, and constipation, were tested on IMQ-induced psoriasis-like mice (Li et al., 2020). The purpose of this study was to (1) assess the beneficial effects of various probiotic strains on the pathological characteristics of psoriasis; (2) evaluate the inhibitory effects of various probiotic strains on inflammatory cytokine levels associated with psoriasis; (3) investigate the modulating effects of various probiotic strains on gut microbiota; (4) conduct correlation analysis to understand how probiotics ameliorate psoriasis.

14.2 MATERIAL AND METHODS

14.2.1 MICROORGANISM STRAINS

The strains used in this experiment have been stored in the Collection of Food Microorganisms Cultures (CCFM). Lactobacillus strains have been cultured at 37C for 16 hours under aerobic conditions with (MRS) broth. *Bifidobacterium* strains have been cultured at 37°C for 30 hours under anaerobic conditions with modified MRS broth containing 0.05% (w/v) L-cysteine-HCl. Detailed information on the probiotics is shown in Table 14.1. The strains have been cultured for 3 generations and centrifuged at 8,000 revolutions per minute for 10 minutes to remove the supernatant. The strains were washed with phosphate-buffered saline 3 times and then resuspended in normal saline at a concentration of 5×10^9 CFU/mL, or colony-forming units.

TABLE 14.1 Information of Strains CCFM (Culture Collection and Food Microorganism)

Strain Number	Strain Original Number	Genus/Species	Origin
Culture collection and food microorganism 667	CCFM667	*Bifidobacterium adolescentis*	CCFM
Culture collection and food microorganism 1078	JSWX17M1	*Bifidobacterium breve*	
Culture collection and food microorganism 1148	JSWX23M8	*Bifidobacterium animalis*	
Culture collection and food microorganism 1074	FJSWX1M3	*Lacticaseibacillus paracasei*	
Culture collection and food microorganism 1147	VCQQJ4174M3		
Culture collection and food microorganism 1032	FZJTZ20M3	*Limosilactobacillus reuteri*	
Culture collection and food microorganism 1040	FYNDL13		

14.2.2 ANIMAL EXPERIMENTS

Bagg albino (inbred research mouse strain) / C mice females (6 to 8 weeks, 18 to 20 grams) are being kept in a barrier-free environment. The temperature is set at 23°C and the humidity at 55%. All animal procedures have been performed. They are maintained in a space without obstacles and have been separated into 10 groups: control group, IMQ positive control group, and probiotic groups (seven groups). Six mice are included in each group. The probiotic groups are orally administered 200 µL of bacterial suspension daily for two weeks, while the other mice receive intragastric administration of the same volume of sterile saline. After two weeks, the dorsal fur is shaved, and 62.5 mg of IMQ cream is applied to the skin and 20 mg to the right ear daily for seven consecutive days, while mice in the control group receive the same volume of Vaseline (Vander et al., 2009). During this period, probiotic groups receive bacterial suspensions, the control, and IMQ groups receive sterile saline, and the MTX group receives methotrexate dissolved in normal saline at 1 mg/kg/day (Zhao et al., 2016; Baker et al., 2016). Mice are sacrificed on the eighth day (Figure 14.1).

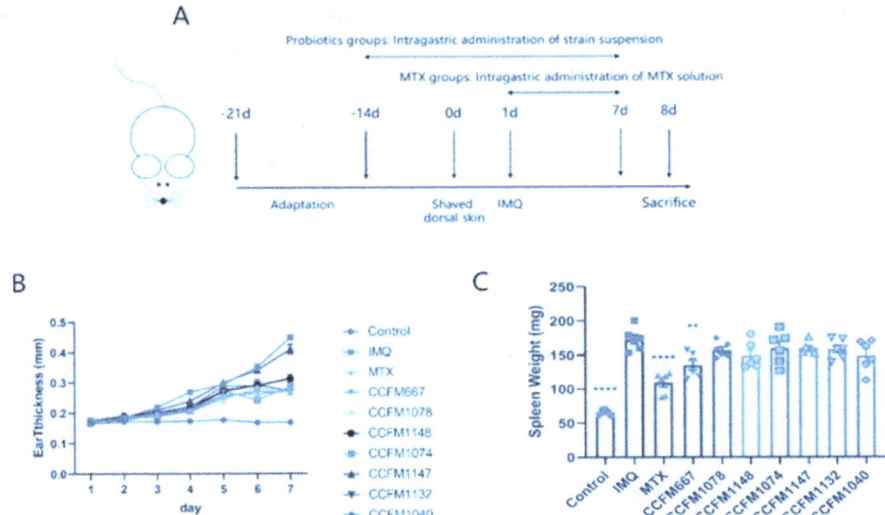

FIGURE 14.1 Effects of probiotics on pathogenic traits similar to psoriasis. (**A**) design of animal experiments; (**B**) mice's ear thickness; (**C**) mice's spleen weight at day seven [**p 0.01 and ****p 0.0001].

14.2.3 EAR THICKNESS DETERMINATION AND DORSAL SKIN SCORE

The size of the mice's ears is measured with a virtual vernier caliper every day during the receiving period. The lesion pores and skin of mice are scored in terms of the clinical psoriasis area and severity index (PASI). Scores are given for the degree of thickness, scaling, and erythema separately on a scale from 0–4: 0, none-1, slight-2, moderate-3, marked-4, and very marked. Cumulative rating is the sum of the ratings of the three.

14.2.4 SKIN HISTOPATHOLOGY

After mice have been sacrificed, the skin is removed, diced, and embedded in paraffin wax, then hematoxylin-stained and eosin for further microscopic examination. A digital scanner is used to scan photomicrographs (20×).

14.2.5 ANALYZES OF SKIN CYTOKINES

Dorsal pores were crushed with skin samples (100 mg) in 900 μl lysis buffer for the radioimmunoprecipitation experiment containing 2% (v/v) protease inhibitor combination and 2% (v/v) phosphatase inhibitor combination with the grinder for 30 s at 60 Hz, 5 times. As per manufacturer instructions, IL-22, IL-23, and IL-17 levels were measured using an enzyme-linked immunosorbent assay, and overall protein levels were measured using an enhanced bicinchoninic acid protein assay kit.

14.2.6 SCFA ANALYSIS

SCFA levels in the caecum (50 mg) were measured by gas chromatography-mass spectrometer using a previously published method (Mao et al., 2016).

14.2.7 16S RRNA FROM FECAL SAMPLES SEQUENCED

A swab was used to collect skin microbes. Samples taken from swabs and feces were collected the day before euthanasia and frozen at $-80°C$. According to the manufacturer's instructions, DNA from fecal samples was extracted using a Fast DNA spin kit for feces. The extracted DNA was then amplified by Polymerase Chain Reaction (PCR). The V4 region of fecal samples of the 16S ribonucleic Acid gene was amplified using the primers 341F and 806R. The detailed protocol has been described previously (Tian et al., 2019). PCR products were purified using a TIAN gel mini purification kit and then sequenced using the Illumina sequencing platform.

14.2.8 BIOINFORMATICS ANALYSIS

All sequences have been analyzed using Statistical Analysis of Microbial Ecology. Alpha and beta diversity analyses have been additionally done using QIIME2. The records have been normalized through the median, converted through log transformation, and scaled through the targeted mean. Heat tree analysis and linear discriminant analysis (LDA) effect size have been done using the. The low recall filter was a 20% incidence filter, whereas the low-variance filter was based on the inter-quantile range. The records have been normalized using total sum scaling. Differences have been deemed significant at $p < 0.05$.

14.3 RESULT

14.3.1 CCFM667, CCFM1078, CCFM1074, AND CCFM1132 PATHOLOGICAL FEATURES SIMILAR TO AMELIORATED PSORIASIS

In previous experiments, it was determined that *B. adolescentis* CCFM667 reduced IL-17 levels in psoriasis and was effective in mice. Meanwhile, *B.*

animalis CCFM1148 and *L. paracasei* CCFM1147 did not reduce IL levels. Therefore, in the selection of strains for this experiment, we chose strains that could or could not reduce the IL-17 level in other animal pathological models, such as mice with asthma, constipation, and rheumatoid arthritis (Li et al., 2020). Continuous application of IMQ resulted in thickening of the ears, swelling of spleens, and dorsal pores showing erythema, scaling, and thickening of the skin in mice. These effects are consistent with literature reports (Van Der Fits et al., 2009; Ru et al., 2020; Zeng et al., 2020). All probiotics, except for *L. paracasei* CCFM1147, effectively reduced ear swelling. In the spleen, only MTX and *B. adolescentis* CCFM667 effectively ameliorated spleen swelling.

With regard to the pathological traits of dorsal pores and MTX, *B. adolescentis* CCFM667, B. breve CCFM1078, *L. paracasei* CCFM1074, and *L. reuteri* CCFM1132 effectively reduced erythema, scaling, and thickening, but *B. animalis* CCFM1148, *L. paracasei* CCFM1147, and *L. reuteri* CCFM1040 had almost no impact (Figure 14.2). Despite the skin's thickening and pores in the *B. animalis* CCFM1148 institution were not critical, this institution had very critical erythema. Pathological sections confirmed that the epidermal structure of the control group consisted of only one or more layers of cells, while the epidermal structure of the IMQ group was significantly thickened. Consistent with the pathological characteristics, MTX, *L. paracasei* CCFM1074, and *L. reuteri* CCFM1132 efficiently decreased epidermal thickness. Therefore, *B. adolescentis* CCFM667, B. breve CCFM1078, *L. paracasei* CCFM1074, and *L. reuteri* CCFM1132 have been considered effective in relieving psoriasis-like pathological characteristics, while *B. animalis* CCFM1148, *L. paracasei* CCFM1147, and *L. reuteri* CCFM1040 have been considered to be ineffective strains.

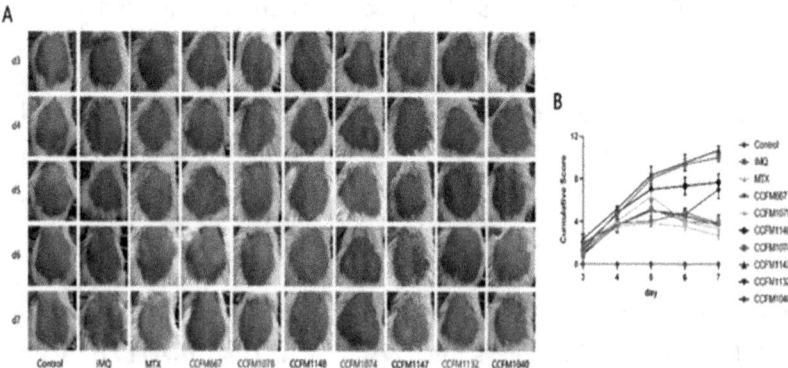

FIGURE 14.2 Probiotic effect on the dorsal skin. (A) Typical images of a mouse's back skin D3 to D7. (B) PASI of several types of mice. Cumulative total score is the scores of intensities of thickening, scaling, and erythema.

14.3.2 CULTURE COLLECTION AND FOOD MICROORGANISM (667, 1078, 1074, 1132) SUPPRESSED THE PSORIASIS-LIKE IMMUNE RESPONSE

Being immune-mediated, psoriasis is a skin disease, and the interleukin-23/T helper cell 17 axis takes part in its progression (Griffith et al., 2007; Greb et al., 2016). Therefore, levels of Interleukin-23, Interleukin-22, and Interleukin-17 in skin lesions were identified. The ongoing use of IMQ led to increased levels of IL-23, IL-22, and IL-17, while MTX significantly halted this trend (Figure 14.5). The probiotic strains including *B. breve* CCFM1078 substantially suppressed the expression of all three cytokines, while *B. adolescentis L. paracasei* CCFM1074, *L. reuteri* CCFM1132, and CCFM667 substantially suppressed the expression of cytokines. In addition to having no effect on reducing psoriasis-like symptoms, *B. animalis* CCFM1148, *L. paracasei* CCFM1147, and *L. reuteri* CCFM1040 no longer inhibit the psoriasis-like immune response (Figure 14.3). It was therefore determined that *B. adolescentis* CCFM667, *B. breve* CCFM1078, *L. paracasei* CCFM1074, and *L. reuteri* CCFM1132 were effective in reducing psoriasis via the IL-23/Th17 axis on levels of inflammatory cytokines connected to the IL-23/Th17 axis (Figure 14.4).

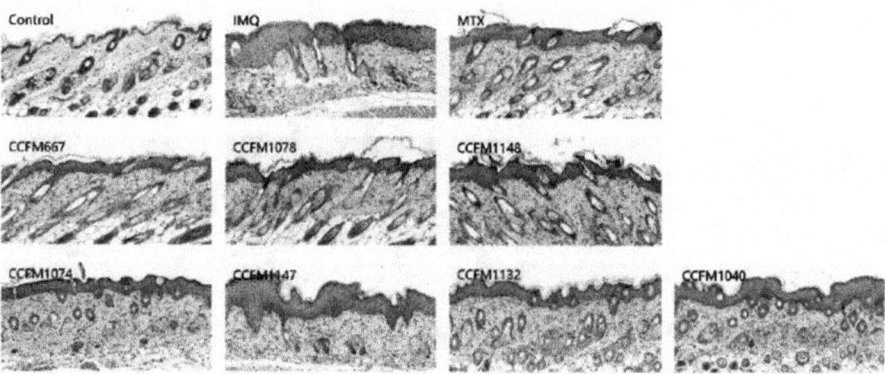

FIGURE 14.3 Hematoxylin and eosin photomicrographs of representative dorsal skin tissue.

14.3.3 THE SCFA METABOLISM WAS AFFECTED DIFFERENTLY BY PROBIOTICS

The primary metabolites of gut microbes ferment acetate, propionate, and butyrate, which are the primary SCFAs (Koh et al., 2016). Compared to the

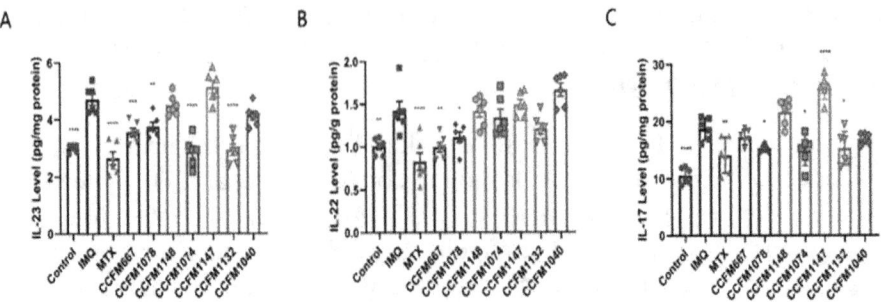

FIGURE 14.4 Outcomes of probiotics on levels of IL-23/Th17 axis-associated inflammatory cytokines. Levels of IL-23 in (A) (n = 6); levels of IL-22 (B) (n = 6); and levels of IL-17 (C) (n = 6). [**p 0.01, ***p 0.001, ****p 0.0001, *p 0.05, and **p 0.01].

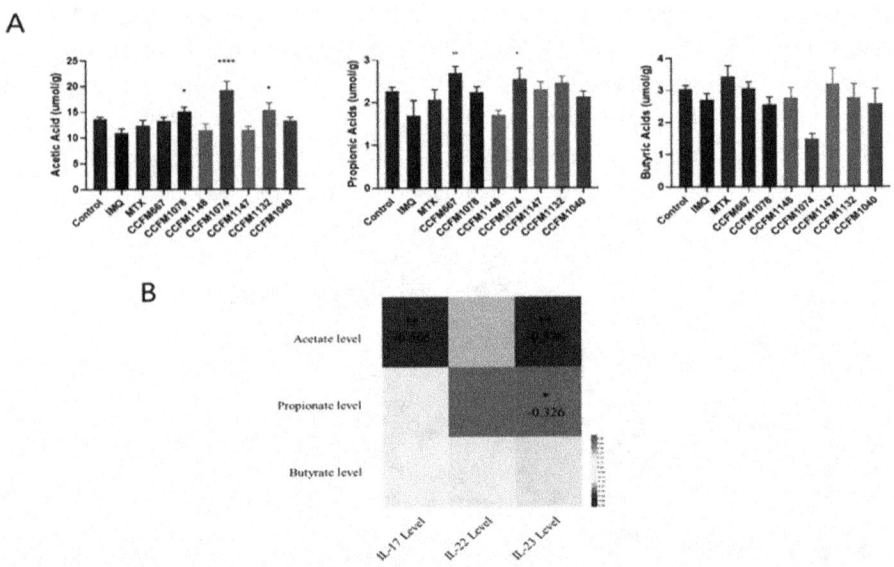

FIGURE 14.5 Results of probiotics on short-chain fatty acid metabolism. (**A**) Different groups' levels of propionate, butyrate, and acetate (n = 6). (**B**) Spearman correlation analysis of the relationship between inflammatory cytokines linked to the IL-23/Th17 axis and SCFA levels. [*** p 0.0001, ** p 0.01 and * p 0.05, respectively].

IMQ groups, the acetate levels in the B. breve CCFM1078, L. paracasei CCFM1074, and L. reuteri CCFM1132 groups were significantly increased, while propionate levels in the B. adolescentis CCFM667 and L. paracasei CCFM1074 groups were significantly increased. However, the butyrate levels in all groups showed no significant difference.

Additional correlation evaluation was performed between the levels of SCFAs in the colon content and the levels of inflammatory cytokines in the skin tissue; the result showed that the level of acetate was significantly negatively correlated with the levels of IL-17 and IL-23, and the level of propionate was significantly negatively correlated with the levels of IL-23. It was concluded that probiotics that effectively alleviated psoriasis could inhibit the release of IL-23/Th17 axis inflammatory cytokines by promoting the production of SCFAs.

14.3.4 KEY DISTINCTIONS BETWEEN PROBIOTICS THAT TREAT PSORIASIS AND THOSE THAT DON'T

To further discover the impact of probiotics on gut microbial composition, the gut microbiota at the genus level in different groups of mice was analyzed using heatmap analysis. Although the control and IMQ groups were clustered into the same category, the abundance of some gut microbiota in the IMQ group was significantly decreased. Additionally, Bifidobacterium CCFM1078, CCFM1148, and CCFM667, *L. reuteri* CCFM1040 and CCFM1132, *L. paracasei* CCFM1074 and CCFM1137, and *L. paracasei* CCFM1074 and CCFM1137 were clustered into the same category. Therefore, it was speculated that the effects of probiotics of the same genus or species were similar in gut microbial composition overall, but there should be some key differences that made certain probiotics effective in ameliorating psoriasis, while others were ineffective. To explore the key differences that made certain probiotics effective in ameliorating psoriasis, a heatmap analysis was performed (Foster et al., 2017). Differential gut microbiota between the control and IMQ, as well as *L. reuteri* CCFM1040 and CCFM1132, *L. paracasei* CCFM1074, and CCFM1137, *Bifidobacterium* CCFM1148, and CCFM667, and *Bifidobacterium* CCFM1148, and CCFM1078).

14.4 DISCUSSION

Psoriasis is an immune-mediated skin disease, and the IL-23/Th17 pathway plays an important role in its progression. IL-23 inhibitors, such as Guselkumab, risankizumab, and tildrakizumab, among others, are used to treat psoriasis as well as other Th17-mediated inflammatory disorders (Roberti et al., 2020; Dattola et al., 2020). Additionally, IL-17 inhibitors, including secukinumab, ixekizumab, and brodalumab, are widely used to treat psoriasis (Kmata et al.,

2018). Probiotics can impact T lymphocytes through their metabolites, influencing the number of Th17 cells in the host and consequently affecting IL-17 levels. Research has shown that obese adults who consumed probiotic-rich yogurt had lower blood levels of IL-17 (Zarrati et al., 2013). Based on this, specific probiotic strains that may decrease IL-17 levels to varying degrees in different animal models, such as mice with asthma, constipation, and rheumatoid arthritis, were selected and applied to IMQ-induced psoriasis-like mice to evaluate the strain's effects on psoriasis (Li et al., 2020). This aligns with a study suggesting that gut flora directly influences skin inflammation triggered by imiquimod. Probiotics have been demonstrated in various studies to reduce levels of inflammatory cytokines related to the Interleukin-23/T helper cell 17 axis (Leccese et al., 2020; Chen et al., 2015).

In recent years, growing interest has been paid to the connection between human health and intestinal microbiota. SCFAs, specifically acetate, propionate, and butyrate, are the primary products of intestinal microbial fermentation (Koh et al., 2016). It has been suggested that SCFAs could promote the differentiation of Treg cells and then influence the balance of Th17/Treg, which could alleviate the occurrence of psoriasis (Hidalgo-Cantabrana et al., 2019). Reduced levels of acetate and propionate have been found in the serum of psoriasis patients (Khyshiktuev et al., 2008). *B. breve* CCFM1078, *L. paracasei* CCFM1074, and *L. reuteri* CCFM1132 increased acetate levels, and *B. adolescentis* CCFM667 and *L. paracasei* CCFM1074 increased propionate levels, while the inactive *B. animalis* CCFM1148 strain, *L. paracasei* CCFM1147 strain, and *L. reuteri* CCFM1040 strain did not. It was suggested that acetate and propionate played a role in the treatment of psoriasis. Additionally, the levels of acetate and propionate were significantly negatively correlated with the levels of IL-23/Th17 axis-related inflammatory cytokines. It was concluded that probiotics that effectively alleviated psoriasis could inhibit the release of IL-23/Th17 axis inflammatory cytokines by promoting the production of SCFAs.

Human fitness is closely associated with the adjustments of intestinal microbiota, and a huge quantity of research has mentioned the adjustments of intestinal plant life variety in sufferers with psoriasis (Cheng et al., 2018; Doaa et al., 2016; Rinninella et al., 2019). Much research has additionally mentioned that there is a big lower in intestinal microbial variety (Hidalgo-Cantabrana et al., 2019; Scher et al., 2015). In this study, the α and β variety of the intestinal microbiota in psoriasis-like mice reduced, and the relative abundance changed. Some research documents an expanded ratio of F/B in sufferers with psoriasis, which is related to altered SCFA in relation to carbohydrates, while others have located that the F/B ratio is definitely correlated with the PASI rating. However, in this study, the F/B ratio in the control and IMQ groups showed no significant difference but was expanded in the CCFM1074 group, which both relieved similar pathogenic features to psoriasis. However, reduced abundance of Bacteroidetes in sufferers with psoriasis. Therefore, the function of the F/B ratio in the development of psoriasis needs further study.

Some research has pronounced strain-unique consequences of probiotics in ameliorating disease. Within this research, heatmap evaluation confirmed that the same genus or species of probiotics had comparable consequences in modulating gut microbiota, even though the consequences of those probiotics in ameliorating psoriasis were different. Consequently, the abundance of gut microbiota was compared between the effective and ineffective probiotic groups, and some key differential gut microbiota were identified. The abundance of the family Rikenellaceae in the IMQ group significantly increased, while the effective strains showed a decrease in abundance by *B. adolescentis* CCFM667, *L. paracasei* CCFM1074, and *L. reuteri* CCFM1132. Meanwhile, the abundance of the family Rikenellaceae was positively correlated with psoriasis-like pathological traits and inversely associated with propionate levels. This suggests that the development of psoriasis may have a correlation with the increase in the abundance of the family Rikenellaceae. Similarly, it has been determined that the Th1 reaction inside the colon of mice is stronger after receiving antibiotics, while the abundance of the family Rikenellaceae increased, indicating that Rikenellaceae diversity is associated with immunity. A subset of the *L. paracasei* CCFM1147 group is *L. paracasei* CCFM1074, which increased the Lachnospiraceae's abundance, strongly associated with IL-23 levels. This suggests that the development of psoriasis may lead to a decrease in the abundance of the Lachnospiraceae, which is linked to inflammatory responses. The key differential gut microbiota was not identified, but the *B. breve* CCFM1078 strain largely ameliorated psoriasis and was highly effective in reducing inflammatory reactions in all probiotic groups. Therefore, it was speculated that psoriasis was ameliorated directly through the IL-23/IL-17 axis rather than exerting effects on gut microbiota. Due to strain-specificity, this study believes that effective strains could be developed into products to help patients increase the intake of these strains to treat psoriasis. Furthermore, probiotics should only alleviate psoriasis to a certain extent and cannot replace medication. Probiotic consumption should be used as a supplement to medication.

In this study, we found that probiotics could ameliorate the pathological traits of psoriasis in mice by inhibiting the IL-23/Th17 axis-associated inflammatory reaction and regulating gut microbiota, providing a new opportunity for the treatment of psoriasis. However, there are still shortcomings in this study, such as the lack of repeated experiments to confirm the results. Additionally, tests of immune cells were lacking to strengthen the link between gut microbial composition and immunological changes in the skin. These will be the direction of future research. In the future, this study will further verify whether the effective strains have the same phenomenon and effects in the human body, and further explore the mechanisms.

14.5 CONCLUSION

In summary, in psoriasis-like mice that had been provoked by IMQ, the effects of 7 probiotic strains on treating psoriasis had been investigated. *L. paracasei* CCFM1074, *B. breve* CCFM1078, *B. adolescentis* CCFM667, and *L. reuteri* CCFM1132 ameliorated psoriasis by suppressing the discharge of IL-23/Th17 axis-related inflammatory elements by promoting the content of SCFAs, while *L. paracasei* CCFM1147, *B. animalis* CCFM1148, and *L. reuteri* CCFM1040 did not have such effects. *B. breve* CCFM1078 demonstrated the most anti-inflammatory effects among them. The improvement of psoriasis may also result in an increase in the abundance of the Rikenellaceae family, while the effective strains *B. adolescentis* CCFM667, *L. paracasei* CCFM1074, and *L. reuteri* CCFM1132 reduced its abundance. These results revealed differences in the regulation of immune response and gut microbiota by strains, confirming that the effects were strain-specific. This study demonstrated the potential of probiotics in the treatment of psoriasis.

KEYWORDS

- gut microbiota
- imiquimod
- interleukin
- Lactobacillus strains
- polymerase chain reaction
- psoriasis area and severity
- short-chain fatty acids

REFERENCES

Baker, H., & Ryan, T. J. (1968). Methotrexate in psoriasis. *The Lancet, 2*(7576), 1395.
Barrea, L., Megna, M., Cacciapuoti, S., Frias-Toral, E., Fabbrocini, G., Savastano, S., & Muscogiuri, G. (2022). Very low-calorie ketogenic diet (VLCKD) in patients with psoriasis and obesity: An update for dermatologists and nutritionists. *Critical Reviews in Food Science and Nutrition, 62*(2), 398–414.
Chen, L., Sun, M., Wu, W., Yang, W., Huang, X., Xiao, Y., & Chen, Z. (2019). Microbiota metabolite butyrate differentially regulates Th1 and Th17 cells' differentiation and function in the induction of colitis. *Inflammatory Bowel Diseases, 25*(8), 1450–1461.
Chen, L., Zou, Y., Peng, J., Lu, F., Yin, Y., Li, F., & Yang, J. (2015). Lactobacillus acidophilus suppresses colitis-associated activation of the IL-23/Th17 axis. *Journal of Immunology Research, 2015*, 909514.
Chen, Y. H., Chao, Y. H., Lin, C. C., Tsai, H. Y., Li, Y. R., Chen, Y. Z., & Chen, Y. K. (2017). Lactobacillus pentosus GMNL-77 inhibits skin lesions in imiquimod-induced psoriasis-like mice. *Journal of Food and Drug Analysis, 25*(3), 559–566.
Chen, Y. J., Ho, H. J., Tseng, C. H., Lai, Z. I., Shieh, J. J., & Wu, C. Y. (2018). Intestinal microbiota profiling and predicted metabolic dysregulation in psoriasis patients. *Experimental Dermatology, 27*(11), 1336–1343.
Christophers, E. (2001). Psoriasis–Epidemiology and clinical spectrum. *Clinical and Experimental Dermatology, 26*(4), 314–320.
Codoner, F. M., Ramirez-Bosca, A., Climent, E., Carrion-Gutierrez, M., Guerrero, M., Perez-Orquin, J. M., & Genoves, S. (2018). Gut microbial composition in patients with psoriasis. *Scientific Reports, 8*(1), 3812.
Cosme-Silva, L., Dal-Fabbro, R., Cintra, L. T. A., Ervolino, E., Plazza, F., Bomfim, S. M., & Gomes-Filho, J. E. (2020). Reduced bone resorption and inflammation in apical periodontitis evoked by dietary supplementation with probiotics in rats. *International Endodontic Journal, 53*(8), 1084–1092.
Dattola, A., Silvestri, M., Tamburi, F., Amoruso, G. F., Bennardo, L., Nisticò, S. P., & Romanelli, M. (2020). The emerging role of anti-IL23 in the treatment of psoriasis, when humanized is very promising. *Dermatologic Therapy, 33*(6), e14504.
Di Cesare, A., Di Meglio, P., & Nestle, F. O. (2009). The IL-23/Th17 axis in the immunopathogenesis of psoriasis. *Journal of Investigative Dermatology, 129*(6), 1339–1350.
Diani, M., Altomare, G., & Reali, E. (2016). T helper cell subsets in clinical manifestations of psoriasis. *Journal of Immunology Research, 2016*, 7692024.
Doaa, M., Dalia, M., & Ahmed, F. S. (2016). Gut bacterial microbiota in psoriasis: A case-control study. *African Journal of Microbiology Research, 10*(41), 1337–1343.
Dominguez-Bello, M. G., Godoy-Vitorino, F., Knight, R., & Blaser, M. J. (2019). Role of the microbiome in human development. *Gut, 68*(6), 1108–1114.
Eppinga, H., Sperna Weiland, C. J., Thio, H. B., van der Woude, C. J., Nijsten, T. E., Peppelenbosch, M. P., & Konstantinov, S. R. (2016). Similar depletion of protective *Faecalibacterium prausnitzii* in psoriasis and inflammatory bowel disease, but not in hidradenitis suppurativa. *Journal of Crohn's and Colitis, 10*(9), 1067–1075.
Fang, Z., Li, L., Liu, X., Lu, W., & Zhao, J. (2019). Strain-specific ameliorating effect of *Bifidobacterium longum* on atopic dermatitis in mice. *Journal of Functional Foods, 60*, 103426.

Ferreli, C., Pinna, A. L., Pilloni, L., Tomasini, C. F., & Rongioletti, F. (2018). Histopathological aspects of psoriasis and its uncommon variants. *Giornale Italiano di Dermatologia e Venereologia, 153*(2), 173–184.

Foster, Z. S., Sharpton, T. J., & Grunwald, N. J. (2017). Meta coder: An R package for visualization and manipulation of community taxonomic diversity data. *PLoS Computational Biology, 13*(2), e1005404.

Greb, J. E., Goldminz, A. M., Elder, J. T., Lebwohl, M. G., Gladman, D. D., Wu, J. J., & Gottlieb, A. B. (2016). Psoriasis. *Nature Reviews Disease Primers, 2*, 16082.

Griffiths, C. E., & Barker, J. N. (2007). Pathogenesis and clinical features of psoriasis. *The Lancet, 370*(9583), 263–271.

Hidalgo-Cantabrana, C., Gomez, J., Delgado, S., Requena-Lopez, S., Queiro-Silva, R., Margolles, A., & Coto-Segura, P. (2019). Gut microbiota dysbiosis in a cohort of patients with psoriasis. *British Journal of Dermatology, 181*(6), 1287–1295.

Kamata, M., & Tada, Y. (2018). Safety of biologics in psoriasis. *Journal of Dermatology, 45*(3), 279–286.

Khyshiktuev, B. S., Karavaeva, T. M., & Fal'ko, E. V. (2008). Variability of quantitative changes in short-chain fatty acids in serum and epidermis in psoriasis. *Klinicheskaia Laboratornaia Diagnostika, 8*, 22–24.

Koh, A., De Vadder, F., Kovatcheva-Datchary, P., & Bäckhed, F. (2016). From dietary fiber to host physiology: Short-chain fatty acids as key bacterial metabolites. *Cell, 165*(6), 1332–1345.

Leccese, G., Bibi, A., Mazza, S., Facciotti, F., Caprioli, F., Landini, P., & Paroni, M. (2020). Probiotic *Lactobacillus* and *Bifidobacterium* strains counteract adherent-invasive *Escherichia coli* (AIEC) virulence and hamper the IL-23/Th17 axis in ulcerative colitis, but not in Crohn's disease. *Cells, 9*(8), 1824.

Li, L., Fang, Z., Lee, Y. K., Zhao, J., Zhang, H., Lu, W., & Chen, W. (2020). Prophylactic effects of oral administration of *Lactobacillus casei* on house dust mite-induced asthma in mice. *Food & Function, 11*(10), 9272–9284.

Li, X., Hu, D., Tian, Y., Song, Y., Hou, Y., Sun, L., & Zhang, W. (2020). Protective effects of a novel *Lactobacillus rhamnosus* strain with probiotic characteristics against lipopolysaccharide-induced intestinal inflammation in vitro and in vivo. *Food & Function, 11*(12), 5799–5814.

Mao, B., Li, D., Ai, C., Zhao, J., Zhang, H., & Chen, W. (2016). Lactulose differently modulates the composition of luminal and mucosal microbiota in C57BL/6J mice. *Journal of Agricultural and Food Chemistry, 64*(32), 6240–6247.

Myers, B., Brownstone, N., Reddy, V., Chan, S., Thibodeaux, Q., Truong, A., & Liao, W. (2019). The gut microbiome in psoriasis and psoriatic arthritis. *Best Practice & Research Clinical Rheumatology, 33*(5), 101494.

Parisi, R., Symmons, D. P., Griffiths, C. E., & Ashcroft, D. M. (2013). Global epidemiology of psoriasis: A systematic review of incidence and prevalence. *Journal of Investigative Dermatology, 133*(2), 377–385.

Paust, H. J., Turner, J. E., Steinmetz, O. M., Peters, A., Heymann, F., Holscher, C., & Stahl, R. A. (2009). The IL-23/Th17 axis contributes to renal injury in experimental glomerulonephritis. *Journal of the American Society of Nephrology, 20*(5), 969–979.

Rather, I. A., Bajpai, V. K., Huh, Y. S., Han, Y. K., Bhat, E. A., Lim, J., & Park, Y. H. (2018). Probiotic *Lactobacillus sakei* proBio-65 extract ameliorates the severity of imiquimod-induced psoriasis-like skin inflammation in a mouse model. *Frontiers in Microbiology, 9*, 1021.

Rinninella, E., Raoul, P., Cintoni, M., Franceschi, F., Miggiano, G., Gasbarrini, A., & Mele, M. (2019). What is the healthy gut microbiota composition? A changing ecosystem across age, environment, diet, and diseases. *Microorganisms, 7*(1), 14.

Scher, J. U., Ubeda, C., Artacho, A., Attur, M., Isaac, S., Reddy, S. M., & Clemente, J. C. (2015). Decreased bacterial diversity characterizes the altered gut microbiota in patients with psoriatic arthritis, resembling dysbiosis in inflammatory bowel disease. *Arthritis & Rheumatology, 67*(1), 128–139.

Schn, M. P. (2019). Adaptive and innate immunity in psoriasis and other inflammatory disorders. *Frontiers in Immunology, 10*, 1764.

Sun, L., Zhang, X., Zhang, Y., Zheng, K., Xiang, Q., Chen, N., & He, Q. (2019). Antibiotic-induced disruption of gut microbiota alters local metabolomes and immune responses. *Frontiers in Cellular and Infection Microbiology, 9*, 99.

Tan, L., Zhao, S., Zhu, W., Wu, L., Li, J., Shen, M., & Peng, C. (2018). The *Akkermansia muciniphila* is a gut microbiota signature in psoriasis. *Experimental Dermatology, 27*(2–3), 144–149.

Thursby, E., & Juge, N. (2017). Introduction to the human gut microbiota. *Biochemical Journal, 474*(11), 1823–1836.

Tian, P., Wang, G., Zhao, J., Zhang, H., & Chen, W. (2019). *Bifidobacterium* with the role of 5-hydroxytryptophan synthesis regulation alleviates the symptoms of depression and related microbiota dysbiosis. *Journal of Nutritional Biochemistry, 66*, 43–51.

Tyagi, A. M., Yu, M., Darby, T. M., Vaccaro, C., Li, J. Y., Owens, J. A., & Jones, R. M. (2018). The microbial metabolite butyrate stimulates bone formation via T regulatory cell-mediated regulation of WNT10B expression. *Immunity, 49*(6), 1116–1131.

Wolters, M. (2005). Diet and psoriasis: Experimental data and clinical evidence. *British Journal of Dermatology, 153*(4), 706–714.

Zarrati, M., Salehi, E., Mofid, V., Hosseinzadeh-Attar, M. J., Nourijelyani, K., Bidad, K., & Shidfar, F. (2013). Relationship between probiotic consumption and IL-10 and IL-17 secreted by PBMCs in overweight and obese people. *Iranian Journal of Allergy, Asthma and Immunology, 12*(4), 404–406.

Zeng, J., Lei, L., Zeng, Q., Yao, Y., Wu, Y., Li, Q., & Zhou, J. (2020). Ozone therapy attenuates NF-kappaB-mediated local inflammatory response and activation of Th17 cells in treatment for psoriasis. *International Journal of Biological Sciences, 16*(10), 1833–1845.

Zhao, J., Di, T., Wang, Y., Wang, Y., Liu, X., Liang, D., & Li, P. (2016). Paeoniflorin inhibits imiquimod-induced psoriasis in mice by regulating Th17 cell response and cytokine secretion. *European Journal of Pharmacology, 772*, 131–143.

INDEX

A

Acacia senegal, 34
Acetylcholinesterase (ACE/AChE), 209, 234, 239, 273, 279
Achyranthes bidentata, 114
Acitretin, 174, 251
Activating protein-1 (AP-1), 59, 120, 123
Active topical psoriasis therapy, 166
Adaptive immune systems, 57
Adhesion molecules, 51, 52
Aggrecan, 15, 50, 117
Akebia saponin D, 106
Akkermansia muciniphila, 287
Albeit modest, 10
Alcohol
  consumption, 171, 211
  related disorders, 210
Algae, 33, 89, 90, 94, 142, 146, 147, 153, 154, 157, 191–199, 201, 211, 212, 215
  extracts, 33
Alkaline, 92, 117
Aloe
  barbadensis Miller, 269
  chemical diversity, 269
  linnaeus, 269
  vera (AV), 231, 268–270
Alpha-linolenic acid (ALA), 56, 72–74, 76–79, 196
Amino
  acids, 36, 39, 101, 103, 191, 192, 195, 231, 254, 268, 274
  sugar, 16
Aminosaccharide, 15
Anabolic processes, 4
Anacardiaceae, 36, 37
Anacardic acids, 28, 37
Anemia, 101, 175, 276
Angelica sinensis, 99, 102
  polysaccharide (ASP), 102, 103
Angiosperms, 193
Animal experiments, 289

Ankylosing spondylitis (AS), 3, 27, 89, 91, 137–140, 143, 183, 205, 263
Anorexia, 47, 115
Anthocyanin, 198
Anthralin, 229, 264
Anthraquinones, 231, 269
Anti-aging, 103, 110, 120, 166
Anti-apoptotic
  properties, 102
  proteins, 116
Anti-arthritic
  effects, 36
  properties, 108, 232
Antibiotic medications, 247
Anticancer, 53, 155, 236, 237, 249, 277
Anti-citrullinated protein, 30
Anticoagulant pills, 80
Anti-diabetic properties, 275, 278
Antigliadin antibodies (AGA), 176
Anti-heart-disease effects, 53
Anti-inflammatory, 3, 4, 12–14, 28, 34–39, 45, 48, 50, 53–56, 58, 59, 69, 78, 81, 90, 92, 93, 95, 100, 102–106, 109–111, 113–115, 117–123, 140–143, 146–149, 152–157, 166, 175–177, 188, 195, 196, 205, 207, 209, 214, 215, 218, 231–233, 236, 237, 250, 251, 253, 255, 256, 258, 269, 270–273, 277, 287, 288, 298
  agent, 28, 35, 103, 105, 148, 157
  component, 36
  cytokines, 109, 250
  effect, 38, 90, 106, 148, 153, 155, 252, 255, 256
  markers, 250
  nutraceuticals, 45, 53
  supplement, 51
Anti-lipid peroxidation, 269
Antimalarial, 205, 209
  medications, 188
Antimicrobial peptides, 267
Anti-nociceptive, 102, 269, 270
  actions, 106

Anti-osteoarthritis, 28, 40, 107, 114
  efficacy, 104
Antioxidant, 48, 55, 79–81, 89, 93, 109, 110, 175, 191, 198, 250, 255, 257
  defenses, 101
  effects, 109, 269, 272
  response element (ARE), 113, 123
Antioxidative properties, 117
Antiphlogistic agent, 155
Antiplatelet pills, 80
Anti-proliferative effects, 233, 275
Antipsoriatic
  characteristics, 274
  effectiveness, 231
  medications, 234, 277
  properties, 236
  systemic drugs, 268
Antipyretic qualities, 270
Anti-rheumatic mechanism, 35
Anti-tumor, 110
Anti-ulcer, 269
Apigenin, 59
Apoptosis, 49, 51, 100, 102, 106–109, 114, 116, 118, 120, 121, 175, 249
  initiating effects, 249
  signal-regulating kinase (ASK-1), 49
Appetite, 139, 257
Aquatic botanicals, 191
Arabinogalactan proteins, 250
Arabinose, 31, 37
Arachidonic acid (AA), 30, 36, 54, 55, 69, 73, 74, 77, 93, 95, 120, 145, 153, 190, 191, 235, 255
Archaeal cytology, 193
Archaebacteria, 193
Arthritic joints, 117
Arthritis, 3, 4, 6, 10, 16, 27–31, 34–36, 38–40, 45–59, 67, 68, 71, 74, 75, 77–82, 89, 90–95, 99, 100, 104–106, 108, 110, 111, 118, 119, 121, 137–144, 146, 147, 149–153, 157, 165, 168, 169, 174, 176, 183, 189, 205, 206, 227–230, 245, 263, 278, 279, 285, 286, 288, 292, 296
  diet, and activity promotion trial (ADAPT), 10
  treatment, 89
Arthrospira platensis, 93

Articular
  erosion, 104
  ligament, 4, 7
  space, 150
Artificial substances, 33
Ascorbic acid, 55
Astaxanthin, 92, 94, 154
Asteraceae family, 237, 276
Asthma, 13, 58, 103, 112, 288, 292, 296
Asymptomatic celiac disease, 255
Atherosclerosis, 58, 74, 75, 248
Atherothrombosis, 75, 76
Atopic dermatitis, 168, 254
Autoimmune
  disease, 48, 138, 139, 150, 166, 238
  disorder, 29, 45, 100, 140, 264
Autoimmunity action, 69
Ayurvedic
  drug, 112
  system, 35, 111
Azadirachta indica, 232, 270
Azadirachtin, 232, 271

B

B cells, 30, 59, 215
Bacillus coagulans, 56
Bacterial fermentation, 57
Bacteroidetes, 287, 297
Bagg albino, 289
Baicalin (BA), 114
Bakuchalcone, 237, 277
Bakuchiol, 237, 277
Benthic
  algae, 194
  zone, 194
Beta boswellic acid, 36
Beta-blockers, 188, 205, 209
Beta-carotene, 53, 89, 215
  shield, 53
Betamethasone
  17-valerate, 234, 273
  dipropionate, 253
Bifidobacterium
  adolescentis, 285, 291–294, 296–298
  bifidum, 57
  strains, 288
Bile acids, 39
Biliary digestive disorders, 115

Bioactive
  compound, 89, 92, 95, 108, 109, 112–115, 141, 147, 154, 195, 218, 274
  lipids, 249
  molecules, 69, 184
  principle, 112
  secondary metabolites, 195
  substances, 89, 137, 157, 184
Bioceuticals, 90, 91
Bioinformatics analysis, 291
Biological
  activities, 37, 106, 150
  agents, 174
  effects, 99
  mechanisms, 268
  processes, 53, 101
  target, 101
Biologics, 81, 82, 287
Biomarkers, 17, 109, 110
Biosynthesis, 15, 68
Biotic crusts, 213
Black cumin, 236, 268, 274
Blood
  serum, 93, 248, 257
  vessels, 74, 75
Blue
  green algae (BGA), 211, 212
  lagoon kelp extract, 249
Body surface area marker, 248
Bone
  demineralization, 253
  marrow suppression, 174
Boswellia serrata, 28, 35, 36, 39, 99, 102–104
  extract (BSE), 36, 104
  gum resin, 28, 39
Boswellic acid (BA), 28, 36, 103
Botanicals, 113, 141, 200, 268
Broad spectrum, 37
Brodalumab, 287, 295
Brown
  algae, 90
  coloration, 213
Buccal films, 32
Bug chomps, 246
Burseraceae, 35, 38, 103, 104
Butyrate, 28, 34, 35, 57, 58, 293, 294, 296

C

Caffeine, 250
  consumption, 250
Calcineurin inhibitors, 229, 264
Calcipotriene, 234, 277
Calcium, 28, 35, 57, 142, 188, 192, 209, 235, 252, 253, 276
  phosphate disease, 28
Calendula officinalis, 277, 278
Camellia sinensis, 116
Cancer, 29, 48, 53, 58, 74, 92, 105, 110, 112, 118, 120, 122, 185, 229, 236, 238, 265, 270, 271, 279
Candida
  albicans, 188, 210, 237, 276
  species, 214
Carbohydrate, 33, 57, 147, 195, 250, 256, 268, 269, 296
  digestion products, 287
Carbon dioxide, 89, 212
Cardiovascular
  disease, 46, 56, 58, 68, 74, 81, 141, 215, 247
  gamble, 14
  gambling, 14
  health, 53
  problems, 79–81
  risk factors, 14, 46
  system, 254
Carotenoids, 48, 51, 55, 92–94, 109, 194, 245, 248
Carpometacarpal joint, 12
Cartilage, 3, 4, 15, 16, 29–31, 35, 46, 50, 74, 90, 100, 104–123, 138, 139, 149
  cells, 90, 122
  degeneration, 4, 106, 121
  metabolism, 4, 107
Cartilaginous extracellular matrix, 114
Carvacrol, 236, 274
Cashew gum, 28, 33, 37, 39
Catabolic genes, 15
Catabolism, 15, 39, 114
Catechins, 116
Caulerpa racemosa, 137, 151, 152
Celecoxib, 14
Celiac disease, 94, 255
Cell
  communication, 8

death, 35, 59
division, 51, 193
matrix synthesis, 114
mediated immunity, 270
proliferation, 30, 49, 53, 58, 59, 101, 208, 235, 237, 250
wall structure, 193
Cellular
energy production, 199
senescence, 7
Cereals, 55, 255
Ceruloplasmin, 246
Chemical
components, 37, 141
fertilizers, 29
structure, 32
Chemokines, 109, 112, 215, 264
Chinese version of the arthritis impact measurement scale 2-short form (CAIMS2-SF), 143
Chitin, 33, 149
Chlorella vulgaris, 93
Chlorophyll, 89, 92, 194, 215
Chlorophyta, 183, 193, 194, 200
Cholecalciferol, 276
Cholesterol, 39, 48, 75, 92, 93, 108, 192, 257
Chondrocyte, 15, 50, 100, 102, 103, 106, 107, 109, 114–123
Chondroitin, 3, 16, 18, 19, 101
group, 19
sulfate, 3, 16, 18, 19
Chondroprotective effects, 4, 117, 123
Chondrus crispus, 198, 215
Chronic
diseases, 28, 37, 102, 118, 121
inflammation, 50, 215
diseases, 45, 48, 103, 151, 256
illness, 45, 46, 53, 57
polyarthritis, 48
process, 247
knee pain, 11
plaque
psoriasis, 234, 251
type psoriasis, 167
Cigarette smoking, 188
Cladosiphon
okamuranus, 199
species, 199

Clinical
investigations, 71, 172
medicine, 76
research, 74, 271
severity of lesions, 264
symptoms, 39, 118, 251
Coal tar, 185, 238
Cochrane, 11, 13, 16, 17
Codeine, 18
Coenzyme Q10, 254
Colitis, 58, 190, 278, 279
Collagen, 3, 50, 92, 107, 108, 117, 119, 143
hydrolysate, 3
induced arthritis (CIA), 92, 106, 119, 143, 144
Collagenase, 108, 111
Collection of food microorganisms cultures (CCFM), 288
Colonic bacterial aerobic fermentation, 34
Commiphora
mukul, 99, 104, 105
wightii, 37–39
Comorbidity, 11, 165, 278
Complete Freund's adjuvant (CFA), 150
Conventional treatment, 100, 275
Copper, 192
Coral reef, 194
Cortex, 32
eucommiae (CE), 107
Corticosteroids, 75, 102, 168, 172, 173, 188, 229, 247, 264
Corticotrophin-releasing hormone (CRH), 210, 218
Cortisol synthesis, 255
Corynebacteria, 213
Cosmeceuticals, 191
Cosmetics, 115, 191, 192, 195, 269, 271
C-reactive protein (CRP), 75, 93, 109, 143, 146, 157, 246, 250
Crotalaria juncea Linn., 276
Crystal accumulation, 27
Cucurbitaceae family, 275
Culture collection and food microorganism (CCFM), 288, 289
Curcuma longa, 115, 116, 232, 271
Curcumin, 50–52, 114–116, 232, 233, 271, 272
Cutaneous disorders, 166

Cyanobacteria, 183, 200, 201, 211, 212
Cyclic endoperoxides, 55
Cyclin adenosine monophosphate (cAMP), 250, 258
Cyclooxygenase, 30, 39, 51, 54, 59, 69, 108, 116, 146, 147, 152, 155
   2 (COX-2), 13, 14, 30, 51, 59, 105, 107, 108, 112, 115, 117–119, 122, 140, 147, 152
Cyclophosphamide, 140
Cyclosporine, 140, 174, 234, 257, 273
Cytokine, 45, 49–54, 57–59, 71, 74, 75, 81, 90, 107, 109, 111, 112, 116, 118, 119, 142, 144, 146, 157, 172, 174, 189, 190, 208, 211, 215, 231, 233, 248, 250–252, 254, 264, 267, 270, 272, 285, 286, 288, 293–296
   interferon-alpha, 189

D

Daily calorie intake (DEI), 56
Dairy products, 175, 248, 249, 255
Deleterious effects, 100
Dementia, 74
Depression, 48, 74, 150, 192
Dermatocorticosteroids, 238
Dermatologist, 183, 239
Dermatology, 238
Dermis, 29, 172, 189, 190, 196, 227, 230, 231, 251, 287
Dexamethasone, 150
Diabetes, 48, 58, 74, 94, 111, 112, 247–249, 267, 270
Diacerein, 18, 19
Diarylheptanoids, 112
Diclofenac, 14
Diet
   regimen, 78
   rich, 53, 56, 255
Dietary
   fiber, 48, 58, 175, 249, 256
   modifications, 249
   supplement, 35, 53, 72, 79, 101, 107, 140, 141, 184, 228, 230, 265, 268, 276
   extracts, 265
Digestive tract microorganisms, 285
Dimethyl sulfoxide (DMSO), 18, 19
Dipsacus asper, 105, 106

Diseasemodifying OA drugs (DMOADs), 5, 19
Disintegrating agents, 32
Dispersing agents, 32
Distal interphalangeal (DIP), 29, 40, 168
   joints, 168
Diterpenes, 35, 103, 250
Diterpenoids, 38
Dithranol stains skin, 174
Dithymoquinone, 236, 274
Dizygotic twins, 170, 206
Docosahexaenoic acid (DHA), 56, 68, 69, 71, 73, 74, 79, 81, 90, 93, 95, 145, 146, 273
Docosapentaenoic acid (DPA), 74, 273
Double-blind, 19, 77, 112, 145, 150, 231–234, 236, 271, 272, 274
Dried rhizomes, 112
Drug, 5, 13, 29, 31, 52, 54, 75, 76, 78, 101, 110, 111, 113, 137, 140, 146, 174, 183, 189, 200, 209, 211, 231, 238
   diet treatment, 78
   aggravated psoriasis, 168
   auranofin, 78
   induced psoriasis, 188
   provoked psoriasis, 168
Dunaliella salina, 94

E

Echinoderms, 199
Efalizumab, 175
Effect size (ES), 10, 11, 13, 15–18
Ehrlich, 6, 7
Eicosa pentaenoic acid (EPA), 56, 68, 69, 71–74, 76, 78–81, 93–95, 143, 145–147, 153, 154, 273
Eicosanoid, 69, 73, 74, 81, 82, 93, 146
   immunomodulatory functions, 74
   metabolic pathways, 54
Eicosatetraenoic acid, 143, 145, 146
Elastin, 50
Endogenous retinoids, 251
Endothelial cells, 75, 175
Energy transmission, 193
Enterocyte proliferation, 57
Environmental factors, 49, 169, 205, 208, 239, 246
Enzyme-linked immunosorbent assay, 291

Epidemiological data, 5
Epidermal
  differentiation, 232, 236, 270, 275
  keratinocytes, 171, 227, 286
Epigallocatechin 3-gallate (EGCG), 114, 116, 117
Epigenetic alterations, 7
Epithelial differentiation, 251
Erosive erythematous plaques, 265
Erythema, 168, 234, 235, 273, 286, 290, 292
Erythematous patches, 166
Erythrocyte sedimentation rate (ESR), 39, 143, 157
Erythrodermic psoriasis, 168, 186, 266
Espresso, 249
Etiology, 137, 187, 264, 287
Eubacteria, 193
Eucommia ulmoides (EU), 99, 102, 106, 107
Euglenoids, 212
Eukaryotic photoautotrophic protists, 211
Euphorbiaceae family, 275
Evening primrose oil (EPO), 77, 235, 236, 268, 274
Ex vivo organotypic culture method, 211
Excimer laser, 265
Excoriation, 205, 209
Exercise therapy, 8
Extracellular matrix, 4, 50, 107, 114, 117–119
  components, 117
Exudate gums, 32

F

Fabaceae, 34, 233, 237, 272, 277
  plant family, 233
Faecalibacterium prausnitzii, 287
Fat-soluble nutrient, 258
Fatty acids (FA), 36, 37, 48, 51, 53, 55–57, 59, 67–74, 76–82, 89, 92–94, 101, 142, 143, 145, 154, 175, 177, 184, 191, 195, 196, 215, 232, 236, 255–258, 271, 273, 274, 285, 287, 298
Fibroblast-like synoviocytes (FLS), 49–51
Fibromyalgia, 137, 138, 140, 150
Fibronectin, 50
Fibrotic ligaments, 100

Fish oil, 56, 71, 73, 76, 78–81, 146, 235, 268, 273, 274
  therapy, 273
  treatments, 235, 274
Flagella structure, 193
Flavonoids, 38, 39, 51, 58, 59, 109, 116, 245
Flavonol, 116, 118
Fluid film, 7
Folate, 75
Folliculitis, 174
Food and Drug Administration (FDA), 80, 113, 174, 238, 239
Formosa soft coral, 152
Fortified foods, 184
Free unsaturated fats, 248
Freshwater environments, 89
Fucoidan, 153, 199–201, 249
Fucoxanthin, 89, 92, 153, 215
Fucus vesiculosus, 199
Fumaric acid esters, 174
Fungi, 32, 58, 137, 140, 143, 194

G

Galactose, 31, 35, 37
Gammalinolenic acid, 235
Gamma-linolenic acid (GLA), 77, 154, 235, 236, 239, 274
Gastric damage, 111
Gastro, 115
Gastrointestinal (GI), 13, 14, 48, 57, 116, 255, 257
  bleeding, 101
  villous atrophy, 255
Gel, 31, 32, 198, 231–233, 237, 265, 269–271, 276, 277, 291
Gelling agents, 32
Gene
  expression, 15, 16, 53, 101, 111, 117, 215, 218
  mutations, 189, 205
  transcription, 52, 174
Generalized pustular psoriasis, 266
Generally recognized as safe (GRAS), 113
  effective (GRASE), 238
Genetic
  predisposition, 166
  vulnerability, 187, 206
Genipin (GNP), 119

Genkwanin, 59
Genome-wide association
   scans, 187
   studies (GWAS), 208, 218
Geographic tongue, 168
Georgi plant, 114
Ginger
   extract, 113
   supplementation, 112, 113
Gingerol analogs, 112
Givotia rottleriformis, 275
Global
   economic burden, 5
   nutraceutical sector, 48
Glucosamine, 3, 15, 16, 18, 19, 101, 149, 150
   chondroitin arthritis intervention trial (GAIT), 16, 18
   hydrochloride, 16, 18
   preparations, 16
   salts, 19
   sulfate (GS), 3, 15, 16, 18, 19, 149
Glucose, 37
Glucuronic acid, 31, 35, 37
Glucuronides, 120
Gluten
   containing cereals, 255
   free diet, 175, 176, 255, 258
   intolerance, 176
   sensitivity, 176
Gluteus, 166, 229
Glycosaminoglycan, 15–17
   chains, 15
Goeckerman
   therapy, 265
   treatment, 229
Golimumab, 140
Gout, 27, 38, 91, 111, 137–139
Gracilaria, 196
   algae, 196
Green
   algae, 194, 212
   lipped mussel (GLM), 18, 19, 143, 144
Gripatoms, 248
Guar gum, 33
Guggul, 104
Guggulu, 28, 38, 39
   extract, 38

Guideline development group (GDG), 153, 166, 178
Gum, 28, 31–34, 39, 57
   Arabic, 28, 31, 33–35, 39, 40
   disadvantages, 33
   resins, 32, 35
Gummy fluid, 32
Gut
   homeostasis, 287
   microbial
      composition, 295, 298
      diversity, 287
   microbiota, 56–58, 177, 249, 287, 288, 295, 297, 298
Guttate psoriasis, 167, 186, 188, 191, 209, 229, 266, 286

H

Haematococcus pluvialis, 94
Hair follicle density, 213
Halichondria sitiens, 137, 154, 155
Hard gum, 34
Hartley guinea pigs, 15
Health
   assessment questionnaire, 77
   benefits, 37, 48, 68, 72, 92, 101, 116, 140, 141, 157, 184, 267, 270, 271
   issues, 74
Healthcare, 5, 28, 99
Heart disease, 67, 74, 94, 170, 270
Helicobacter pylori, 210
Hepatic, 39, 115, 174
Hepatitis, 270
Hepatoprotective activities, 110
Herbal
   compounds, 114
   extracts, 101, 110, 238, 263, 268, 279
   medications, 172
   nutraceuticals, 27
   plants, 124
   shampoos, 231
Herbicides, 29
Heterogeneity, 11, 14, 16, 17
Heteropolysaccharide compound, 37
High
   bioavailability property, 32
   temperature receptor A1 (HTRA1), 110
Hip OA, 11, 12, 15, 17

Histone deacetylase (HDAC), 34
Homeopathy systems, 211
Homocysteine levels, 75, 76, 256
Hormones, 49, 210
Host-microbe interaction, 58
Human
   chondrocytes, 103, 120
   health, 32, 74, 287, 296
   leukocyte antigen (HLA), 171, 178, 207, 246
   organs, 114
Humira, 29
Hyaline cartilage, 31
Hyaluronan, 7
Hyaluronic acid, 3, 17
Hydration, 7, 34
   grease, 7
   lubrication mechanism, 7
   oil system, 7
Hydrocarbons, 31
Hydrochloride, 16, 18, 19, 121, 122
Hydrogels, 32
Hydrolysis, 31, 35
Hydrophilic polymer, 31
Hydrotherapy, 11
Hydroxy
   carboxylic acid receptor 2 (HCAR-2), 177
   genkwanin, 59
Hydroxycarbamide, 174
Hydroxychloroquine, 140
Hydroxymethyl, 143, 144
Hypercalcemia, 173, 253
Hyperhomocysteinemia, 247
Hyperkeratosis, 168, 174
Hyperproliferation, 171, 210, 227, 231, 251, 264, 271, 287
Hypertension, 101, 107, 192, 247, 257, 268
Hypertrophy, 100
Hypervitaminosis, 257
Hypocalcemia, 168
Hypolipidemia representative, 39

I

Ibuprofen, 140
Imiquimod (IMQ), 209, 233, 285, 288, 289, 292–298
   induced psoriasis, 233

Immature dendritic cell maturation, 270
Immune
   cells, 74, 188, 189, 264, 267, 286, 298
   disorders, 246
   mediated disease, 230, 286
   regulatory effects, 59
   structure, 29
   system, 54, 59, 67, 94, 138, 171, 172, 183, 187–189, 198, 199, 207, 210, 230, 231, 237, 249, 273, 276, 286
   development, 249
   disorder, 183, 286
Immunomodulatory
   effects, 115, 288
   properties, 68, 237, 277
Immunosuppressant, 140, 271
   drugs, 172
Immunosuppressive effect, 250
Indomethacin, 14, 108, 234, 273
Inducible nitric oxide synthase (iNOS), 58, 59, 107–109, 112, 117–119, 122, 148
Infections, 28, 29, 101, 166, 198, 206, 209, 210, 213, 214, 271, 275
Inflammation, 3, 5–7, 27, 29, 30, 34, 37–39, 46, 49–51, 54, 56, 57, 59, 67–71, 73–78, 81, 90–94, 99, 100, 103, 104, 107, 111–114, 118, 119, 121, 122, 138–140, 146, 147, 151, 155, 172, 175, 177, 184, 186, 189, 195, 196, 199, 201, 205, 206, 214, 215, 218, 228, 229, 231–233, 236, 238, 250, 254, 255, 265, 269–273, 275, 277, 286, 296
   activity, 37
   related signaling pathways, 218
Inflammatory
   arthritis, 48, 56
   bowel
      disease (IBD), 58, 68, 70, 103, 190, 218, 206, 278
      illnesses, 58
   cell infiltration, 264
   cellular infiltration, 227
   cytokine, 29, 51, 52, 109, 121, 189, 233, 246, 251, 288, 293, 295, 296
   diseases, 58, 94
   disorders, 47, 52, 53, 73, 176, 295
   hyperplasia, 211
   mediators, 58

metastatic processes, 54
milieu, 51
OA, 6
pathway, 52, 119, 258
process, 30, 250
skin
　conditions, 166, 215
　disorders, 218
substances, 49, 76, 251
Infliximab, 140, 188, 279
Innate lymphocyte cell (ILC), 267
Insulin-like growth factor-1 (IGF-1), 8
Intercellular communication, 7
Interferon, 59, 71, 112, 118, 188, 189, 251, 258
　gamma (IFN-γ), 71, 109, 120, 246, 251, 258
Interleukin (IL), 45, 49–51, 53, 54, 56, 57, 71, 74–76, 81, 103, 106–109, 111, 112, 114, 116–118, 120–123, 142, 148, 154, 157, 188–190, 207–211, 215, 233, 246, 248, 250, 252, 254, 264, 267, 272, 279, 285–288, 291–298
　1 (IL-1), 45, 49–51, 53, 54, 57, 71, 74, 76, 81, 103, 106–109, 111, 112, 114, 116–118, 120, 122, 123, 142, 154, 157, 189, 190, 207, 208, 210, 211, 233, 250, 254, 267, 272, 286–288, 291–297
　1 beta (IL-1 beta), 74, 76, 81
　17 (IL-17), 50, 71, 190, 208, 233, 267, 286–288, 291–297
　1ß (IL-1β), 45, 51, 53, 54, 71, 106, 107, 109, 112, 114, 116–118, 120, 122, 123, 142, 157, 189, 272
　22 (IL-22), 190, 293
　23 (IL-23), 208, 233, 264, 286, 288, 291, 293–298
　6 (IL-6), 45, 50, 51, 53, 57, 71, 75, 107, 109, 116, 121, 122, 148, 154, 189, 209, 210, 233, 248, 250, 254, 272
　8 (IL-8), 50, 109, 211, 215, 233, 272
International units (IU), 80
Intestinal
　homeostasis, 58, 287
　immune cells, 285
　microbial
　　community, 286
　　fermentation, 296

Intestine microbiota, 287
Intra-articular corticosteroid injections, 17
Intragastric administration, 288, 289
In-vitro, 15, 34, 35, 37, 39, 51, 107–109, 111, 112, 117, 120, 122, 123, 142, 144, 151, 156, 210, 211, 237, 253, 254, 276
In-vivo, 35, 37, 39, 51, 105, 112, 115, 122, 123, 144, 172, 237, 277
Iodine, 192
Iron, 36, 192
Ischemic coronary illness, 14, 248
Isoflavones, 233
Isoforms, 30
Isopsoralen, 237
Isostichopus badiontus, 137, 149
Ixekizumab, 287, 295

J

Janus kinase (JAK), 49, 51, 52, 121, 208
　phosphorylation, 52
　STAT signaling, 49, 52
Japanese, 145, 169
　Knee Osteoarthritis Measure (JKOM), 145
　Orthopedic Association score (JOA), 145
Jelly diffuses, 32
Joint, 3, 4, 6–8, 10, 12, 15, 17–19, 27, 29–31, 36, 45, 46, 48–52, 56, 57, 68, 72, 74, 78, 81, 90–93, 99–101, 104, 106, 109, 110, 116, 117, 119, 121, 123, 137–140, 146, 148, 149, 168, 184, 189, 229, 278
bones, 139
capacity, 8
capsule, 100, 121
cartilage, 103, 104, 149
cavity, 121
damage, 49
degeneration, 46, 107
diameter, 106, 115
disease, 90, 99, 100
disorder, 3, 36
function, 36, 99, 104, 116
　treatments, 36
health, 81, 123
inflammation, 7, 27, 49, 51, 57, 119, 229
issues, 78, 99
motion, 100
movement, 4

pain, 6, 10, 72, 100, 116, 137, 138, 146
replacement, 6
sickness, 6, 278
space, 18, 19, 100, 104
   loss reduction, 18
   narrowing, 18, 19
   width (JSW), 18, 19
structure, 4
torment, 8
Jurisdiction, 28
Juvenile
   arthritis (JA), 137, 138, 140
   rheumatoid arthritis (JRA), 29

K

Kaempferol, 114, 118, 119
Karaya gum, 33
Kefir, 249
Kelp forests, 194
Keratinocyte, 171, 172, 189, 190, 210, 227, 230, 246, 251, 264, 267, 286
   cytokine secretion, 214
   differentiation, 208, 252, 264
   dysfunction, 228
   hyperproliferation, 210
   proliferation, 210, 211
Ketoconazole medication, 214
Ketogenic diet (KD), 177, 178, 256
Ketone bodies, 177, 256
Key
   products, 34
   risk factor, 6
   symptoms, 5
Kidney, 29, 139, 150
   stones, 150
Kinases, 49
Knee, 4–6, 10–13, 15–19, 91, 100, 104–106, 108, 110, 112, 113, 116, 121, 138, 139, 143, 145, 150, 157, 166, 167, 184, 185, 229, 264
   joint, 12, 106
   OA, 5, 10–13, 15–17, 19, 143
   pain, 11, 12, 104, 113, 145
   replacement, 138
   supports, 12
   torment, 12
Krill, 137, 145
   oil, 145

L

Lachnospiraceae, 297
Lactic acid bacteria (LAB), 57
Lacticaseibacillus paracasei, 285
Lactobacillus
   acidophilus, 57
   casei, 56
   pentosus, 288
   rhamnosus, 56
   strains, 288, 298
Lagoons, 194, 212
Laminaria
   hyperborea, 90
   japonica, 92, 199
Laminin, 50
Langerhans cells, 230
L-ascorbic acid, 245
Leguminosae, 269, 276
   family, 269
Leprosa graecorum, 185
Leprosy, 166, 237, 270, 275, 277, 278
Lequesne index, 16
Leukocytoclastic vasculitis (LCV), 29
Leukotriene synthesis, 103
Lichens, 194, 213
Lifestyle assessment, 5
Ligament
   annihilation, 18
   grease, 7
Liliaceae family, 231, 269
Limosilactobacillus reuteri, 285
Linear discriminant analysis (LDA), 291
Linoleic acid (LA), 56, 68, 69, 72, 77–79, 82, 138, 140, 154, 171, 235, 236, 274
Lipid digestion, 248, 249
Lipo polysaccharide (LPS), 50, 118, 119, 215, 216
Lipoxygenase, 36, 39, 51, 54, 69, 146, 156
Liquor utilization, 247
Lithium, 205
Lithothamnion corallioide, 137, 142
Long
   chain
      fatty acids (LCT), 256, 258
      sugar molecule, 90
   term effects, 11
Low-energy diet, 10, 245
Lubrication, 7, 8, 195

Index 313

Lubricin, 7
Lumps, 46, 138
Lungs, 29
Lupus arthritis (LA), 137, 138, 140
Lutein, 53, 89, 92
Luteolin, 59
Lycopene, 53, 94
Lymphocytes, 54, 120, 121, 143, 172, 246, 248, 270, 296
Lymphopenia, 174

M

Macroalgae, 92, 193–195
Macrophages, 30, 50, 75, 119, 120, 152, 189, 215, 270
Magnesium, 35, 57, 142, 192
Major histocompatibility complex (MHC), 71, 170, 187, 188, 207, 218
Malabsorption, 47
Malalignment, 12
Malarial medications, 247
Malassezia spp., 188
   yeasts, 214
Mammalian tissues, 121
Mangroves, 193, 194
Mannose, 31
Marine
   botanical, 141, 183, 184, 187, 191, 194, 200, 201
   botany, 193
   ecology
   habitats, 193
   meadows, 32
   organisms, 141, 191
Maritime invertebrates, 184
Matrix
   metalloprotease
      13 (MMP-13), 110
   metalloproteinase (MMP), 50, 108, 117, 144, 152
   9 (MMP-9), 152
   systems, 32
Mechanical stress, 171
Medication, 8, 78, 79, 81, 141, 168, 173, 183, 187, 237, 238, 256, 257, 263, 276, 277, 287, 297
   intervention, 8
   toxicity, 183, 263
      profiles, 183

Medicinal
   food, 101
   plants, 99, 101, 102, 112, 118
Mediterranean
   diet, 175, 176, 256
   eating regimen, 245, 255
Medium-chain fatty acids (MCT), 256, 258
Melanin synthesis, 249
Meliaceae family, 232, 270
Membrane
   bound organelles, 193
   phospholipids, 55
   receptors, 49
Menadione, 254
Menisci, 100
Menopausal females, 6
Menorrhagia, 276
Mental stress, 166
Mesokaryotes, 212
Meta-analysis, 11, 13–17, 110, 113, 116, 171, 210, 255
Metabolic
   connection, 6
   disorder, 247
   factors, 10
   homeostasis, 8
   regulation, 273
   syndrome, 170, 247, 267
      disorders, 267
Metacarpophalangeal (MP), 29, 40, 46, 50, 121, 123, 168
   joints, 46, 168
Metalloproteinase (MMP), 15, 50, 105, 107, 109, 110, 117, 119, 120, 123, 124, 144, 152
Metatarsophalangeal joints, 46
Methanolic extract, 38, 151, 152
Methodical survey, 14
Methotrexate, 75, 140, 174, 246, 250, 256, 257, 278, 289
Methylsulfonylmethane (MSM), 18, 19
Micro traumata, 4
Microalbuminuria, 247
Microalgae, 89, 90, 92, 93, 95, 151, 153, 154, 157, 193, 195, 206, 211–215, 218
   diversity, 213
Microbes, 51, 213, 291, 293
Microbial
   impurity, 33
   sources, 32

Microbiota composition, 249
Micro-CT, 107, 114
  scanning, 107
Microemulgel-treated patients, 233
Microemulsions, 116
Micrograms, 80
Microorganism strains, 288
Microparticles, 32
Microphytes, 89
Minerals, 32, 53, 92, 93, 101, 105, 142, 191, 192, 195, 198, 199, 231, 250, 254, 256, 268, 269, 274
Minocycline, 140
Mitochondria, 193
Mitochondrial
  dysfunction, 7
  integrity, 53, 101
Mitogen-activated protein kinase (MAPK), 49, 50, 59, 120
  activated protein kinase (MAPKAPK), 49, 50
  interacting serine/threonine kinase (MNK), 49
Mitogenand stress-activated protein kinase (MSK), 50
Molecular
  biology study, 212
  mass, 31
  mechanism, 45, 53, 117
Momordica charantia, 275
Monoclonal antibodies, 174
Monosaccharide, 37, 231
  units, 31, 33
Monosodium iodoacetate (MIA), 106, 115
Monoterpenes, 35, 103
Monoterpenoids, 38
Monotherapy, 251–253
Monounsaturated fatty acids (MUFAs), 36, 37, 175
Monozygotic twins, 170, 206
Mood swings, 74
Morphine, 18
Mucilage, 32–34, 269
  gums, 32
Mycosis fungoides, 237, 277
Myocardial infarction, 68, 247
Myrrhanone, 38
Mytilidae, 147

Mytilus edulis, 137, 147, 148

N

Nannochloropsis oculata, 93
Nanotechnology, 117
Naproxen, 14, 140
Narcotics, 17
Narrowband UVB phototherapy, 265
National
  Institutes of Health (NIH), 16
  Psoriasis Foundation (NPF), 172, 176, 186
Natural
  blood-cleansing function, 270
  killer (NK), 50, 208
Naturopathy, 211
Nausea, 174
Necrosis factor-alpha, 56, 59, 71, 73, 82, 189, 233, 252, 272
Neem oil, 232, 271
Nephron, 115
Nephrotoxicity, 13, 174, 268
Neuroendocrine system, 192
Neurological system, 67
Neuromuscular pain relief, 270
Neuroprotective activities, 110, 118
Neurotransmitters, 49
Neutrophil
  accumulation, 208
  attracting cytokines, 190
  elastase, 234, 273
Niacin, 48, 93
Nigella sativa (NS), 236, 274, 275
Nigella sativa Linn., 236, 274
Nitric oxide (NO), 38, 58, 59, 107–109, 112, 117–119, 121, 122, 147, 152, 270
  synthase, 59, 107, 108, 117, 147, 152
Nitrogen species, 109, 124
Non-acidic components, 28
Non-alcoholic fatty liver disease, 247
Noncorrosive blocker, 40
Non-enzymatic antioxidant, 253
Non-histone proteins, 35
Non-inflammatory arthritis, 27
Non-poisonous food, 28
Non-reactive tocopherol
  dimers, 55
  quinones, 55

Nonsteroidal
  anti-inflammatory
    drugs (NSAID), 3, 12–15, 17, 18, 45, 54, 56, 78, 100–102, 110, 113, 114, 116, 137, 142, 188
    medicines, 78
  calming drugs, 247
Novel methodologies, 8
Nuclear, 8, 15, 39, 49, 51, 55, 59, 112, 113, 117, 174, 177, 215, 232, 252, 272, 279, 286
  factor (NF), 8, 15, 34, 49, 51, 54, 55, 59, 71, 92, 103, 105, 109–118, 120, 122, 123, 144, 177, 207, 208, 215, 232, 233, 252, 272, 279
    erythroid-derived 2 (NF-E2), 177
    kappa B/active protein-1 (NF-κB/AP-1), 15, 49, 51, 55, 59, 92, 103, 110, 112, 114–118, 120, 122, 123, 144, 215, 232, 233, 252, 272, 279
Nutraceutical, 3, 27, 28, 35, 40, 45, 47, 48, 50–55, 67, 81, 89–95, 99, 101, 102, 104, 110, 114, 116, 119, 122–124, 137, 140–142, 147, 149, 157, 165, 183, 184, 192, 200, 205, 211, 227, 228, 230, 238, 245, 263, 265, 267, 268, 279, 285
Nutrient, 28
  cycles, 193
  supplementation, 258
Nutrition, 48, 101, 140, 166, 184, 194, 227, 256, 258, 267
Nutritional
  benefits, 28, 53, 184
  functions, 101
  supplements, 53, 101, 178, 191, 238, 263, 265, 268, 279
  value, 45, 89, 101

O

Obesity, 4, 6, 10, 35, 38, 46, 48, 58, 91, 92, 105, 110, 138, 166, 170, 177, 178, 188, 205, 208, 211, 278
Ochrophyta phylum, 194
Odontella aurita, 94
Ointments, 173, 238
Olea europaea, 50
Oleic acid, 72
Oleo-gum resins, 32
Oleoresin, 39
Oligosaccharides, 57
Olive oil, 68, 72, 175, 255, 256
Omega-3
  fatty acids (OMG-3-FA), 55, 56, 67–74, 76–82, 101, 142, 175, 195, 196, 255
  polyunsaturated fatty acids (OMG-3-PUFA), 68, 70–72, 215, 273
  unsaturated fats, 249, 256
Ophthalmic solutions, 32
Opioid, 18
  analgesia, 17
Oral vitamin D supplements, 176, 253
Organic
  extracts, 231, 270
  remineralization, 192
Osteoarthritic
  chondrocytes, 114
  involvement, 12
Osteoarthritis (OA), 3–19, 27–29, 31, 36, 38–40, 46, 50, 72, 90–92, 94, 99–124, 137, 138, 142, 143, 145, 149, 150, 168
  global burden, 5
  knees, 112
  patients, 5, 7, 99, 109
  symptoms, 3, 17, 100, 101, 119
  treatment, 3, 7, 8, 36, 99, 101–103, 106, 110, 117, 121, 143
Osteophyte, 104
  arrangement, 8
  formation, 4
Osteoprotective effects, 106
Oxford knee score (OKS), 143, 157
Oxidative stress, 53, 54, 90, 103, 108, 111–114, 116, 120, 122, 177, 215, 233, 272
Oxycodone, 18
Oxygen, 57, 72, 94, 215

P

P38-regulated/activated protein kinase (PRAK), 50
Palmaria palmata, 215
Palmoplantar psoriasis, 251, 286
Panniculus, 187
Paphia malabarica, 137, 156
Paracetamol, 13, 143
Paraffin treatment, 235, 273

Parakeratosis, 264
Passive treatments, 10
Patella, 12
Patellar realignment, 12
Patellofemoral joint, 10
Pathogen, 37, 51, 205, 215, 287
Pathogenesis, 4, 5, 47, 103, 115, 171, 208, 228, 245, 246, 252, 267, 286
Pathological conditions, 99
Pathophysiological processes, 108
Pathophysiology, 5, 49, 72, 102, 138, 165, 171, 189, 201, 228, 230, 233, 267, 279
Patient-driven treatments, 10
Pavlova lutheri, 215
Pentacyclic
   triterpene acids, 103
   triterpenic acids, 35
Peptic ulcer disease, 14
Peptides, 89, 149, 155, 184
Periarticular
   bone, 3, 4
   muscle, 31
Periostitis, 168
Peritoneal macrophages, 38, 250
Perna canaliculus, 137, 143, 144
Peroxisome proliferator activated receptor-gamma (PPAR-γ), 177
Pestalotiopsis species, 137, 143
Pesticides, 29
Phaeodactylum tricornutum, 92
Phaeophyceae, 191, 194
Phaeophyta, 183, 193, 199, 200
Pharmaceutical, 28, 101, 205, 209
   agents, 28
   reactions, 205
Pharmacodynamics, 19
Pharmacokinetics, 19
Pharmacologic agent, 13
Pharmacological
   therapies, 13, 268
   treatments, 113
Pharyngitis, 186, 188, 247
Phenolic compounds, 48, 51, 53, 55, 106, 195, 250, 269
Phenols, 36, 103
Phosphatidylcholine lipid, 7
Phosphatidylinositol 3-Kinases (PI3K/Akt), 106, 107, 144

Phosphocholine groups, 7
Phospholipid complexes, 116
Phosphotransferase (PhK), 271, 272, 279
Photoactive furocoumarin psoralen, 277
Photosynthetic pigments, 193
Phototherapy, 174, 229, 238, 264, 265
Phycobilins, 194
Phycobiliprotein, 89, 92
Phylogenetic diversity, 212
Physical therapy, 5
Physicochemical properties, 39
Physiotherapy, 100
Phytochemicals, 51, 111, 184, 228, 263, 268, 279
Phytomedicine, 268
Phytoplankton, 194
Phytosterols, 48, 51, 53, 55, 93
Pimecrolimus, 229, 264
Pityriasis rubra pilaris (PRP), 168
Placebo, 12, 13, 15–19, 36, 77, 110, 112, 116, 143, 145, 150, 176, 231–236, 271, 272, 274, 275, 277
   controlled clinical
      experiment, 231
   trial, 233, 272
Plant
   based gums, 32
   exudates, 33
   seed endosperm, 33
Plantae kingdom, 193
Plaque, 75, 167, 168, 172, 173, 186, 214, 229, 231, 264–266, 279
   irritation, 235
   psoriasis, 184–186, 196, 206, 207, 228, 229, 233, 234, 236, 251, 265, 266, 272, 274, 277
   thickness, 273
   type psoriasis, 167, 286
Plasma lipoproteins, 55
Plasmacytoid dendritic cells, 264
Pleura, 29
Polycyclic aromatic hydrocarbons, 238
Polygonum cuspidatum, 120
Polymerase chain reaction (PCR), 291, 298
Polymeric micelles, 116
Polymers, 32, 89, 199
Polyphenols, 109, 175, 250

Polysaccharide, 32, 35–37, 89, 90, 103, 107, 149–151, 153, 184, 195, 199, 231, 249, 269
Polyunsaturated
　fatty acids (PUFA), 48, 51, 53, 55, 56, 68–74, 76, 81, 89, 92, 93, 145–147, 195, 215, 257, 273
　　dietary composition, 73
　　unsaturated fats, 245
Pomegranate peel extract (PPE), 108, 124
Pongamia pinnata, 269
Pongamia seed oil, 269
Porphyra dioica, 215
Portal vein, 120
Prebiotics, 48, 55, 57, 58
Primary
　algal metabolites, 195
　rat chondrocytes (PRCs), 108
Probiotic, 48, 55–58, 285–288, 290, 292, 294–298
　consumption, 297
　effects, 58
　microorganisms, 249
　rich yogurt, 296
　supplementation, 249
Prognosis, 90, 258
Proinflammatory
　biomarker, 233, 234, 272
　cells, 214
　cytokine, 45, 50, 54, 57, 59, 107, 112, 118, 119, 211, 250, 272
　　production, 246
　genes, 55, 117, 177
　interferons, 59
Proliferator-activated receptor-gamma, 178
Prostaglandin, 15, 56, 73, 76, 104, 116, 274
　E2 (PGE2), 15, 56, 73, 76, 104, 109, 117–119, 122, 147
　synthesis, 274
Protectins, 69
Protein-coding gene, 115
Proteoglycans, 15, 16, 116
Proteostasis, 7
Proton-pump inhibitor (PPI), 14
Proximal interphalangeal (PIP), 12, 29, 40, 46
Pseudogout, 27
Psora leprosa, 185

Psoralea corylifolia, 237, 277
Psoralen, 237, 277
　photoactivation, 237
　ultraviolet A (PUVA), 189, 201, 229, 234, 239, 265, 273
Psoraliacorylifolia, 237
Psoriasis, 3, 27, 45, 67, 89, 99, 137, 140, 150, 165–178, 183–191, 195, 196, 198, 200, 201, 205–211, 213, 214, 227–239, 245–258, 263–279, 285–288, 290–293, 295–298
　area severity index (PASI), 176, 178, 232, 233, 236, 252, 258, 271, 272, 275, 286, 290, 292, 297, 298
　etiology, 187
　momordica charantia, 275
　nigella sativa, 274
　nutraceuticals, 183, 231
　pathogenesis, 245, 246, 252, 267, 286
　pathophysiology, 228, 233, 279
　pharmacological treatment, 250
　pongamia pinnata, 269
　potential causes/triggers, 206
　psoralea corylifolia, 277
　pustulosa palmoplantar (PPP), 266, 279
　severity, 176, 250, 287
　susceptibility, 170, 187
　vulgaris, 184, 185, 228, 232, 233, 253, 265, 271, 272
Psoriatic
　arthritis (PA), 27, 46, 56, 90, 93, 137, 138, 140, 168, 169, 174, 176, 189, 206, 278, 286
　gut enterobacteria, 267
　injuries, 248
　lesional skin, 213
　phenotype, 169
　plaques, 228, 231, 235, 246, 251, 253, 273
　skin
　　irritation, 214
　　lesions, 214
Psychological stress, 205, 208, 210
Punica granatum L, 108, 119
　peel (PGP), 108
Punicalagin, 108, 119
Purple sea moss gel, 198
Pustular psoriasis, 168, 186, 208, 229, 266, 286

Q

Qualitative decision making, 45
Quality, 11, 18, 32, 45, 46, 56, 99, 100, 168, 183, 195, 199, 228, 233, 263, 264, 268, 272, 288
Quantitative decision making, 45
Questions, 19

R

Radical events, 55
Radiographic progression, 81
Radioimmunoprecipitation, 290
Radiotherapy, 171
Randomized controlled trials (RCTs), 11–13, 18, 19, 36, 110
Ranunculaceae family, 236, 274
Reactive oxygen, 45, 54, 55, 58, 59, 109, 113, 117, 124, 146, 166, 205, 215, 218
   nitrogen species (RONS), 109
   species (ROS), 45, 54, 55, 58, 59, 113, 115, 117, 123, 146, 166, 205, 215, 218
   induced oxidative stress, 215
Reciprocal treatments, 18
Rehabilitation, 5
Relative risk (RR), 13, 14, 56
Remicade, 29
Remission myelosuppression, 173
Resistin, 211
Resolvins, 56, 69, 146
Respiratory tract infection, 167
Resveratrol
   injection, 120, 121
   intra-articular injection, 120
Retinoid, 174, 229, 251, 257
Rhamnose, 37
Rhein, 18
Rheumatic
   diseases, 72
   illnesses, 48
Rheumatism, 35, 38, 112, 275
Rheumatoid, 29, 30, 34, 36, 46–49, 51, 91, 137, 138, 279
   arthritis (RA), 6, 27–31, 35, 36, 40, 45–59, 68, 71, 74, 75, 77–82, 90, 91, 93, 94, 100, 105, 108, 112, 137–139, 143–146, 151, 153, 157, 168, 230, 279, 288, 292, 296
   factor, 29, 30, 78, 146
   nodules, 29, 46, 139
   vasculitis, 46
Rhodophyta, 183, 193, 194, 196, 197, 200, 201
Rikenellaceae, 297, 298
Rofecoxib, 14
Rosa canina, 109, 110
Rosehip powder (RHP), 109, 110
Rosmarinic acid (RA), 108
Ruminococcus, 287

S

Sacrum, 166, 229
S-adenosylmethionine (SAMe), 18
Salicylic acid, 37, 172, 231, 232, 238, 271
Saline, 17, 89, 119, 288, 289
   injections, 17
Salt marsh, 194
Saponins, 106, 149, 231
Sargassum wightii, 137, 146, 147
Scaliness, 235, 274
Scan photomicrographs, 290
Scavenging peroxyl radicals, 55
Schizochytrium sp., 93
Scientific intelligence, 101
Sclerosis, 8, 68, 104, 249
Scutellaria baicalensis, 110, 114, 122
Sea grass, 193, 194
Seawater, 191
Seaweed, 137, 142, 153, 157, 191, 193–196, 199–201, 215, 249
Sebaceous glands, 254
Seborrheic dermatitis (SD), 168
Secukinumab, 287, 295
Seed gums, 32
Self-greasing system, 7
Semilunar cartilage, 31
Septic arthritis, 28
Serum, 198, 272
   malondialdehyde, 236, 275
Sesquiterpenoids, 38
Sezary syndrome, 168
Short-chain fatty acid (SCFA), 34, 56–59, 285, 287, 293–296, 298
Silibinin, 237, 276
Silicristin, 237, 276
Silidianin, 237, 276

Silvery-white
  patches, 184
  plaques, 228
Silybum marianum, 237, 276
Silymarin, 237, 276
Single-nucleotide polymorphism (SNP), 102, 208, 211, 218
Sinomenine, 121, 122
  hydrochloride, 121
Sinomenium acutum, 121
Sinularia querciformis, 137, 152, 153
Skin
  cell proliferation, 171, 172, 229, 230
  disease, 165, 177, 183, 185, 201, 206, 215, 228, 236, 246, 269, 270, 275, 278, 293, 295
  histopathology, 290
  irritation, 154, 229
  medicines, 247
  microbiomes, 198
  pathology, 253
  pigmentation, 249
  sicknesses, 247
Slow-acting antirheumatic drugs (SAARDs), 78
Small pink scaly papules, 167
Social care systems, 5
Sodium, 102, 192, 257
  nitroprusside (SNP), 102
Soft gelatin capsule, 230, 265
Sorbicillactone, 155
Spectroscopy, 156
Spirulina platensis, 92, 95
Spondylosis deformation, 150
Staphylococcus aureus, 188, 209
Stearidonic acid (SDA), 74, 153, 154
Stem cell exhaustion, 7
Steroid, 38, 39, 75, 107, 110, 111, 253
  formulations, 17
  injections, 17
Steroidal anti-inflammatory drugs, 13, 54, 140, 142, 205
Sterol, 89, 93, 105, 149, 156, 195, 231
Stiffness, 10–13, 29, 36, 46, 56, 77, 78, 90, 100, 105, 116, 138, 140, 145
Stilbenoid, 120
Stratum corneum, 254
Streptococcal
  pharyngitis, 186, 247
  throat infections, 209

Streptococcus, 167, 209, 213, 214
  bacteria, 266
  pyogenes, 209
  tonsillitis, 214
Subchondral bone, 8, 31, 100, 107, 114
Subcutaneous fat tissue, 248
Sunflower oil, 76
Supplements, 3, 19, 75, 76, 78–81, 92, 141, 184, 230, 257, 268
Surfactants, 32
Swelling, 4, 46, 74, 90, 100, 103, 104, 139, 140, 146, 157, 186, 292
Swollen jelly, 32
Symbiotics, 55, 57, 58
Symmetric effect, 140
Symptomatic progression, 6
Synergetic treatment, 8
Synovial
  effusion, 104
  fluid, 4, 17, 56, 111
  histology, 81
  inflammation, 114, 121
  joints, 31
  membrane, 3
Synoviocytes, 30
Synovitis score, 114
Synovium, 4, 30, 31, 50–52, 100, 140

T

T-cell, 30, 71, 155, 172, 175, 187, 189, 210, 213, 214, 231, 252, 264, 287
  activation, 175, 231
Tacrolimus, 173, 229, 264
Tartrate-resistant acid phosphatase (TRAP), 152
Tattoos, 205, 209, 246
Taxanthin, 89
Tazarotene, 172, 232, 236, 251, 270, 275
  gel, 236, 275
Telomere attrition, 7
Teratogenicity, 174
Terpene, 36, 103, 105
  compounds, 112
Terpenoids, 39
Tetracyclic
  triterpene acids, 103
  triterpenic acids, 35
Tetracyclines, 205, 209

Tetrahedral framework nucleic acid (TFNA), 123
  wogonin complex (TWC), 123
Thalassotherapy, 191, 192, 201
Therapeutic, 7, 8, 111
  effect, 15, 34, 38, 68, 78, 81, 101
  intervention, 4
Thromboembolic events, 247
Thromboxane, 56, 73, 76
Thymohydroquinone, 236, 274
Thymol, 236, 274
Thymoquinone, 236, 274
Tissue, 4, 31, 46, 50, 51, 74, 75, 113, 117, 121, 138, 139, 149, 192, 231, 248, 293, 295
  mast cells, 121
Tobacco smoking, 247
Tocopherols, 48, 51, 53, 55, 254
Tocopheroxyl radical, 55
Toll-like receptor (TLR), 51, 59, 215, 252, 253
Tonsillectomy, 191
Tonsils, 214
Toxic homocysteine, 256
Toxins, 89, 214
Traditional Chinese medicine (TCM), 102, 105, 107
Traditional systemic medicines, 174
Tragacanth, 32, 33
Tramadol, 18
Transforming growth factor-β1 (TGF-β1), 8, 110
Translucent colloidal solution, 31
Triglyceride levels, 108, 257
Triterpenes, 35, 103
Triterpenoids, 38
Tumor necrosis factor (TNF), 29, 34, 35, 49–51, 55–57, 59, 71, 73–76, 81, 82, 93, 101, 104, 107, 109, 111, 112, 115–117, 120, 140, 142, 143, 152, 157, 188, 189, 209, 211, 233, 246, 248, 250–252, 254, 264, 267, 272, 279
  alpha (TNF-α), 34, 35, 50, 51, 56, 57, 59, 71, 73–76, 81, 82, 101, 104, 107, 109, 112, 115–117, 120, 142, 152, 157, 189, 211, 233, 246, 248, 250–252, 254, 272
Turbinaria ornate, 137, 150, 151
Turmeric, 51, 115, 232, 268, 271
  microemulgel, 233, 272

U

Ultraviolet (UV), 53, 155, 171, 178, 185, 189, 195, 201, 229, 234, 237, 239, 246, 265, 271, 277, 279
  ray protector, 155
Umbilicus, 229
Unanimous expert, 12
Undaria pinnatifida, 92, 137, 153, 154, 199
Unhealthy coronary artery disease, 248
Unicellular photosynthetic microorganisms, 89
Unique, 45, 104, 119, 121, 141, 285, 297
United
  Kingdom (UK), 5
  States (US), 4, 5, 48, 79, 169, 206, 228, 238
  economy, 5
Uric acid, 139

V

Valgus stress, 12
Varus malalignment, 12
Vascular space, 54
Vasculitis, 139
Very low-calorie ketogenic diet (VLCKD), 177, 178
Viruses, 49, 140
Viscosity, 32, 34
  changes, 34
  reduces, 34
Vision, 74
Visual analog scale (VAS), 143, 157
Vitamin, 53, 56, 79, 80, 92, 93, 101, 109, 175, 184, 191, 192, 195, 198, 228, 230, 231, 250, 254, 256, 263, 268, 269, 274, 279
  A, 251, 257
  C, 80
  D, 173, 176, 183, 196, 234, 245, 252, 276
  E, 55, 80, 232, 245, 253, 254, 271
  K, 254
Volatile oils, 237, 277

W

Waer column, 194
Wage loss, 138
Walker, 186

Walking
  aids, 12
  distance, 16, 104
  stick, 12
War, 109
Warm, 29, 191
Warrant, 273
Water, 191, 192
  insoluble, 31
  molecules, 32
  retention, 231
  solubility, 31
  soluble, 31, 37, 269
Waxy gum, 35
Weaker opioids, 18
Wear, 4, 100
Weather patterns, 34
Wedge, 12
Weed, 120
Weight, 4–6, 10, 11, 17, 29, 35, 46–48, 72, 91, 110, 199, 211, 245, 256, 290
  bearing joints, 6
  control plans, 245
  endurance joints, 4
  loss, 10, 11, 29, 46, 47, 72, 110, 211
  technique, 177
  reduction, 10
Welcome discovery, 271
Welfare, 27, 191
Western
  blot
    analysis, 113
    study, 118
  diet, 73
  hemisphere, 48
  nations, 69
  Ontario and McMaster Universities Osteoarthritis Index (WOMAC), 10, 13, 16, 17, 150
  world, 190
Wheat germ, 248
White
  blood cells, 75
  European descent, 190, 191
  people, 169
  plaques, 168, 228, 230
  scales, 229, 264
Whitish-silver, 184

Whole grain, 76, 248, 257
Wholesome foods, 81
Wide
  applications, 33
  forefoot, 12
  geographic distribution, 194
  range, 7, 93, 103, 109, 115, 205, 212, 215, 265, 275, 277
Widespread, 32, 90, 175, 184, 190, 191, 265, 266
  accessibility, 32
  autoimmune disease, 171
Wild fish, 79
Willian's lepra, 185
Wine, 120, 175, 255, 256
Winter, 209
Wistar rats, 108
Withania somnifera, 111
Withanolides, 111
Wogonin, 114, 122, 123
  exerts chondroprotective effects, 122
  induced oxidative stress, 123
Women, 6, 10, 12, 46, 56, 74, 108, 139, 190, 211, 267, 274, 278
World Health Organization (WHO), 5, 7, 56, 168, 246
Worldwide
  disability, 5
  nutraceuticals industry, 90
Wounds, 32, 275
Wrists, 46, 139, 140, 166

X

Xanthan, 32, 33
  gum, 33
Xanthophylls, 94
X-rays, 18
Xu-duan, 105

Y

Yang-tonifying medicine, 105
Yeast, 57, 214
  species, 214
Yellow, 37, 38, 248, 269
  color, 115
  flowers, 276
  plant, 271
Yellowing gum, 38

Yellowish substance, 105
Yield, 35, 72, 99, 199, 212
Yoga, 211
Yogurt, 249, 296
Young
  age, 248
  child, 80
  women, 267
Youth, 91

Z

Zero, 8
Zinc, 192
Zingiber officinale, 112, 113
  roscoe, 112
Zingiberaceae, 112, 115
  family, 112
Zwitterions, 7

For Product Safety Concerns and Information please contact our EU
representative GPSR@taylorandfrancis.com
Taylor & Francis Verlag GmbH, Kaufingerstraße 24, 80331 München, Germany

www.ingramcontent.com/pod-product-compliance
Lightning Source LLC
Chambersburg PA
CBHW070954240526
45469CB00016B/385